Disabling Barriers - Enabling Environments

SAGE has been part of the global academic community since 1965, supporting high quality research and learning that transforms society and our understanding of individuals, groups and cultures. SAGE is the independent, innovative, natural home for authors, editors and societies who share our commitment and passion for the social sciences.

Find out more at: **www.sagepublications.com**

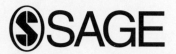

Disabling Barriers - Enabling Environments

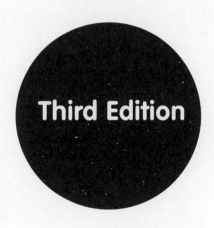

Third Edition

edited by
John Swain, Sally French, Colin Barnes & Carol Thomas

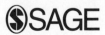

Los Angeles | London | New Delhi
Singapore | Washington DC

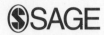

Los Angeles | London | New Delhi
Singapore | Washington DC

SAGE Publications Ltd
1 Oliver's Yard
55 City Road
London EC1Y 1SP

SAGE Publications Inc.
2455 Teller Road
Thousand Oaks, California 91320

SAGE Publications India Pvt Ltd
B 1/I 1 Mohan Cooperative Industrial Area
Mathura Road
New Delhi 110 044

SAGE Publications Asia-Pacific Pte Ltd
3 Church Street
#10-04 Samsung Hub
Singapore 049483

Editor: Kate Wharton
Assistant editor: Emma Milman
Production editor: Katie Forsythe
Copyeditor: Sharon Cawood
Proofreader: Neil Sentance
Indexer: Anne Fencott
Marketing manager: Tamara Navaratnam
Cover designer: Wendy Scott
Typeset by: C&M Digitals (P) Ltd, Chennai, India
Printed in India at Replika Press Pvt Ltd

Editorial arrangement and intro-duction © John Swain, Sally French, Colin Barnes and Carol Thomas 2014
Chapter 1 'A Critical Condition' © Paul Hunt 1966
Chapter 1 'The Helped/Helper Relationship' © Vic Finkelstein 1981
Chapter 2 © Carol Thomas 2014
Chapters 3 and 6 © Colin Barnes 2014
Chapter 4 © Colin Cameron 2014
Chapter 5 © Colin Goble 2014
Chapter 7 © John Swain and Sally French 2014
Chapter 8 © Bill Hughes 2014
Chapters 9 and 18 © Dan Goodley 2014
Chapters 10, 23 and 42 © Alison Sheldon 2014
Chapter 11 © Steve Robertson sand Brett Smith 2014
Chapter 12 © Liz Crow 2014
Chapters 13 and 33 © Donna Reeve 2014
Chapter 14 © Mark Priestley 2014
Chapter 15 © Robert Williams-Findlay 2014
Chapter 16 © Alison Wilde 2014
Chapter 17 © Yasmin Hussain 2014
Chapter 19 © Selina Bonnie 2014

Chapter 20 © Dawn Benson and Sarah Keyes 2014
Chapter 21 © John M. Davis 2014
Chapter 22 © Laura Hemingway 2014
Chapter 24 © Alan Hewitt and Carole Pound 2014
Chapter 25 © Michele Moore 2014
Chapter 26 © Sally French 2014
Chapter 27 © Hannah Morgan 2014
Chapter 28 © Donna Marie Brown, Pauline Gertig, Maureen Gillman, Joyce Anderson, Cathy Clarke and Simon Powell 2014
Chapter 29 © Brett Smith and Anthony Papathomas 2014
Chapter 30 © Ann Macfarlane 2014
Chapter 31 © Alan Roulstone 2014
Chapter 32 © Sarah Woodin 2014
Chapter 34 © Peter Beresford 2014
Chapter 35 © Maria Berghs 2014
Chapter 36 © Sally French and John Swain 2014
Chapter 37 © Rob Imrie 2014
Chapter 38 © Alice Maynard 2014
Chapter 39 © Bill Ahmer 2014
Chapter 40 © Pam Thomas 2014
Chapter 41 © Marcia Rioux and Bonita Heath 2014

First edition published 1992, reprinted in 2002 and 2003.
Second edition published 2004, reprinted in 2007, 2008, 2009, 2010 and 2011.
This edition first published 2014

Library of Congress Control Number: 2013934995

British Library Cataloguing in Publication data

A catalogue record for this book is available from the British Library

ISBN 978-1-4462-5898-9
ISBN 978-1-4462-5899-6 (pbk)

To Vic Finkelstein – an inspiration to us all

Contents

Notes on the Editors and Contributors

Joyce Anderson is a visually impaired member of the project. A retired Library Assistant, Joyce is also actively involved as a RNIB Volunteer and a Director of Eye Wish Access.

Bill Armer gained his PhD from Leeds University, where he later lectured in Social Policy and was associated with the Centre for Disability Studies. He is now an independent researcher/lecturer in Disability Studies (email: bill@gmx.ca).

Colin Barnes is Professor of Disability Studies at the Centre for Disability Studies, University of Leeds (email: c.barnes@leeds.ac.uk).

Dawn Benson is a Senior Lecturer in Disability Studies and Inclusive Education at Northumbria University and a parent of disabled children.

Peter Beresford, OBE, is Professor of Social Policy and Director of the Centre for Citizen Participation at Brunel University. He is Chair of Shaping Our Lives, the national disabled people's and service users organisation and network and has long-term experience as a mental health service user.

Maria Berghs is a Research Fellow at the University of York. Her particular research interests centre on disability, social justice and gender (email: maria.berghs@york.ac.uk).

Selina Bonnie is an Indian/Irish disabled woman who holds a Masters Degree in Disability Studies from the University of Leeds. She has been an activist, lecturer and trainer in the international disabled people's movement for the past 20 years. Her particular research interests centre on sexuality and reproductive rights for disabled people (for further information, visit www.sexualcitizens.com).

Dr Donna Marie Brown is a Senior Lecturer of Social Research in the Faculty of Health and Life Sciences at the University of Northumbria.

Colin Cameron is a Senior Lecturer in Disability Studies at the University of Northumbria, Newcastle upon Tyne. His research interests include the affirmation model, disability arts and identity. He is a disabled person.

Cathy Clarke has been visually impaired since her teens, and is now also hearing and mobility impaired. She is an active member of disability groups since the early 1990s and currently a Director of Eye Wish Access.

Liz Crow is an artist-activist and founder of Roaring Girl Productions (www.roaring-girl.com), working with text, audio, film and performance as a means to trigger social and political change (email: info@roaring-girl.com).

John M. Davis is Professor of Childhood Inclusion at the School of Education, University of Edinburgh. His research promotes creative and innovative approaches to inclusion, integrated working, participation and social justice.

Vic Finkelstein (1938–2011) was a disabled South African disability activist and writer, and a principal architect of the redefinition of disability as social oppression and the social model of disability. Following his imprisonment for anti-apartheid activities he came to Britain in 1965. In 1972 he joined Paul Hunt in the formation of the Union of the Physically Impaired Against Segregation (UPIAS) and the redefinition of disablement. Also in 1975 he was a driving force behind the Open University's 'Handicapped Person in the Community' course; widely regarded as the UK's first Disability Studies course.

Sally French is an Associate Lecturer at the Open University. She has researched and written extensively in the area of Disability Studies particularly for healthcare professionals.

Pauline Gertig is a Senior Lecturer in Social Work in the Faculty of Health and Life Sciences at the University of Northumbria.

Dr Maureen Gillman is a visually impaired member of the project. She is a retired Principal Lecturer and disability researcher and also Chair of Eye Wish Access, a DPULO that provides Vision Awareness Training.

Colin Goble is Senior Lecturer in Childhood, Youth and Community Studies at the University of Winchester. His interests include exploring psycho-social and cultural factors influencing the health and well-being of children and young people with learning difficulties, and 'so-called' neuro-developmental conditions, especially autism.

Dan Goodley is Professor of Disability Studies and Education, University of Sheffield. Recent publications include *Disability Studies: An Interdisciplinary Introduction* (London: SAGE, 2011).

Bonita Heath is a PhD candidate in Critical Disability Studies at York University, Toronto, Canada. Her research focus is social policy in poverty and disability and injured workers and workers' compensation.

Laura Hemingway received her PhD in the School of Sociology and Social Policy, University of Leeds in 2011. Her research interests include housing, disability and social policy (email: laura.j.hemingway@gmail.com).

Alan Hewitt has aphasia and works for the organisation Connect as the London Group Coordinator. He founded Aphasia News, a quarterly national newsletter by and for people with aphasia (email: alanhewitt@ukconnect.org).

Bill Hughes is Professor of Sociology in the Glasgow School for Business and Society at Glasgow Caledonian University. He is author of number of articles on disability, co-author of *The Body, Culture and Society: An Introduction* (Open University Press, 2000) and co-editor (with Dan Goodley and Lennard Davis) of *Disability and Social Theory* (2012).

Paul Hunt (1937–1979) was a disabled activist and writer and a key figure in the formation of Britain's disabled people's movement. He bagan campaigning for disabled people's rights whilst living in residential homes for 'the disabled' during the 1950s. In 1972 he was primarily responsible for the formation of the Union of the Physically Impaired Against Segregation (UPIAS) and the redefinition of disability as a form of social oppression on a par with racism and sexism.

Yasmin Hussain is Senior Lecturer in the School of Sociology and Social Policy at the University of Leeds. Her research interests include ethnicity, gender, disability and terrorism (email: y.hussain@leeds.ac.uk).

Rob Imrie's research and writing focuses on design and disabling spaces, and looks to evaluate the relevance of specific design discourses that purport to overcome the disabling nature of our designed environments.

Sarah Keyes is a Researcher in Ageing and Dementia at the University of Edinburgh. Her current work focuses on developing inclusive research and support for people living with dementia.

Ann Macfarlane, OBE, is an Independent Living and Disability Equality Consultant.

Alice Maynard takes a broad interest in the building blocks of a fair society. She has a DBA from Cranfield and was a member of the Human Genetics Commission.

Michele Moore is Professor of Inclusive Education at Northumbria University and Editor of the leading international journal *Disability & Society*. Her current research is concerned with understanding international perspectives on disability to advance the global agenda for inclusion.

Hannah Morgan is a lecturer in Disability Studies and member of the Centre for Disability Research (CeDR) at the University of Lancaster. Her research and teaching are concerned with the experiences of disabled people who use social care and other welfare services.

Dr Anthony Papathomas specialises in the psychology of sport, exercise and health. His work involves the application of psychological principles to disability physical activity promotion. He is a member of Loughborough University's Peter Harrison Centre for Disability Sport.

Carole Pound is a disabled speech and language therapist. Co-founder of Connect, the communication disability network, she is currently based at Brunel University researching experiences of friendship with people who live with aphasia.

Simon Powell is a visually impaired member of the Project since its inception. He is actively involved in a number of Social and Community groups including Eye Wish Access.

Mark Priestley is Professor of Disability Policy at the University of Leeds and Scientific Director of the European Commission's Academic Network of European Disability experts (ANED).

Donna Reeve is an Honorary Teaching Fellow at Lancaster University with research interests in psycho-emotional disablism, identity, the body, social theory and disability.

Marcia Rioux is a Distinguished Research Professor in the School of Health Policy and Management; on the MA/PhD in Critical Disability Studies and the MA/PhD in Health Policy and Equity programmes; and the Director of the Institute of Health Research at York University, Toronto, Canada.

Steve Robertson is Professor of Men, Gender and Health at Leeds Metropolitan University and Editor-in-Chief of the *International Journal of Men's Health*.

Alan Roulstone is Professor of Disability Studies at the University of Leeds. Alan has written and researched widely on disability issues, especially institutional and social barriers faced by disabled people.

Alison Sheldon is Director of the Centre for Disability Studies at the University of Leeds and runs the Centre's postgraduate Disability Studies programme.

Dr Brett Smith, PhD, works within the Peter Harrison Centre for Disability Sport at Loughborough University. His interests include physical activity, men's health and narrative inquiry. He is Editor of the journal *Qualitative Research in Sport, Exercise, and Health*.

John Swain is Professor of Disability and Inclusion at Northumbria University where he has worked as a tutor and researcher for over 30 years. He began his work in the area of disability studies at the Open University and has made numerous contributions to this area.

Carol Thomas is a Professor of Sociology at Lancaster University. She is best known for her publications in Disability Studies – including her books *Female Forms: Experiencing and Understanding Disability* (1997, Open University Press) and *Sociologies of Disability and Illness: Contested Ideas in Disability Studies and Medical Sociology* (2007, Palgrave Macmillan).

Pam Thomas is a freelance researcher and consultant in disability equality. She has written and researched on disablist hate crime, inclusive design and independent living.

Alison Wilde is currently Lecturer in Special Educational Needs and Inclusion in the School of Education, Bangor University, Wales. Her teaching and research is primarily in the areas of SEN and inclusion, disability studies and in cultural/media representations of impairment and disability.

Robert Williams-Findlay is the Equality Training Officer for the University of Wolverhampton. His central academic interest is disabled people's representation in the mass media. He was a former Chair of the British Council of Disabled People (BCODP).

Sarah Woodin is a Research Fellow in Sociology and Social Policy at the University of Leeds. Her research interests focus on independent living in its broadest sense (email: s.l.woodin@leeds.ac.uk).

Publisher's Acknowledgements

The two extracts in Chapter 1 have been abridged by the editor Sally French and appeared in previous publications.

Vic Finkelstein's 'Disability and the helper helped relationship: an historical view' was first published in Finkelstein, V. (1981) 'Disability and the helper helped relationship: an historical view', in A. Brechin, P. Liddiard and J. Swain (eds), *Handicap in a Social World*. Sevenoaks: Hodder and Stoughton and Milton Keynes: The Open University. Republished with kind permission of The Open University.

Paul Hunt's 'A critical condition' was first published in Hunt, P. (1966) 'A critical condition', in P. Hunt (ed.), *Stigma: The Experience of Disability*. London: Geoffrey Chapman. Republished with kind permission of Judy Hunt.

Introduction

The first edition of this book was compiled as a reader for the Open University (OU) course, 'The Disabling Society'. Between 1975 and 1994, the OU team produced a wealth of material that provided the basis for the development of disability studies courses and professional training schemes at both the undergraduate and post-graduate levels in mainstream colleges and universities across the UK, including the course readers *Handicap in a Social World* (Brechin et al., 1981) and *Disabling Barriers – Enabling Environments* (1993). The latter became, arguably, the most widely used reader in disability studies, both in the UK and internationally.

The second edition of *Disabling Barriers – Enabling Environments* was published in 2004. Only two chapters were retained in slightly revised form from the first edition, the other chapters being entirely new. At that time, the editors pinpointed three key themes of social change, recognising that each held its own controversies and tensions:

1 The most obvious changes in the ten years after the first edition, in the UK and internationally, were embodied in relevant policy relating to disabled people, particularly as expressed within legislation. Anti-discrimination laws had been passed in numerous countries and, on a broader front, human rights legislation.
2 The second change was not simply the quantitative growth of disability studies literature, but the variety of voices that could be found in journals, books and on the Internet – almost a cacophony of personal experiences, research and analysis.
3 Perhaps above all was the changing social context and, in particular, the impact of the escalating processes of 'globalisation' and the political, economic, social and cultural interdependence of nation-states. The reverberations were multiple and complex, including the rise in political activism by disabled people's organisations at the international level.

Given the passage of almost a further ten years, this third edition attempts to update again and to capture the continuing processes of social change which reverberate through disabled people's lives, experiences and opportunities. In relation to the book itself, some key characteristics have been retained:

1 The main assumptions underlying this compilation remain unchanged – encapsulated by the title. The focus is on disabling barriers faced by people with impairments in their interactions with a physical and social world designed for non-disabled living. It is also on the establishment of enabling environments and the control by disabled people of their own lives and their participation in the community.

2 Disability impacts on and finds expression in every aspect of contemporary social life. Disabling barriers permeate the physical and social environment: organisations and institutions; language and culture; the organisation and delivery of services; and the power relations and structures of which society is constructed. Thus, a wide range of topics is covered – though we would not claim that it is comprehensive. As in the first edition, this is a collection of quite short, pithy and, we hope, challenging analyses of disability issues.

3 The contributors, and editors, are predominantly disabled academics and activists. Some chapters are written by well-established authors, but the book also provides a forum for new voices within this burgeoning arena.

The aims of this volume are also carried forward from the first two editions – that is to:

- increase knowledge about the more active role that disabled people play in the community and how this can be supported
- develop a greater understanding of the experiences and situation of disabled people from their own perspective
- further the involvement of disabled people in controlling their lives through the development of an understanding of citizenship and empowerment.

So how did we put together this third edition? First, we would like to recognise our debt to Vic Finkelstein who died in 2011. Vic is an inestimable loss to disabled people, the disabled people's movement, disability arts and disability studies. The first edition of *Disabling Barriers – Enabling Environments* came out of work led by Vic at the Open University and even the title came from Vic, in discussions with Sally French, Mike Oliver and John Swain. The present volume, then, begins with an historical piece from the work of Vic and Paul Hunt, with whom he was closely involved. We have done this in the belief that the continuing development of disability studies needs to be grounded in the foundations that disabled people themselves have put in place over the years and as a mark of respect for their seminal work. Word-length restrictions limited what we could include, and we would recommend anyone with an interest in such early disability studies documents to go to the Leeds Archive website at www.disability-studies.leeds.ac.uklibrary.

So what are the social changes over the past ten years that have underpinned this third volume? Any succinct summary of social change is exceedingly challenging to encapsulate, particularly when looking globally. Change is certainly recognised in simple content terms by 15 completely new chapters (new topics and/or new authors) and a substantial update of the remaining chapters. Clearly, the themes of change summarised above remain. We would tentatively suggest three further themes, none of which could be deemed new but which have come to the fore in different ways:

1 The first is technological change which seems to advance at an increasing rate. It is there in every aspect of present-day life, in Western society at least, being dominant in leisure, communication, the media and work. Technology is commonplace in

our homes and on our streets. It is even there in life and death decisions, not least with developments in genetics.

2 Violence, too, is manifest in many forms – sexual abuse, physical abuse and hate crimes – or at least awareness of violence. The very existence of people with impairments is brought into question through practices such as genetic testing, genetic counselling, the abortion of impaired foetuses, genetic engineering and the euthanasia of disabled people.

3 The economic context still plays an overarching role. A global recession is being experienced through cuts in funding and an increase in poverty. Globally, disabled people still remain the poorest of the poor and poverty is the main cause, or underlies causes, of impairment. In the minority world, too, the disabled people's movement is floundering with organisations of disabled people being slowly decapitated through lack of funding.

Within the disability studies academic discipline, the passing years have also seen a continued debate around the social model of disability. Arguments range, at one end, from a rejection of this way of understanding disability to, at the other, a strengthening of it through, for instance, the affirmative model (see Chapter 5). We hope some of the arguments are reflected in this volume. For us as editors, however, the social model of disability remains the fundamental stance for the critique of changing theory, policy and practice. It is rooted in the history of the oppression of disabled people – a history of elimination, segregation, marginalisation, enforced dependency and social death – rationalised on the grounds of progress for disabled people.

The structure of the book remains much the same as in the earlier editions:

Part I: Perspectives on Disability and Impairment

Part I charts the continuing development of a social approach to understanding disability and impairment that emanates from the lived experience of injustice and the establishment of a collective identity of disabled people. These chapters set the scene by providing a conceptual map for exploring the tensions inherent in understanding disability and impairment, approaching the issues from different directions.

Part II: In Our Own Image

This section addresses 'image' in its broadest sense – as encompassed by the notion of identity. The chapters contribute to the growing literature by disabled people and their supporters in writing their own history, creating their own images in literature and art, and developing their own accounts of disability that reflect their experiences and vested interests. Two related themes are apparent. The first is power in determining and controlling identities. Disabling images, themselves created and controlled by non-disabled people, are essentially founded on concepts of dependency, abnormality, individual tragedy and the colonisation of disability by professionals and policy makers as gatekeepers of services and support. 'In our own image' encapsulates disabled people's direct opposition to the dominant ideologies that would reduce, determine and stereotype disabled people. The second, and related, theme is commonality and diversity, and the politics of difference. This collection of chapters concerns the diversity of disabled people, different forms of oppression – and the affirmation of disabled identity in terms of gender, ethnicity, sexuality and impairment. Inherent in these analyses, and explicitly addressed by some authors, are questions of fragmentation and unity, commonality and difference that have taken on a particular significance in contemporary disability studies.

Part III: Controlling Lifestyles

The disabling barriers analysed in Part III are those that prevent the full participative citizenship of disabled people, that marginalise and segregate people in every aspect of social life, that deny access to and participation in organisations and that preclude equal rights. 'Enabling' is crucially founded on disabled people's control in their day-to-day lives in the community, and the chapters in this section are essentially concerned with processes of social inclusion. The range of topics covered is an expression of the broadening of disability studies within a changing social context: including technology, communication, family life and childhood.

Part IV: In Charge of Support and Help

The fourth section turns to the help and support provided for and by disabled people. Disabling barriers here are those faced by disabled people within service-providers' models (such as the medical model) for understanding, planning and evaluating services, and the views of disability in which these are grounded. The chapters included here represent some ostensibly significant developments over the past decade. The primary concern, however, is the continuing critical analysis of the health and welfare services.

Part V: Looking to the Future for Disabled People

The title of this section has been adapted. This, in part, reflects the history of this book in that we see this as the final edition with this particular group of editors. We wanted to look forward as well as back in time, as in the first chapter. The chapters address the key themes of social change over the past ten years to engage with future possibilities for disabled people, possibilities for the dismantling of disabling barriers and the establishing of enabling environments – and the study of such possibilities within disability studies.

Overall, we hope that this third edition continues to take forward thinking in understanding and analysing disabling barriers and the development of practice in creating enabling environments.

Reference

Brechin, A., Liddiard, P. and Swain, J. (eds) (1981) *Handicap in a Social World*. London: Hodder and Stoughton.

Part 1

Perspectives on Disability and Impairment

1

An Historical Overview

The following abridged chapters by Paul Hunt and Vic Finkelstein aim to give an historical perspective to the field of disability studies. Both of these authors were leading figures within this field and have contributed to it hugely.

A Critical Condition

Paul Hunt

(Hunt, P. (1966) 'A critical condition', in P. Hunt (ed.), *Stigma: The Experience of Disability*. London: Geoffrey Chapman. Abridged by Sally French.)

All my adult life has been spent in institutions amongst people who, like myself, have severe physical disabilities. So naturally this personal experience forms a background to the views on disability that follow. But apart from the obvious value of writing from my own direct knowledge, it is also true that the situation of 'the young chronic sick' (as we are officially and rather unpleasantly termed) highlights that disabilities like ours, which often prohibit any attempt at normal living in society, almost force one to consider the basic issues, not only coping with a handicap, but with life itself.

I want to look at this special situation largely in terms of our relations with others, our place in society. This is essentially related to the personal aspect of coping with disablement since the problem of disability lies not only in the impairment of function and its effects on us individually, but also, more importantly, in the area of our relationship with 'normal' people. If everyone were disabled as we are, there would be no special situation to consider.

I think the distinguishing mark of disabled people's special position is that they tend to 'challenge' in their relations with ordinary society. The challenge takes five main forms: as *unfortunate, useless, different, oppressed and sick*. All of these are only facets of one situation, but here it seems worth taking each in turn.

The first way we challenge others is by being unfortunate. We do not enjoy many of the 'goods' that people in our society are accustomed to. The opportunity for marriage and having children, authority at home and at work, the chance to earn money, independence and freedom of movement, a house and a car – these things, and plenty more, may be denied us.

But set against this common-sense attitude is another fact, a strange one. In my experience, even the most severely disabled people retain an ineradicable conviction that they are still fully human in all that is ultimately necessary. This becomes fully operational when those with severe disabilities live full and happy lives in defiance of the usual expectations. It is they who present the most effective challenge to society.

When confronted with someone who is evidently coping with tragic circumstances, able-bodied people tend to deny the reality of the adjustment. The disabled person is simply making the best of a bad job, putting a good face on it. But when it becomes obvious that there is also a genuine happiness, another defensive attitude is taken up. The 'unfortunate' person is assumed to have wonderful and exceptional courage. This devalues other disabled people by implication, and leaves the fit person still with his original view that disablement is really utterly tragic. Such reactions appear to be caused by the need to safeguard a particular scale of values, where someone's sense of security depends on this being maintained. So if those of us who are disabled live as fully as we can, we can communicate to others an awareness that the value of the human person transcends his social status, attributes or possessions or his lack of them.

A second aspect of our special position in society is that we are often *useless*, unable to contribute to the economic good of the community. As such, again, we cannot help posing questions about values, about what a person is, what he is for, about whether work is the most important contribution anyone can make to society. Obviously, we who are disabled are deeply affected by the assumptions of our use-lessness that surround us. But it is vital that we should not accept this devaluation of ourselves. We do not have to prove anything. We can act as a symbol for the pre-eminent claims of non-utilitarian values, a visible challenge to anyone who treats his job as a final end in itself. Those who lead active lives are perhaps especially inclined to ignore man's need to accept passivity in relation to so many facets beyond his control. They may need reminding sometimes of our finiteness, our feminine side in the hands of fate or providence. We are well placed to do this job at least.

The next challenging characteristic of the disabled is that we are *different*, abnormal, marked out as members of a minority group. Normality is often put forward as the goal for people with handicaps. But it is doubtful if this is what we should really fix our sights on. If it means simply trying to be like the majority, then it is hardly a good enough ideal at which to aim. People need something more than this to work towards if they are to contribute to society and grow in maturity.

We face more obviously than most the universal problem of coming to terms with the fact of man's individuality and loneliness. The disabled person's 'strangeness' can manifest and symbolise all differences between human beings and demonstrate the unimportance of these differences compared to what we have in common.

The fourth challenging aspect of our situation follows inevitably from our being different. Disabled people often meet prejudice which expresses itself in discrimination and even oppression. Whatever we do people put it down to our being disabled. You may produce the most logical and persuasive arguments only to have them dismissed as products of our disability. The frustrating thing is that there is no appeal against this. If you point out what is happening you are assured it isn't, that you are imagining a prejudice that does not exist. And immediately you know you are branded again as being unrealistic and impossibly subjective. So many people take it for granted that what you say can be explained by a crude theory of compensation. And they tell themselves that you can't really help having these ideas, poor thing.

In the hospitals and homes I have lived in one rarely sees any physical cruelty. But there are administrators and matrons who have had people removed on slight pretexts, who try to break up ordinary friendships if they don't approve of them. There are staff who bully those who cannot complain, who dictate what clothes people should wear, who switch the television off in the middle of a programme, and will take away 'privileges' (like getting up for the day) when they choose. Then there are the visitors who automatically assume an authority over us and interfere without regard for our wishes. In the wider community employers turn away qualified and competent workers simply because they are disabled. Restaurants and clubs give excuses for refusing our custom. Landladies reject disabled lodgers. Parents and relations fight the marriage of a cripple into their family.

The last aspect of our challenge to society as disabled people is that we are sick, suffering, diseased, in pain. For the able-bodied, normal world we are representatives of many of the things they most fear – tragedy, loss, dark and the unknown. Contact with us throws up in people's faces the fact of sickness and death in the world. People do not want to acknowledge what disability affirms – that life is tragic and that we shall all soon be dead. Closely associated with death and dark is the idea of an evil body and mind and a warped personality. Disabled people find that the common assumption of good health often carries with it undertones of a moral failure on our part. 'If only you had enough will-power ...'. Sometimes people are trying to reassure themselves that they are 'saved', justified, in a state of grace – a satisfaction got from their 'good' selves juxtaposed with the 'unclean', the untouchables, who provide them with an assurance that they are all right, on the right side. Such attitudes, whether in ourselves or others, have to be rooted out.

Nowadays many disabled people will have nothing to do with resignation as it used to be understood. Now we reject any view of ourselves as being lucky to be allowed to live. We reject too all the myths and superstitions that have surrounded us in the past. We are challenging society to take account of us, to listen to what we have to say, to acknowledge us as an integral part of society itself. We do not want ourselves, or anyone else, treated as second-class citizens and put away out of sight and mind. Many of us are just beginning to *refuse* to be put away, to insist that we are part of life.

Disability and the Helper Helped Relationship: An Historical View

Vic Finkelstein

(Finkelstein, V. (1981) 'Disability and the helper helped relationship: an historical view', in A. Brechin, P. Liddiard and J. Swain (eds), *Handicap in a Social World*. Sevenoaks: Hodder and Stoughton. Abridged by Sally French.)

In this short essay attempts have been made to draw attention to a long neglected area of study: the historical origins of the relationship between disabled people and those who may work with them in a helping role. For convenience the discussion is centred around the disablement of those who have physical impairments although it applies equally to all disabled people. It is hoped that this essay will encourage practitioners to take a more positive attitude towards supporting physically impaired people.

There can be no doubt that over the last two decades there has been a radical improvement in the situation of disabled people in the United Kingdom. Twenty years ago few disabled people were to be seen in public. Probably the most significant measure of this changing and improving situation is the number of physically impaired people who have come forward to express their views and describe their *problems*. It is this trend which is particularly significant in the history of disability and in the relationship between helpers and helped.

Traditionally disabled people have been viewed as passive, unable to cope with normal social relations and dependent on others. The professions came into being with this assumption. 'Disabled people cannot do things' goes the idea 'and therefore we intervene to help'. Central to this idea is the notion that disabled people possess the 'problems'.

Now as disabled people have become more active in defining the 'problem' the traditional helper/helped relationship has come under strain. The suggestion is that in addition to their physical problems disabled people are placed in an oppressive relation to able-bodied people. This is particularly so when as a result of physical impairment they are assumed to be socially passive, inadequate and helpless. Since some of these assumptions underlie the evolution of the professions it has become imperative that traditional restrictive professional practice give way to a new helper/helped relationship. To do this it is necessary to take another look at the assumptions handed down to us by history and, until recently, only interpreted through the eyes of active able-bodied helpers.

Phase 1

It is convenient to take our starting point with the emergence of the British capitalist system. In its earliest period, prior to the Industrial Revolution, the population was overwhelmingly rural with production essentially agricultural with limited craft production. In these conditions 'cripples' can be assumed to have lived not very differently to the cripples under feudalism. In the small communities of early capitalism everyone knew each other and had a relatively fixed social status with its attendant family and social obligations. Those who survived severe physical impairments would have lived as cripples within their communities. It is this proximity between able-bodied and disabled people which explains the ease with which writers could include crippled characters within the literature when writing about the common people. Conditions of life were extremely harsh for cripples, but in a context where life was harsh for all the common people.

Apart from performing domestic duties for their families cripples unable to perform agricultural work could have supplemented the family income by spinning and weaving. The work was carried out in their home and cripples had no need to seek employment beyond the family. However, the rural population was being increasingly pressed by the new capitalist market forces and when families could no longer cope the crippled members would have been most vulnerable and liable to turn to begging and church protection in special poor houses. Market forces soon favoured machinery which was more efficient and able to produce cheaper more plentiful woven material. Those working larger looms would more likely survive and cripples would have had greater difficulty working such equipment.

The physically impaired people living in early capitalism were just as crippled by capitalist production as they were by the physical condition of their bodies. It took the Industrial Revolution to give the machinery of production the decisive push which removed crippled people from social intercourse and transformed them into disabled people.

Phase 2

By the late eighteenth century, highly complex mechanical devices were in use. The size of the equipment necessitated special buildings and the increasing need for workers to travel to their place of employment. At this time, the manufacture of machinery became an important economic development. Machines were for use by average human beings and workers could not have any impairment which would prevent him or her from operating the machine. Thus production for profit undermined the position of physically impaired people within the family and the community.

Unemployed workers mingled with unemployable disabled people in the growing towns. The need to control population mobility became necessary as well as the need to control civil discontent among those out of work. So it was that the next step was taken and civil authorities began building special secure places for disabled people and others who had no permanent home or source of income, and staffed these places with wardens and attendants.

In a climate of great productive activity those who did not work were regarded with abhorrence and held to be responsible for their poverty and afflictions. But the work ethic made it necessary to distinguish between those who were able-bodied but did not work and those who were physically impaired. The latter were to be accepted as rightful recipients of charity and the former as indolent wasters to be hounded and punished for their sins. Thus the final segregation process occurred which set disabled people apart from all others. Even in unemployability physically impaired people were to be removed from their fellow citizens. By the end of the 1880s and into the twentieth century it had come to be accepted that disabled people ought to be 'protected' by being placed in large institutions or, when families refused to abandon their members, to be hidden out of sight. The only source of income for the disabled population was charity. Following the Second World War there was a tremendous development of professionalisms and an isolated disabled population available for intensive treatment.

There have always been a few physically impaired people who managed to avoid the disabling pressures of the social system and find a place within the society where they have achieved recognition as fellow human beings. The movement of this group into the community, however, has confronted them with the experience of disability as a form of social discrimination and oppression. The successful disabled integrators have found that society, unaccustomed by their presence for centuries, has designed a world which does not recognise their existence. Such people have been forced to protest, first individually and then collectively about their social situation. This protest has not been confined to the material world of buildings and streets but includes a rejection of the now well established view that disability means passivity in organising one's own life.

Centuries of isolation have been followed by help to counteract this situation and disabled people have begun articulating their own interpretations of their social situation as well as defining the roles and limitations of the professional and lay workers. It is clear that professional practice which grew up on the basis of the social exclusion of physically impaired people led professionals into a set of practices which has now become a barrier to further development of their client group. What should be clear from the above historical sketch is that it is not professional practice, as such, which impedes the flow of disabled people back into the community but that aspect of their relationship which places them in an active controlling role over a passive patient or client.

Phase 3

It will be clear that we have only started entering the new phase whereby the helper/helped relationship will become reformed into one of equality. Exactly what the requirements are lies in the future but it is clear that any future relationship between physically impaired people and those who help them will have to encourage the utmost activity of the client in the decision-making process and access to all records, plans and planning meetings will be necessary. If disability was a social imposition of physically impaired people, the reintegration of disabled people will not only remove their disabilities but introduce a new era of cooperative work between helpers and helped.

2

Disability and Impairment

Carol Thomas

Introduction

Disability studies (DS) in the UK continues to grapple with the meaning of two key concepts in its lexicon: disability and impairment. Debates about what each term means, and about the relationship between disability and impairment, occupy many pages in DS books and journal articles. In my view, this ongoing consideration of foundational concepts is testimony to the growing strength and richness of disability studies, as it attracts writers who bring a variety of theoretical perspectives and experiential knowledge to bear.

This chapter briefly reviews the conceptual landscape associated with disability and impairment. Although these two concepts are allocated separate sections in what follows, I am sensitive to the argument that such a structure sustains what some see as an unhelpful disability/impairment dualism and binary separation in DS thinking (Corker and Shakespeare, 2002b; Goodley et al., 2012). Nevertheless, I find this analytical separation to be a useful explanatory device, but one to be made in the context of a discussion where the overriding interest is in the relationship between disability and impairment.

Disability and disablism

The social model of disability

In the UK, the emergent disabled people's movement of the 1970s was the force behind the reclaiming of the term 'disability' from professionals in medicine and social care (UPIAS, 1976; Campbell and Oliver, 1996; Barnes, 2012). In wrenching this term from the powerful grip of doctors and social workers who believed that disability either *was* the impairment itself or resided in restrictions of activity *caused by* impairment, disabled activists like Paul Hunt and Vic Finkelstein set about entirely reconstructing its meaning in the light of the social exclusions encountered in their own lived experience (UPIAS, 1976; Barnes, 2012: Chapter 1). In a radical move, they severed the presupposed causal link between impairment and disability, asserting instead that *being disabled* was an entirely socially caused phenomenon. In this way, disability was reformulated to mean the social disadvantages and exclusions that people with impairment face in all areas of life: employment, housing, education, civil rights, transportation, negotiation of the built environment, and so forth. Traditional medical and welfarist models of disability, together with their individualist *personal tragedy* counterpart, were thrown aside in favour of a social understanding of disability. Mike Oliver (1990, 1996a) coined the phrase 'the social model of disability' to capture this new perspective, and the model became the organising principle of DS in the UK and the banner headline of the UK's disabled people's movement.

Adopting the social model understanding of disability allowed socially created barriers and exclusions to be readily observed. For example, despite the presence of anti-discrimination legislation, exclusion and inequity occur if a wheelchair user or a person with visual impairment cannot access public transport systems, or cannot obtain a quality education that would enable them to compete for well-paid jobs in the labour market, or if a disabled individual is represented as a person of lesser value in films and other media (Swain et al., 2003). The disabling social barriers in the lives of people with impairments can be identified *and challenged* because such barriers are not immovable and can be dismantled. On a personal level, too, the social model of disability has had a transformative effect:

> It has enabled a vision of ourselves free from constraints of disability (oppression) and provided a direction for our commitment to social change. It has played a central role in promoting disabled people's individual self worth, collective identity and political organisation. I don't think it is an exaggeration to say that the social model has saved lives. (Crow, 1996: 207)

Disablism

Writing in the second decade of the twenty-first century, it is evident that the adoption of the social model of disability unleashed a powerful but contradictory drive for social and political change in the UK (Morris, 2011), and that parallel and linked political shifts have occurred in other nations and regions of the world (Priestley, 2001; Barnes et al., 2002; United Nations, 2006). The term *disablism* has come into use to capture the wide range and types of social exclusions and disadvantages encountered by disabled people. Disablism has been recognised by many to be a form of *social oppression* that sits alongside dimensions of oppression associated with gender relations, race relations, sexuality, and other key axes of social diversity. In my own writings in disability studies, I have found it useful to pin down and present the following definition of disablism:

Disablism: refers to the *social* imposition of *avoidable restrictions* on the life activities, aspirations and psycho-emotional well-being of people categorised as 'impaired' by those deemed 'normal'. Disablism is *social-relational* in character and constitutes a form of *social oppression* in contemporary society – alongside sexism, racism, ageism, and homophobia. As well as enacted in person-to-person interactions, disablism may manifest itself in institutionalised and other socio-structural forms. (Thomas, 2012: 211)

Indeed, I have become convinced that it is wise to use the term 'disability' only when referring to general topics and themes, because the term has been invested with a rather confusing mix of imprecise and varying meanings both within disability studies and in society more broadly. Within disability studies, I now prefer to describe my own writings as focused on understanding disablism.

So, what brings disablism into being?

Theorising disablism – like theorising gender or 'race' relations – is a challenging endeavour that involves applying and developing philosophical and theoretical traditions in the social sciences and humanities (Thomas, 2007). In disability studies, there are two dominant theoretical traditions at work:

1 *Marxism/materialism*. Social modellist thinkers like the late Vic Finkelstein (1980), Mike Oliver (1990, 2009) and Colin Barnes (1991, 2012; Barnes et al., 2002) understand disability and disablism to reside principally in the socio-structural barriers that serve to disadvantage and exclude people who live with impairments. This perspective draws upon, and sits comfortably within, a Marxist and materialist interpretation of the world. Capitalist social relations of production, and particularly industrial capitalism, are understood to lie at the root of the social exclusion of people with impairments by medically defined 'normal' people (Oliver, 1990; Gleeson, 1999; Thomas, 2007). In late eighteenth- and early nineteenth-century Britain, the imperatives of the system of generalised commodity production demanded that the non-owners of the means of production sell their labour-power as a commodity – to be consumed in the service of a fast-moving and exhausting industrial labour process. This meant that those who could not sell their labour-power on 'normal' and 'average' terms faced exclusion from the opportunity to obtain, independently, the means of subsistence. Living independently was the source of social standing, merit and approved personal identity in modern society (Oliver, 1990; Gleeson, 1999; Barnes, 2012). On this economic basis, and with the assistance of an ascendant medical profession, an ideology of the 'devalued difference' represented by 'cripples', 'imbeciles', 'the disabled' took hold in all quarters of society. The rest is history: workhouses, enforced dependency, 'special' education, 'sheltered' workshops and community care – in other words, the whole paraphernalia of

institutionalised care and 'welfare services' which constitute philanthropic and professional control in disabled people's lives.

2 *Poststructuralism/postmodernism.* Since the 1990s, the materialist perspective on what brought disability and disablism into being has been viewed as too limiting, or as downright wrong, by some writers in DS. Those informed by postmodernist and poststructuralist theoretical perspectives – the late Mairian Corker and Margarit Shildrick in particular – rejected the Marxist focus on socio-structural determinants of disablism and turned instead to cultural and linguistic theory for answers (Corker and Shakespeare, 2002a; Tremain, 2005; Goodley et al., 2012; Shildrick, 2012). Many have been drawn towards the French philosophical ideas of Foucault (1980) or Derrida (1978, 1993), and in recent years have begun to locate their contributions in what they prefer to call *critical disability studies*. From these perspectives, disability has no 'fixed', 'absolute' and 'essential' qualities; rather, disablist practices stem from the operation of powerful systems of *knowledge* in society – particularly biomedical knowledge. Biomedicine provides the authoritative reference points for what is deemed 'normal' and 'acceptable' in society, and gives rise to cultural practices in the population that reject and/or despise the 'abnormal' and the 'other'. Thus, those who wield power through the authority and status of their specialist knowledge – doctors, state administrators and legislators – construct and impose the category 'disabled' upon selected individuals in their purview. The person who is socially constructed as 'disabled' in this way may often come, in turn, to view him- or herself as 'abnormal'. That is, people with features and differences marked out as impairments often reflexively construct themselves as 'pitiable' or 'useless' – because 'disabled'. Any hope for resistance – and it is a slim hope – lies in a disabled person's ability to reject and resist the medical and associated categories imposed upon them, and to break free from the discursive bonds in which they are held.

Today, as well as Marxist/materialist and postmodernist/poststructuralist perspectives in disability studies, there are others in use, especially those drawing on phenomenology (Goodley et al., 2012) or critical realism (Watson et al., 2012); and all traditional and contemporary theoretical perspectives have strong feminist variants (Thomas, 2007). For a minority of writers, these conceptual developments have meant that the continued existence of the social model of disability is questioned, for example:

> the British social model has been an excellent basis for a political movement, but is now an inadequate grounding for a social theory. This social model was a modernist project, built on Marxist foundations. The world, and social theory, has passed it by, and we need to learn from other social movements, and from new theoretical perspectives, particularly those of post-modernism and post-structuralism. (Shakespeare and Watson, 2001: 44)

For other writers, the social model of disability retains its conceptual centrality (Barnes, 2012) or its importance as a political or disciplinary organising principle and banner headline (Thomas, 2007).

Impairment and impairment effects

In severing any causal link between impairment and disability, social modellists of a Marxist/materialist hue relegated impairment to a theme of little theoretical or political concern. As Oliver (1996b: 41–2) famously put it: 'disability is wholly and exclusively social ... disablement has nothing to do with the body'. Indeed, to dwell on impairment in DS or the disabled people's movement was viewed as hazardous because to do so gave credence to the medical preoccupation with bodily matters, deflecting attention away from disablist social barriers (Finkelstein, 1996; Oliver, 1996a).

Interestingly, critiques of this theoretical and political avoidance of impairment were first heard in the materialist camp when the late Paul Abberley (1987) argued that most impairments should be recognised as *socially* produced – by, for example, industrial accidents, environmental pollution, wars and medical practices. However, other criticisms of the avoidance of impairment gathered pace on different grounds in the 1990s. First, feminist writers such as Jenny Morris (1991) argued that experiences of the body should have a place in DS and disability politics, and that the exclusion of such experiences was tantamount to a patriarchal rejection of 'personal' experiences:

> there is a tendency within the social model of disability to deny the experience of our own bodies, insisting that our physical differences and restrictions are entirely socially created. While environmental barriers and social attitudes are a crucial part of our experience of disability – and do indeed disable us – to suggest that this is all there is is to deny the personal experience of physical and intellectual restrictions, of illness, of the fear of dying. (Morris, 1991: 10)

Second, the disabled activist and writer Sally French (1993) wrote about her own experiences as a person with visual impairment, noting that some restrictions of her activity *were* indeed 'caused by' her impairment. Put another way, not all restrictions could be explained by the presence of social barriers, and some restrictions would remain if all disabling social barriers in society were removed. A third set of criticisms began to be presented by writers who drew on phenomenological theoretical perspectives. Thus, Bill Hughes and Kevin Paterson argued that the social modellist desire to leave impairment out of account effectively colluded with medical ideas that impairment constituted a fixed, pre-social, 'biological abnormality':

> there is a powerful convergence between biomedicine and the social model of disability with respect to the body. Both treat it as a pre-social, inert, physical object, as discrete, palpable and separate from the self. The definitional separation of impairment and disability which is now a semantic convention for the social model follows the traditional, Cartesian, western meta-narrative of human constitution. (Hughes and Paterson, 1997: 329)

Moreover, poststructuralists added the argument that the social model's impairment/disability dualism is problematic because it fails to appreciate that *both* sides of this conceptual dualism are socially constructed and culturally specific. That is, both impairment and disability are powerful socially generated linguistic categories that divide, govern and control disabled people (Corker and Shakespeare, 2002a; Tremain, 2005).

In the face of some of these criticisms, Oliver (1996b: 49) suggested that those who are so inclined should develop a 'social model of impairment', but maintained his own conviction that a focus on disablist social barriers is the overriding priority for DS and the disabled people's movement. In contrast, I have argued that it is important to try to understand the relationship between disablism and impairment (Thomas, 2007), and as a materialist feminist have attempted to contribute to a social model of impairment by introducing the concept *impairment effects*. I define the latter as follows:

> *Impairment effects*: the direct and unavoidable impacts that 'impairments' (physical, sensory, intellectual, emotional) have on individuals' embodied functioning in the social world. Impairments and impairment effects are always bio-social and culturally constructed in character, and may occur at any stage in the life course. (Thomas, 2012: 211)

It is of note that many writers in disability studies have made use of the impairment effects idea because it has allowed them to acknowledge that impairments can and do have a direct or immediate impact on daily life – but without undermining their prioritisation of the importance and centrality of disablism in everyday experiences (Thomas, 2007: 135). My own view is that in any social setting, impairment effects and disablism are thoroughly intermeshed with the social conditions that bring them *both* into being and give them meaning. Further, I have argued that a materialist ontology of impairment and impairment effects is required – an ontology that is neither biologically reductionist nor culturally determinist (Thomas, 1999, 2007). To put it another way, we should not give the bio-medics exclusive rights over the concept of impairment, nor perform the poststructuralist 'vanishing act' involved in treating *real bodily variations from the average* as entirely linguistically or culturally constructed differences. What is required, I suggest, is a theoretical framework that recognises the *social dimensions of the biological* and the irreducibly *biological dimensions of the social*.

Conclusion: Ways forward?

In my view, the social model of disability should be acknowledged and celebrated as a powerful tool for political struggle, and as a point of assembly in disability studies. Beyond this, DS requires the enrichment of theoretical work on both disablism and impairment effects, and on the relationship between them. Further empirical research and theoretical development in disability studies will support the ongoing struggle of the disabled people's movement across the globe.

References

Abberley, P. (1987) 'The concept of oppression and the development of a social theory of disability', *Disability, Handicap and Society*, 2 (1): 5–20.

Barnes, C. (1991) *Disabled People in Britain and Discrimination*. London: Hurst.

Barnes, C. (2012) 'Understanding the social model of disability: past, present and future', in N. Watson, A. Roulestone and C. Thomas (eds), *Routledge Handbook of Disability Studies*. London: Routledge. pp. 12–29.

Barnes, C., Oliver, M. and Barton, L. (eds) (2002) *Disability Studies Today*. Cambridge: Polity.

Campbell, J. and Oliver, M. (1996) *Disability Politics: Understanding Our Past, Changing Our Future*. London: Routledge.

Corker, M. and Shakespeare, T. (eds) (2002a) *Disability/Postmodernity: Embodying Disability Theory*. London: Continuum.

Corker, M. and Shakespeare, T. (2002b) 'Mapping the terrain', in M. Corker and T. Shakespeare (eds) *Disability/Postmodernity: Embodying Disability Theory*. London: Continuum.

Crow, L. (1996) 'Including all of our lives: renewing the social model of disability', in C. Barnes and G. Mercer (eds), *Exploring the Divide: Illness and Disability*. Leeds: The Disability Press. pp. 55–72

Derrida, J. (1978) *Writing and Difference*. Chicago: University of Chicago Press.

Derrida, J. (1993) *Memoirs of the Blind: The Self-Portrait and Other Ruins*. Chicago: University of Chicago Press.

Finkelstein, V. (1980) *Attitudes and Disabled People: Issues for Discussion*. New York: World Rehabilitation Fund.

Finkelstein, V. (1996) 'Outside, "inside out"', *Coalition*, April, 30–6.

Foucault, M. (1980) *Power/Knowledge: Selected Interviews and Other Writings, 1972–1977*. Brighton: Harvester.

French, S. (1993) 'Disability, impairment or something in between?', in J. Swain, V. Finkelstein, S. French and M. Oliver (eds), *Disabling Barriers – Enabling Environments*. London: SAGE, in association with the Open University. pp. 17–25.

Gleeson, B.J. (1999) *Geographies of Disability*. London: Routledge.

Goodley, D., Hughes, B. and David, L. (eds) (2012) *Disability and Social Theory: New Developments and Directions*. Buckingham: Palgrave Macmillan.

Hughes, B. and Paterson, K. (1997) 'The social model of disability and the disappearing body: towards a sociology of impairment', *Disability & Society*, 12 (3): 325–40.

Morris, J. (1991) *Pride Against Prejudice: Transforming Attitudes to Disability*. London: The Women's Press.

Morris, J. (2011) Rethinking Disability Policy. Viewpoint paper for the Joseph Rowntree Foundation. Available at: www.jrf.org.uk/sites/files/jrf/disability-policy-equality-summary.pdf [accessed 07/12].

Oliver, M. (1990) *The Politics of Disablement*. London: Macmillan.

Oliver, M. (1996a) *Understanding Disability*. London: Macmillan.

Oliver, M. (1996b) 'Defining impairment and disability: issues at stake', in C. Barnes and G. Mercer (eds), *Exploring the Divide: Illness and Disability*. Leeds: The Disability Press. pp. 39–54.

Oliver, M. (2009) *Understanding Disability: From Theory to Practice* (2nd edn). Basingstoke: Palgrave Macmillan.

Priestley, M. (ed.) (2001) *Disability and the Life Course: Global Perspectives*. Cambridge: Cambridge University Press.

Shakespeare, T. and Watson, N. (2001) 'The social model of disability: an outdated ideology?', in S.N. Barnartt and B.M. Altman (eds), *Exploring Theories and Expanding Methodologies: Where We Are and Where We Need to Go. Research in Social Science and Disability*, Vol. 2. Amsterdam, London, New York: JAI.

Shildrick, M. (2012) 'Critical disability studies: rethinking the conventions for the age of postmodernity', in N. Watson, A. Roulestone and C. Thomas (eds), *Routledge Handbook of Disability Studies*. London: Routledge. pp. 30–41.

Swain, J., French, S. and Cameron, C. (2003) *Controversial Issues in a Disabling Society*. Buckingham: Open University Press.

Thomas, C. (1999) *Female Forms: Experiencing and Understanding Disability*. Buckingham: Open University Press.

Thomas, C. (2007) *Sociologies of Disability and Illness: Contested Ideas in Disability Studies and Medical Sociology*. Basingstoke: Palgrave Macmillan.

Thomas, C. (2012) 'Theorising disability and chronic illness: where next for perspectives in medical sociology?', *Social Theory and Health*, 10 (3): 209–27.

Tremain, S. (ed.) (2005) *Foucault and the Government of Disability*. Ann Arbor: University of Michigan Press.

United Nations (UN) (2006) Convention on the Rights of Persons with Disabilities (CRPD). Available at: www.un.org/disabilities/default.asp?navid=14&pid=150 [accessed 03/12].

UPIAS (1976) *Fundamental Principles of Disability*. London: UPIAS.

Watson, N., Roulestone, A. and Thomas, C. (eds) (2012) *Routledge Handbook of Disability Studies*. London: Routledge.

3

Disability, Disability Studies and the Academy

Colin Barnes

Since the emergence of the disabled people's movement in the latter half of the twentieth century, there has been a steady growth of interest in disability issues amongst social scientists in universities and colleges, referred to collectively as the 'academy' (Delanty, 2001) throughout the world. This has generated a radical critique of conventional thinking and research on disability-related issues, a large and expanding literature from various 'social science' perspectives, and the emergence of a new interdisciplinary area of enquiry generally known as disability studies (recent examples include Davis, 2010; Goodley et al., 2012; Watson et al., 2012). Initially disability activists and scholars played a crucial role in shaping our understanding of disability which sometimes resulted in an uneasy relationship between the disabled people's movement (organisations controlled by disabled people) and the academy (Barnes and Mercer, 1996). In recent years, this relationship has diminished, raising some concern about the future direction of the discipline (Oliver and Barnes, 2012). This chapter will trace the origins of these developments with particular reference to the UK and, to a lesser degree, the USA.

The re-interpretation of disability

Before the 1980s, academic interest in disability within the social sciences was confined almost exclusively to conventional individualistic explanations linked in one way or another to medicine and medical concerns. An important early example is found in the work of the American sociologist Talcott Parsons. Bowing to established wisdom, Parsons (1951) viewed short- and long-term 'sickness' as a deviation from the 'normal' state of being and, therefore, as a threat to economic and social activity or functioning. For Parsons, illness, and by implication, impairment is more than a biological condition; it is a social status and those cast in what he termed the 'sick role' have certain rights and responsibilities. Thus, 'sick people' are relieved of the usual roles and responsibilities associated with non-disabled lifestyles. In return, they are required to view their current status as unacceptable. To this end, they are expected to seek help from those charged with the responsibility of fulfilling this task: namely, medical and rehabilitation professionals. Although Parsons's work has attracted widespread criticism from practitioners and activists alike, mainly for its deterministic tendencies, it has, nonetheless, had an enormous impact on the social sciences and professional thinking in universities and colleges throughout the world.

Following Parsons, the analysis of social responses to impairment or disability was mainly the preserve of academics concerned primarily with the reaction to and management of ascribed social deviance. A notable example is Goffman's (1968) account of the interactions between 'normal' and 'abnormal' people. However, many writers paid particular attention to the social construction of 'mental illness'. A psychoanalyst, Thomas Szasz (1961), went so far as to question the very existence of mental illness, the validity of psychiatry as a legitimate medical discipline and the rehabilitation potential of psychiatric hospitals. He argued that the concept of 'mental illness' represents little more than a mythical substitute for the various problems associated with modern living. Such ideas were given further impetus by the writings of the French philosopher Foucault, who argued that mental illness, and other forms of ascribed social deviance, are social constructs generated by an increasingly dominant and moralistic social order (Foucault, 1975). Foucault's work has been particularly influential in a variety of fields including disability studies (Corker and Shakespeare, 2002).

Within sociology, interest in the general area of disability increased steadily during the late 1960s and 1970s with publications by Scott (1969), Albrecht (1976), Blaxter (1976) and Townsend (1979). Although each of these studies to varying degrees drew attention to the various economic and social consequences of the ascription of a disabled identity, the causes of disabled people's individual and collective disadvantage remained un-theorised and unchallenged.

The challenge to established views came not from within universities and colleges, but from disabled people themselves (see Chapter 1). British activists were especially important as they produced a radical new interpretation of disability that generated a new approach to disability practice and theory, commonly referred to as the social model of disability. Grassroots organisations controlled and run by disabled people, such as UPIAS and the Liberation Network of People with Disabilities, provided fertile ground for disabled activists to explore and reconfigure the concept of 'disability'. These 'organic intellectuals' (Gramsci, 1971) produced an impressive body of work which formed the bedrock for both the politicisation of disability and the development of disability studies in the UK and beyond during the 1990s and early 2000s. Key texts include Hunt (1966), UPIAS (1976), Finkelstein (1980), Sutherland (1981) and Oliver (1990).

Drawing on both personal experience and sociological insights, these writings posed a direct challenge to conventional thinking and practice on disability. Nonetheless, although the emergence of the social model of disability provided the 'big idea' (Hasler, 1993) for the mobilisation of disabled people, it was slow to find acceptance in universities and colleges in the UK.

The coming of disability studies

Until the 1990s, studies of 'disability' in British universities were typically located within a narrow range of academic disciplines including medicine, psychology, special educational needs and social work. Sociologists, despite their traditional focus on social inequality, were content to situate the analysis of disability within medical sociology and sociologies of health and illness perspectives. These are characterised by a largely a-theoretical tradition of socio-medical research driven by practical medical, health service concerns and interactionist, phenomenological perspectives. The outcome is an extensive literature that documents the extent and nature of chronic illness, its consequences for daily living and its impact on social relationships, the sense of self and identity (Barnes and Mercer, 2010).

Consequently, the UK's first disability studies course was not developed within a conventional university setting. It was conceived and developed by an interdisciplinary team at the Open University (OU) in 1975. A key figure in the production of this programme was a disability activist, Vic Finkelstein. The OU was an appropriate location for this new course as its emergence signalled a new and innovative approach to university education. In its first year, the course recruited over 1200 students, including professionals, voluntary workers and disabled people. As disabled people were increasingly involved in the production of teaching and learning materials, the course was updated twice before its abolition in 1994. The final version of the scheme was re-titled 'The Disabling Society' to reflect its wider content.

Similarly, the social dynamics of the disability experience were introduced on to the mainstream academic agenda in the USA and Canada in the 1970s. Again, the link between disability activism and higher education was the key to this development. Disability rights advocates and scholars concerned with disability came together at several conferences and realised that they shared similar interests and goals. A major catalyst for bringing these two groups together was the 1977 'White House Conference on Handicapped Individuals' which attracted over 3000 delegates. As in the UK, these early activities generated a small but significant body of work, primarily within the field of medical sociology. Important early examples include Bowe (1978) and Zola (1982). These and other studies drew attention to the disabling tendencies of American rehabilitation programmes and American society generally.

Even so, in contrast to the British approach, the literature failed to recognise the theoretical and analytical importance of the distinction between the biological (impairment) and the social (disability). Arguments for inclusion are couched within US traditions of minority group politics and individual consumer rights. These approaches have only a limited utility in capitalist societies characterised by vast inequalities of wealth and power such as the USA (Russell, 1998; Frances and Silvers, 2001; Oliver and Barnes, 2012). However, in recent years a more radical perspective has appeared, spearheaded by a small but vocal band of mainly disabled writers working in the humanities and cultural studies fields in universities in North America, Australia and New Zealand. This has resulted in the demand for a more critical interdisciplinary approach to the study of disability, more in keeping with advocates of social model perspectives (Clear, 2000; Hahn, 2002).

All of this has stimulated important debates about the role and development of the social model of disability within university settings and also relations between disability activists and professional academics. This is because, historically, universities have been a predominantly reactionary rather than a truly radical political force for social change (Delanty, 2001). Furthermore, the coming of the social model and, subsequently, disability studies provide a complete contrast to the kind of orthodox thinking hitherto generated in large part by scholars working in the established disciplines of medicine, sociology and psychology (Barnes et al., 2002).

Disability studies in the academy

When thinking about links between universities and the disabled people's movement, it is useful to consider three distinct strategies. These are the 'outside out', 'inside out' and 'outside in' approaches. The 'outside out' position is the one favoured by most professional 'experts' and academics. It is rooted in the positivist traditions of the nineteenth century and is clustered around the idea that the social world can only be properly understood through the application of the principles of rational thought, the natural sciences and the pursuit of 'objective' knowledge (Giddens, 2006). Since this perspective is widely regarded as value free and politically neutral, it is the one that has sustained universities and colleges and those who work in them for most of their existence (Barnes et al., 2002).

However, in recent years this perspective has increasingly been called into question. This is almost certainly due to the surfeit of information generated from various sources outside universities (Delanty, 2001) and the growing use and misuse of social statistics by politicians and the media. One outcome of this situation is that some universities and subject disciplines are now striving to include lay experiences in their research. Yet in many ways, this amended or 'realist' approach still situates the professional scholar as arbiter of everything that counts for acceptable and meaningful knowledge. For instance, Dyson (1999) refers to himself as a 'professional intellectual' rather than a positivist. He has recently argued that the academy has a role to play as 'instigator and sustainer of rational debate' between academic and lay communities.

Clearly then, the 'outside out' perspective, largely because of its claims to value freedom and political neutrality, does not sit easily with the radical politics of oppressed groups. Moreover, by attempting to incorporate and re-interpret lay knowledge and experiences, academics and researchers are in danger of doing what they have always done: that is, colonising and reproducing in a less radical form the work, ideas and experience of others. Unsurprisingly, therefore, there is a general concern about the role of academics amongst the UK's disabled people's movement (Barnes and Mercer, 1996; Finkelstein, 1996; Germon, 1998; Thomas, 2007). Consequently, attempts to build meaningful working and fruitful relationships between the academy and disabled people and their organisations based on the 'outside out' position should be treated with the utmost caution.

The foundations for the 'inside out' approach are based in the interactionist, phenomenological traditions favoured by medical sociologists mentioned above and, later, the women's movement. Proponents argue that the direct experience of a particular phenomenon is necessary not only to facilitate a thorough and meaningful analysis and understanding, but also to engender an appropriate political response. However, this can easily lead to the claim that only those with direct experience of a phenomenon are entitled to analyse and discuss it. Hence, only women can articulate about women's experiences, black people the black experience, disabled people the disability experience, and so on.

Whilst there is no consensus on this particular issue amongst academics, the same can also be said of the UK's disabled people's movement. Some disabled people's organisations, including members and staff, are exclusive to disabled people. Some groups employ non-disabled people as support workers. Others adopt a more inclusive approach and have 'non-disabled allies' in their membership and in their workforce (Barnes and Mercer, 2006).

It is evident, therefore, that the 'inside out' approach is potentially exclusionary and reductionist. Because of the heterogeneity of the disabled population and the fact that it is not only people with ascribed impairments who encounter oppression, exclusivity can easily lead to the marginalisation of both groups and individuals. Such a position is frequently politically and academically counter-productive. Furthermore, as noted earlier, the 'inside out' position ultimately reduces experience to the individual level and, therefore, negates the production of meaningful analyses and policy recommendations based on collective insights. Finally, studies based entirely on personal experience often read as little more than special pleading and are characteristic of what the disabled activist Hunt (1966: ix) termed 'sentimental biography'.

The alternative, the 'outside in' position, emerged from within disabled people's organisations partly in response to the ways in which experiential accounts have historically been individualised and/or medicalised by social scientists. Advocates do not deny the significance of direct experience but maintain that by itself it is not enough. Disabled people's experiences of disabling barriers (inside) must be located within a political analysis (outside) of why these barriers exist and how to eradicate them (UPIAS, 1976; Finkelstein, 1996). To facilitate such accounts, they must have firm working links between the disabled people's movement and the academy, since the former can provide the experience and the latter a coherent and scholarly political analysis. What is at stake, therefore, is not whether such a relationship should be constituted, but how it should be constructed and maintained (Barnes et al., 2002).

Critics have suggested, however, that this is an essentially masculine account of that political standpoint. Thomas (2007) suggests that the most appropriate solution to this problem is for academics to write themselves into the analysis and be explicit about the relationship between subjective experience (inside) and objective action in the wider world (outside). Others have gone further and argued that this approach is based on what they consider to be an outmoded ideology: a social model of disability that is no longer tenable in the postmodern world of the twenty-first century and is, therefore, in need of revision (Shakespeare and Watson, 2002). Such arguments have led to the emergence of a 'second generation' of academics from a variety of disciplines (Goodley et al., 2012; Watson et al., 2012), who advocate a more holistic 'critical disability studies' agenda that prioritises complex theoretical debates about the body, impairment, identity and discourse over and above those dealing with the economy, politics and social policy. It is an agenda that is more in keeping with the work of medical sociologists and the inside out approach, rather than that advocated by disability activists and their organisations.

Given the recent incorporation of disability issues into government circles and the growing threats to disabled lifestyles posed by recent cuts in disability services due to the ongoing global economic crisis in the UK and elsewhere, it is difficult to see how this agenda will benefit disabled people and their families – all of which raises important questions about the future of disability studies and its relations with disability activists and their organisations.

Conclusion

This chapter has demonstrated how the re-interpretation of disability by disabled activists during the 1970s has had an important impact on the perceptions and analysis of disability within universities and colleges in the UK and the USA. Although slow to become established, this approach has attracted considerable attention in universities in recent years. Whilst this is to be welcomed as it signifies a growing recognition of the importance of the issues, it should also be treated with some caution (Sheldon, 2006). The recent and growing individualisation of disability studies within the academy by some disability scholars signifies nothing less than a reaffirmation of traditional academic values and the effective de-politicisation of the discipline. In view of the enormity of the challenges facing disabled people and their organisations in the coming decades both nationally and internationally, this is the very opposite of what is needed (see Chapter 43).

References

Albrecht, G.L. (ed.) (1976) *The Sociology of Physical Disability and Rehabilitation*. Pittsburgh, PA: University of Pittsburgh Press.

Barnes, C. and Mercer, G. (eds) (1996) *Exploring the Divide: Illness and Disability*. Leeds: The Disability Press.

Barnes, C. and Mercer, G. (2006) *Independent Futures: Creating User-Led Disability Services in a Disabling Society*. Bristol: Policy Press.

Barnes, C. and Mercer, G. (2010) *Exploring Disability* (2nd edn). Cambridge: Polity.

Barnes, C., Oliver, M. and Barton, L. (eds) (2002) *Disability Studies Today*. Cambridge: Polity.

Blaxter, M. (1976) *The Meaning of Disability*. London: Heinemann.

Bowe, F. (1978) *Handicapping America*. New York: Harper & Row.

Clear, M. (ed.) (2000) *Promises, Promises: Disability and Terms of Inclusion*. Leichhardt, NSW: Federation Press.

Corker, M. and Shakespeare, T. (eds) (2002) *Disability/Postmodernity*. London: Continuum.

Davis, L.D. (ed.) (2010) *The Disability Studies Reader* (3rd edn). London: Routledge.

Delanty, G. (2001) *The University in the Knowledge Society*. Buckingham: Open University Press.

Dyson, A. (1999) 'Professional intellectuals from powerful groups: wrong from the start', in P. Clough and L. Barton (eds), *Articulating with Difficulty: Research Voices in Inclusive Education*. London: Paul Chapman. pp. 1–15.

Finkelstein, V. (1980) *Attitudes and Disabled People*. New York: World Rehabilitation Fund.

Finkelstein, V. (1996) 'Outside, inside out', *Coalition*, April, 30–6.

Foucault, M. (1975) *The Birth of the Clinic: An Archaeology of Medical Perception*. New York: Vantage.

Frances, P. and Silvers, A. (eds) (2001) *Americans with Disabilities: Exploring Implications of the Law for Individuals and Institutions*. London: Routledge.

Germon, P. (1998) 'Activists and academics: part of the same or a world apart?', in T. Shakespeare (ed.), *Disability Studies: Social Science Perspectives*. London: Cassell. pp. 245–55.

Giddens, A. (2006) *Sociology* (5th edn). Cambridge: Polity.

Goffman, E. (1968) *Stigma: Notes on the Management of a Spoiled Identity*. Englewood Cliffs, NJ: Prentice Hall.

Goodley, D., Hughes, B. and Davis, L. (eds) (2012) *Disability and Social Theory: New Developments and Directions*. Basingstoke: Palgrave Macmillan.

Gramsci, A. (1971) *Selections from the Prison Notebooks*. London: New Left.

Hahn, H. (2002) 'Academic debates and political advocacy: the US disability movement', in C. Barnes, M. Oliver and L. Barton (eds), *Disability Studies Today*. Cambridge: Polity.

Hasler, F. (1993) 'Developments in the disabled people's movement', in J. Swain, V. Finkelstein, S. French and M. Oliver (eds), *Disabling Barriers – Enabling Environments*. London: SAGE, in association with the Open University. pp. 278–84.

Hunt, P. (ed.) (1966) *Stigma: The Experience of Disability*. London: Geoffrey Chapman.

Oliver, M. (1990) *The Politics of Disablement*. Basingstoke: Macmillan.

Oliver, M. and Barnes, C. (2012) *The New Politics of Disablement*. Basingstoke: Palgrave Macmillan.

Parsons, T. (1951) *The Social System*. New York: Free Press.

Russell, M. (1998) *Beyond Ramps: Disability at the End of the Social Contract*. Monroe, ME: Common Courage.

Scott, R. (1969) *The Making of Blind Men*. London: SAGE.

Shakespeare, T. and Watson, N. (2002) 'The social model of disability: an outmoded ideology', *Research in Social Science and Disability*, 2: 9–28.

Sheldon, A. (2006) Disabling the Disabled People's Movement: The Influence of Disability Studies on the Struggle for Liberation. Keynote address]presented at the Third Disability Studies Association Conference, Lancaster, 18–20 September.

Sutherland, A.T. (1981) *Disabled We Stand*. London: Souvenir.

Szasz, T.S. (1961) *The Myth of Mental Illness: Foundations of a Theory of Personal Conduct*. New York: Dell.

Thomas, C. (2007) *Sociologies of Disability and Illness: Contested Ideas in Disability Studies and Medical Sociology*. Basingstoke: Palgrave.

Townsend, P. (1979) *Poverty in the United Kingdom*. Harmondsworth: Penguin.

UPIAS (1976) *Fundamental Principles of Disability*. London: UPIAS.

Watson, N., Roulstone, A. and Thomas, C. (eds) (2012) *Routledge Handbook of Disability Studies*. London: Routledge.

Zola, L.K. (1982) *Missing Pieces: A Chronicle of Living with a Disability*. Philadelphia, PA: Temple University Press. Also available at The Disability Archive UK: www.leeds.ac.uk/disability-studies/archiveuk/

4

Developing an Affirmative Model of Disability and Impairment

Colin Cameron

In this chapter, I outline the origins and development of the affirmation model, from its suggestion in 2000 by John Swain and Sally French to the proposal of new definitions of impairment and disability in 2010. Countering the dominant cultural view of impairment as personal tragedy, the affirmation model offers a framework for relating to impairment as difference to be expected and respected on its own terms, as an ordinary part of human experience rather than inevitably as misfortune. Grounded in the insights and perspectives of disabled people, the affirmation model is proposed as a tool for identifying ways in which people with impairments are required to become disabled people in everyday interactions and as a tool for resilience in the face of day-to-day disabling encounters.

Critical debate around the social model of disability is not new. It has been a focus for disability studies academics almost since Michael Oliver first used the term as a description of the UPIAS principles in 1983 (Barnes, 2004). Disabled feminists, for example, have argued that the social model over-emphasises socio-structural barriers and ignores personal and experiential aspects of disability (Reeve, 2004). Jenny Morris (1991) suggested that the social model tends to deny the experiences of our own bodies; Liz Crow called for a renewed social model which would allow for 'a more complete recognition and understanding of individuals' experiences of their body' (1996: 210). Carol Thomas (1999: 47) developed a social-relational definition of disability to account for the 'socially engendered undermining of the psycho-emotional well-being of disabled people'. Tom Shakespeare contended that the social model has provided disabled activists with a framework through which they 'could deny that impairment was relevant to their problem' (2006: 33). The response to these criticisms made by social modellists has been that 'the social model is nothing more or less than a tool with which to focus on those forces, structural and social ... that shape our understanding and responses to people with designated impairments'

(Barnes, 2007). The social model, in other words, while illuminating disability as an oppressive, restrictive social relationship, as something 'imposed on top of our impairments' (UPIAS, 1976: 14), has not been premised as a grand theory intended to explain all questions relating to disability in all contexts (Oliver, 2004).

One intervention within the individual/structural, experience/barriers debate was made by John Swain and Sally French in a *Disability & Society* article in 2000 entitled 'Towards an affirmation model of disability'. Rooting their idea within perspectives emerging from the disability arts movement, through which disabled people have retold their individual and collective stories on their own terms and with their own voices, the affirmation model was proposed as a critique of the personal tragedy model corresponding to the social model as a critique of the medical model. The affirmation model was, Swain and French stated, 'essentially a non-tragic view of disability and impairment which encompasses positive social identities, both individual and collective, for disabled people grounded in the benefits of lifestyle of being impaired and disabled' (2000: 569).

In proposing an affirmation model, Swain and French set out a position from which it can be asserted that, far from being necessarily tragic, living with impairment can be experienced as valuable, interesting and intrinsically satisfying. This is not to deny that there can be negative experiences resulting from impairment, but to make the point that this is not all that impairment is about. While Swain and French made it very clear that the affirmation model builds upon, and is a development emerging from, the social model, they suggested that the need for an affirmation model is established in that it is not a purpose of the social model to reject a tragic view of impairment: 'even in an ideal world of full civil rights and participative citizenship for disabled people, an impairment could be seen to be a personal tragedy' (Swain and French, 2000: 571).

In 2006, I was awarded a PhD bursary by Queen Margaret University, Edinburgh, to carry out research exploring ways in which disabled people see themselves in the light of ways they are represented by mainstream media. The research was also to involve exploring tensions for disabled people in the construction of positive identities in contexts in which self-understanding is shaped both by social structural relations of inequality and unique individual experience. Until I carried out my PhD, there had been no major research projects engaging with the affirmation model, which remained a tentative proposition rather than a tested hypothesis. Asking questions about the usefulness and validity of the affirmation model – do we really need the affirmation model when we already have the social model? Is the affirmation model another useful tool or just another academic abstraction? – I aimed to develop a critical reflection on the affirmation model in the light of the everyday lived experience of disabled people.

To this end, I completed a series of interviews, conversations and observations with 16 disabled people from Scotland and England, involving people with a range of physical, sensory, emotional and cognitive impairments; with congenital and acquired impairments; who lived in isolated rural settings as well as town and city environments; black, white, gay and straight disabled people; who had and who did not have religious faith; who came from a variety of class backgrounds; and who were aged from their early 20s to their mid-50s. My initial criteria for identifying participants included those who felt strong and positive about being disabled, those who regarded themselves as just getting on with it but who did not see disability as something to go on about, and those who really hated the experience and who would do anything for a cure. The research involved semi-structured interviews around participants' life experiences and ways in which they had learned about and come to relate to the idea of disability; unstructured interviews about their perceptions of media representations of disabled people as resources to draw on in making sense of the experience of impairment; and go-along observations as participants engaged in a range of ordinary, everyday activities, including, for example, crossing Birmingham New Street railway station, going shopping, going out to a restaurant with a friend, going to a 1960s disco, and watching an episode of *Deal or No Deal*. Interviews and observations were carried out between 2007 and 2009. It should be noted that where participants' words are used in this chapter, names given are those they chose for identification.

It had, I considered, been a weakness of the affirmation model that Swain and French had left it unclarified, had omitted to give it structure. While they had told us what the affirmation model is *about* and what it is *like*, and while they had offered a summary of it (Swain and French, 2000: 580), they had stopped short of specifying what it *is* (Cameron, 2008). One of my research aims was to enquire whether useful affirmation model definitions of impairment and disability might be fashioned. While they had not provided descriptions which would enable us to define this model succinctly, Swain and French had, on the other hand, identified a number of features by which the affirmation model *is* and *is not* characterised. The affirmation model *is*, they stated (Swain and French, 2008: 185), about:

- being different and thinking differently about being different, both individually and collectively
- the affirmation of unique ways of being situated in society
- disabled people challenging presumptions about themselves and their lives in terms of not only how they differ from what is average or normal, but also about the assertion, on their own terms, of human embodiment, lifestyles, quality of life and identity
- ways of being that embrace difference.

Within my PhD research, these descriptions are reflected in the following remarks by Lola, a wheelchair user from London:

> I haven't been terribly well and it's the grey area of impairment that we don't yet feel widely comfortable discussing … it's starting to change, but … I'd rather be me than not be the whole mix … positive, negative, flawed, happy, sad mixture that I am … that makes me *me* … and, you know, you can play the sort of games with yourself, thinking … if you had that or you didn't have that would it still make you who you were … and I don't believe I would be the same person. (Cameron, 2010: 238)

For Lola, being a disabled woman is an experience she would not want to be without. While she acknowledges the uncomfortable reality of her impairment, she rejects the futile pursuit of wishing things could be otherwise, the seductions of the ideology of normality (Oliver, 1996). She regards her impairment as a core part of her person, something without which she would not be who she is.

Swain and French (2008: 185) emphasised that the affirmation model *is not* about:

- all people with impairments celebrating difference
- disabled people 'coming to terms' with disability and impairment
- disabled people being 'can do' or 'lovely' people
- the benefits of living and being marginalised and oppressed in a disabling society.

Roshni, a blind woman from Glasgow, remarked during an interview:

> I've yet to meet anybody who is a hundred per cent happy with who they are ... I don't necessarily think that because you're disabled you are extra unhappy with who you are ... but equally I've yet to meet the person who's jumping up and down, celebrating that they've got dodgy eyesight ... but, having said that, it's certainly not a cause for me to cry and weep and wring my hands and give up on the world ... there are lots of things I'm not happy about ... I'm not happy about the fact that I've got dry rot in the next room and the ceiling needs replacing ... I think my visual impairment is on the same scale as that ... life happens. (Cameron, 2010: 119)

Roshni suggests that impairment is something to live with rather than a source of perpetual distress. Her blindness is something ordinary for her, part of her everyday experience of life. She is realistic about her situation, recognising that to be blind does not make life any easier, but at the same time, she does not regard her life as a blind person as being one long worthless experience. She knows that life is not a rose-strewn path for very many people and that, within the scheme of things, being blind is not the end of the world.

In that it involves a rejection of assumptions of tragedy, yet seeks to build on the social model, the affirmation model requires recognition of the oppressive contexts within which everyday life is experienced by disabled people. If it is to become regarded as a useful tool, it needs to be more than just a 'Pollyanna' model of disability, which involves playing 'the glad game' (Porter, 2011). In my PhD research, this was brought into focus by Charles, a wheelchair-user from Liverpool when he recollected that:

> when I was talking in the pub with Erin and yourself tonight ... with every sentence I wasn't thinking oh, I'm going to say this sentence with a speech impairment ... blah blah blah ... now I'm going to say this with a speech impairment ... blah blah blah ... I'm going to move back, but I'm moving back in my wheelchair ... you know ... you don't think ... but ... when you catch somebody looking at you ... and looking at the effects of your impairment ... concentrating on your impairment ... then you're suddenly aware ... that you're speaking differently. (Cameron, 2011: 19)

Charles's point here is that while impairment is not necessarily experienced as a problem for the person concerned, he finds that it is often made a problem by other people around. It is not the experience of impairment which is negative, but other people's response to impairment. I would suggest that the problematising of impairment by those who identify as normal involves a transactional exchange which validates their own sense of self. Disability is the ontological price paid by people with impairments for the relative security of identity of those occupying what Rosemarie Garland-Thomson has characterised as 'the normate position' (Garland-Thomson, 1997, 2009). At its simplest, the affirmation model makes the point that impairment is not an unfortunate aberration or a deviation from a norm, but is a relatively common and ordinary part of human life. The impression that impairment is unusual is a popular fiction given credence by media and charity objectification, as well as by the continuing societal practices of segregating disabled people within 'special' schools, 'care' homes and 'sheltered' employment, instead of ensuring the physical and cultural accessibility of the general environment.

Analysis of the data I gathered through interviews and observations led me to propose the following affirmation model definitions:

Impairment: physical, sensory, emotional and cognitive difference, divergent from culturally valued norms of embodiment, to be expected and respected on its own terms in a diverse society.

Disability: a personal and social role which simultaneously invalidates the subject position of people with impairments and validates the subject position of those considered normal. (Cameron, 2010: 113)

Conclusion

If we understand narratives as 'claims to see what is going on in any situation' (Carson, 2009: 5), the affirmation model establishes a framework for a subversive narrative that challenges the dominant cultural narrative which can only conceive of impairment in terms of loss or abnormality (Edwards, 2005). In identifying impairment as difference, the affirmation model establishes the rights of people with impairments to feel OK about themselves and to take pride in who they are, even when they are having bad days, and to be able to have bad days as well as great days or ordinary days without having to pretend otherwise. It also establishes their rights to enjoy being who they are as people with impairments rather than regarding impairment as a cloud overshadowing their existence. It demands recognition of impairment as an ordinary rather than an extraordinary characteristic of human experience, and for inclusion in ordinary life on that basis.

In naming disability as role, the affirmation model identifies disability as a productive as well as a restrictive relationship. It is not just about what people with impairments are excluded from and prevented from being, but also about the kind of social actors they are required to become instead. This role may involve performing disability as passive dependency or in terms of strenuous denial of the significance of impairment, but either part negates the lived experience of impairment and signifies the desirability of normality. Identifying disability in this way, the affirmation model can be used as a tool for making sense of what is going on within disabling encounters and interactions, and as a resource for resilience in the face of what Cal Montgomery has described as: 'those little acts of degradation to which others subject us ... those little reminders that we need to know our place in the world' (2006: unpaginated).

When Montgomery tells us that 'every few hours I run up against people who feel free to remind me that I'm their inferior and that I should conform to whatever they've decided "people like [me]" are supposed to be like' (2006: unpaginated), an affirmation model understanding allows us to recognise that what is going on involves other people in meeting their own identity needs. Having understood this, we are strengthened to resist.

During our last discussion Charles laughed as he reflected: 'It's hard to walk through life and constantly experience shit ... constantly experience negative attitudes ... and think ... ah ... that's a social barrier.'

It may well be that the insights given by the affirmation model were already implicit within the social model. However, access is not the same as inclusion. While public space may be being increasingly opened up to disabled people, there is still a gap between being able to be there and being valued there. Whereas the social model has established the rights of disabled people to physical access, perhaps the affirmation model can be used to throw a different light on what happens next.

References

Barnes, C. (2004) 'Reflections on doing emancipatory research', in J. Swain, S. French, C. Barnes and C. Thomas (eds), *Disabling Barriers – Enabling Environments* (2nd edn). London: SAGE. pp. 47–53.

Barnes, C. (2007) Disability Research Archives, April (#76). Available at: www.jiscmail.ac.uk/cgbin/webadmin?A2=ind0704andL=disability-researchandT=OandF=andS=andP=9526 [accessed 30/11/07].

Cameron, C. (2008) 'Further towards an affirmation model', in T. Campbell, F. Fontes, L. Hemingway, A. Soorenian and C. Till (eds), *Disability Studies: Emerging Insights and Perspectives*. Leeds: The Disability Press. pp. 14–30.

Cameron, C. (2010) Does Anybody Like Being Disabled? A Critical Exploration of Impairment, Identity, Media and Everyday Life in a Disabling Society. Available at: http://etheses.qmu.ac.uk/258/1/258.pdf [accessed 21/03/12].

Cameron, C. (2011) 'Not our problem: impairment as difference, disability as role', The *Journal of Inclusive Practice in Further and Higher Education*, 3 (2): 10–25.

Carson, A.M. (2009) 'The narrative practitioner: theory and practice', *International Journal of Narrative Practice*, 1 (1): 5–8.

Crow, L. (1996) 'Including all of our lives: renewing the social model of disability', in J. Morris (ed.), *Encounters with Strangers: Feminism and Disability*. London: The Women's Press. pp. 55–72.

Edwards, S.D. (2005) *Disability: Definitions, Value and Identity*. Abingdon: Radcliffe.

Garland-Thomson, R. (1997) *Extraordinary Bodies: Figuring Physical Disability in American Culture and Literature*. Chichester: Columbia University Press.

Garland-Thomson, R. (2009) *Staring: How We Look*. Oxford: Oxford University Press.

Montgomery, C. (2006) Little Acts of Degradation: Ragged Edge Online Launches Project Cleigh, in *Ragged Edge Online*. Available at: www.raggededgemagazine.com/departments/closerlook/00713.html [accessed 21/07/09].

Morris, J. (1991) *Pride Against Prejudice*. London: The Women's Press.

Oliver, M. (1996) *Understanding Disability: From Theory to Practice*. London: Macmillan.

Oliver, M. (2004) 'The social model in action: if I had a hammer', in C. Barnes and G. Mercer (eds), *Implementing the Social Model of Disability: Theory and Research*. Leeds: The Disability Press. pp. 18–31.

Porter, E.H. (2011) *Pollyanna*. Oxford: Oxford University Press.

Reeve, D. (2004) 'Psycho-emotional dimensions of disability and the social model', in C. Barnes and G. Mercer (eds), *Implementing the Social Model of Disability: Theory and Research*. Leeds: The Disability Press. pp. 83–100.

Shakespeare, T. (2006) *Disability Rights and Wrongs*. London: Routledge.

Swain, J. and French, S. (2000) 'Towards an affirmation model', *Disability & Society*, 15 (4): 569–82.

Swain, J. and French, S. (2008) *Disability on Equal Terms*. London: SAGE.

Thomas, C. (1999) *Female Forms: Experiencing and Understanding Disability*. Buckingham: Open University Press.

UPIAS (1976) *Fundamental Principles of Disability*. London: UPIAS.

5

Dependence, Independence and Normality

Colin Goble

In this chapter, I will examine the concepts of dependence and independence in relation to disability, and their link to the concept of normality. I will explore in particular how these concepts have been shaped by professional thinking and practice in services directed at disabled people, and also explore something of how they relate to wider socio-cultural ideas of personhood in modern societies shaped by dominant 'neo-liberal' political-economic ideology. Alternative ideas shaped by disabled people themselves will also be outlined to explore how they continue to challenge these dominant ideas. I will make particular reference to people with learning difficulties who, in my view, continue to face the greatest challenges of all in relation to these concepts and ideas – even to the extent of being allowed to be born or survive at all!

Ideas about dependence and independence have often been central to the views held about disability from various perspectives, including those of social, political and medical science. In the first edition of this book, Mike Oliver (1993) outlined how disability as we know it was created by an interweaving of these various elements in the emergence of industrialised society. The shift from a rural, agrarian and artisanal form of economic production, to an urban, industrialised environment, with strict new rules about time and speed of production, created a new and often hostile working and social environment for people with physical, sensory and intellectual impairments. They often became economically and socially marginalised as, in a wage-based rather than subsistence-based economy, they became burdensome to families in which they had found at least some level of integration and sustenance in the pre-existing social order. The political response to this marginalisation was to institutionalise the provision of care and support for 'the disabled', first in the workhouse, and later in various specialised institutions, such as schools for the deaf or blind, or 'colonies' for the feeble-minded and/or mentally defective. In these isolated, and often closed and authoritarian worlds, inmates were socialised into a view of themselves as sick, helpless, inferior and dependent on care to survive. Thus, the circle was closed, and many disabled people themselves internalised their role and identity as tragic, dependent on the compassion and benevolence of their social superiors.

It was Oliver's argument in that original chapter that the key to understanding how and why this marginalisation occurred lay in the way that disabled people were forced into roles of dependency in industrial society. This implies that many disabled people had lived independent lives in the pre-existing era. It is probably more accurate to say that, whilst new forms of dependency were indeed created in the shift from pre-industrial to industrialised society, it is unlikely that many disabled people would ever have been independent in that pre-existing social order in the sense that that term is meant in modern industrial and post-industrial societies. The significance of what occurred in the shift to industrialisation wasn't the creation of dependence so much as the rise to dominance of an ideological context in which being dependent on others came to be seen as problematic in ways it had not been before. The rise of capitalism broke down pre-existing systems of solidarity and inter-dependence that had sustained many disabled people in society, including the capacity of subsistence-wage-reliant families to care for and support members living with impairments of various kinds. The loss of those systems and relationships and their replacement with institutionalised and professionalised systems of 'care', steeped in medicalised systems of classification that equated disability with sickness, reshaped the situation of disabled people in the social upheaval of the industrial revolution. It also underpinned many of the assumptions about service systems and professional practice that came to be adopted by the welfare state in the post-Second World War era, and which still persist today in many ways.

Professional conceptions of independence

Professionals working in services for disabled people, including doctors, nurses, social workers, teachers and various therapists, often use the promotion of independence as a central rationale underpinning their interventions (Morris, 1998). Disabled people themselves have also placed issues of dependence and independence at the centre of both individual and collective agendas to reshape services and support systems – the obvious example being the independent living movement. However, as a number of writers have pointed out over the years, these terms mean different things to different people depending on how they conceptualise disability (French, 1993; Oliver, 1993; Finkelstein and Stuart, 1996).

Despite the widespread rhetorical adoption of the social model of disability, many disability professions still work to a personal-deficit-based conception of disability. From this perspective, disabled people are dependent because their bodies, senses or minds are somehow defective and thus don't allow them to function independently. Thus, 'dependence' is characterised as 'abnormal', and the role of professional support and service systems is primarily to mitigate the effects of these people's functional deficits in order to help them achieve a greater level of 'normality', that is 'independence' in their personal or social functioning.

Although there are variations, the general pattern of professional interventions is as follows. The functional capacity of the individual is assessed using scales and assessment tools that measure their performance against 'normative' standards of functioning. Programmes or interventions are then designed which aim to reduce the gap between the performance of the impaired individual and the normative standard as far as possible. Success is achieved when the professional expert judges that the performance of the individual has moved as far as possible in the right direction. The 'programme' or intervention will usually focus on whatever the most senior expert professional regards as the deficit that is most significant in preventing the person from functioning independently. Thus, for a deaf child it might be to learn to lip read, for a child with cerebral palsy it might be to focus on walking or feeding themselves, or for an elderly person recovering from a stroke it might focus on re-teaching them to wash themselves. The assumption usually remains, however, that the problem lies within the person, and the solution is a technical intervention from a professional expert who helps the person achieve a greater level of independence, and thus moves them closer to a more socially and culturally accepted level of normality.

Although there has been a great deal of emphasis placed in recent years on 'person-centred' or even 'personalised' assessments and interventions, there often remains an element of pressure on the disabled person to conform to a passive 'sick role', to go along with the programme or intervention, and to accept the expert verdict on its effectiveness. This includes a subtle pressure to be grateful for this caring attention, and to be as little bother as possible to the busy, caring professional. To step outside the parameters of this role is to risk becoming characterised as awkward and ungrateful, or even to invite further psycho-medical diagnosis, as in the judgement that the person is failing to adjust to, or come to terms with, their condition. In the learning difficulties field, there is a particularly potent version of this pathologisation and psychologisation of resistant and non-conformist behaviour in the classification of 'challenging behaviour', a classification for which the service response is often still institutionalisation and the heavy usage of psychoactive medication.

Although it should be remembered that human service professionals can and do work in alliance with disabled people to achieve emancipatory ends, it is clearly the case that many disabled people continue to experience this professionalised approach to the issue of independence as irrelevant, disempowering or oppressive (French and Swain, 2008).

Disabled people's conception of independence

Some groups of disabled people have challenged this professionalised conceptualisation of independence and the broader socio-cultural view of disability it reflects. They have based their approach to the dependence/independence issue on a fundamentally different conceptualisation derived from the social model of disability, in which disability is defined as a form of social oppression, separate and distinct from the issue of functional difficulty. They have argued that the dependency many people with impairments face is, as Oliver (1993) argued, the creation of a disabilist society.

Brisenden (1998) showed how the definition of disability can have a direct bearing on how issues of dependence and independence are conceived and responded to. A social model definition of disability suggests that people have often been forced into dependency on professional human service systems that segregate them from mainstream education, work, housing and other opportunities. To be independent, it has been argued, disabled people need rights to access these things. The right to a mainstream education, for example, would help to ensure that children with physical, sensory or intellectual impairments would gain the chance to learn and develop knowledge and skills to access mainstream employment, which would in turn allow them to support themselves financially. From this perspective then, independence is about rights, access and control rather than functional capacity.

Morris (1998) argued that in our society the loss, or lack, of capacity in one or more areas of functioning often leads to the assumption that the individual is unable to exercise control over most other aspects of their lives as well. The independent living movement has successfully challenged this view in recent decades by demonstrating that the presence of a functional impairment need not, and should not, be used to undermine individual control and autonomy.

It has been people with physical and sensory impairments, however, who have primarily shaped the social model critique of the deficit-orientated, biomedical model of disability and dependence/independence issues. It has been relatively straightforward for them to argue their case successfully because they are seen as able to exercise sound judgement and to speak with an articulate voice. For people with intellectual impairments, that case continues to be harder to make, however, partly because of the real difficulty they may have in being able to articulate their case, but also because, even when they do, their voice continues to be ignored or severely devalued. It is in fact professionals, working in alliance with people with learning difficulties and other intellectual impairments, who have often been at the forefront of attempts to challenge this devaluation. Usually, however, it is professions with relatively little power in the medical and manager-dominated welfare state, such as learning disability nurses and social workers, who have attempted this. Nonetheless, it is worth making the point again that professionals can and do sometimes work in alliance with, rather than in opposition to, disabled people pursuing emancipatory agendas (e.g. Scott and Larcher, 2002).

Intellectual impairment and independence

For most people with intellectual impairments, the issues relating to dependence and independence are no different than those outlined above for disabled people generally. They are disabled by society in much the same way as people with physical and sensory impairments, albeit by somewhat different disabling practices and environments. The answer to their disablement is much the same too: to establish legal rights to combat disabling discrimination and prejudice, and to manipulate the social and physical environment to enable rather than disable. An example would be the simplification of language and use of alternative symbols and media to convey important information, such as legal information; a manipulation that might be welcomed by many people without intellectual impairments!

Some people with intellectual impairments face a much harder task than other groups of disabled people, however, in struggling to attain, or maintain, independence in the sense of exercising autonomous control over their lives. This is related to both the nature and site of their impairment, and for reasons that are partly cultural as well as biological. In western society, the mind/brain is seen as the seat of individuality and the autonomous self. In these conceptualisations, the self is typically seen as self-contained, self-reliant, unique, separate, consistent and private – a hegemonic model of rationality and independent functioning, close to that idealised by the neoliberal, political economic consensus currently dominant in much of the western-influenced world. Such a view emphasises strongly the independence, autonomy and privacy of the individual (Wetherell and Maybin, 1997). The implication of this is that to experience impairment of the mind/brain is, in this culture at least, to be seen as losing all, or a critical part of, the self, and the autonomy and independence that go with it. The rights of people with intellectual impairments to hold or keep their property, money, freedom of movement, sexuality or even life itself continues to be challenged through the courts, and in public, political and philosophical debate. It is people with intellectual impairments who are most vulnerable, for instance, to utilitarian arguments for legalised infanticide and euthanasia. Eminent philosophers promote the argument that the likelihood that an infant will never become the self-sufficient, independently functioning autonomous individual so idealised in western culture is reason enough in itself to warrant killing him or her at birth (Kuhse and Singer, 2002).

At the same time, intellectual impairment, when severe, profound and/or 'degenerative' in nature, does impact on individuals in ways which challenge all our thinking about issues of dependence and independence. Even the disabled people's movement, not a place that people with intellectual impairments have always found very welcoming (Stevens, 2002), still needs to seek ways to pursue rights, citizenship and enablement that are not necessarily built around the concept of personal independence. There is a need to develop and incorporate models which support those people who are disabled because of the nature of their impairment as much as society's response to it, and who are always going to be dependent on others for control and choice making, as well as managing physical aspects of their daily life.

It continues to challenge human service professionals, too, to find ways in which people with severe and profound intellectual impairments can be 'listened to' using behavioural and subtle non-verbal communicative cues. Accepting and developing these modes of communication as forms of self-advocacy, and building in other sources and models of advocacy as a right, rather than an option, still need to be pursued as strategies in relation to people with intellectual impairments and communication difficulties.

Ultimately, however, the challenge still lies with all concerned citizens in wider society to seek ways and means by which the lives of people with severe or profound intellectual impairments can be valued and granted respect, even when the capacity for autonomy and independence are severely limited, or just not possible. Perhaps a starting point might be to question and challenge the cult of selfish individualism that lies at the heart of the currently dominant neo-liberal ideology invoked by our political and economic elites to justify continuing the erosion of social solidarity and responsibility – thus absolving them of the obligation to redistribute rather than privatise wealth. For this to be accepted requires the suspension of the obvious fact that the 'independence' we all enjoy only comes courtesy of a web of supportive relations and inter-dependencies. We are all who we are because of our interrelationship with others, and we are all 'independent' because we are inter-dependent. Looked at from this perspective, the 'dependency' of some disabled people actually looks a lot less abnormal than it might at first seem.

References

Brisenden, S. (1998) 'Independent living and the medical model of disability', in T. Shakespeare (ed.), *The Disability Reader: Social Science Perspectives*. London: Cassell. pp. 20–7.

Finkelstein, V. and Stuart, O. (1996) 'Developing new services', in G. Hales (ed.), *Beyond Disability: Towards an Enabling Society*. London: Sage.

French, S. (1993) 'What's so great about independence?', in J. Swain, V. Finkelstein, S. French and M. Oliver (eds), *Disabling Barriers – Enabling Environments*. London: SAGE, in association with the Open University. pp. 45–8.

French, S. and Swain, J. (2008) *Disability on Equal Terms*. London: SAGE.

Kuhse, H. and Singer, P. (2002) 'Should all seriously disabled infants live?', in H. Kuhse (ed.), *Unsanctifying Human Life: Essays on Ethics*. Oxford: Blackwell. pp. 233–45.

Morris, J. (1998) 'Creating a space for absent voices: disabled women's experience of receiving assistance with daily living', in M. Allot and M. Robb (eds), *Understanding Health and Social Care: An Introductory Reader*. London: SAGE, in association with the Open University. pp. 163–70.

Oliver, M. (1993) 'Disability and dependency: a creation of industrial society', in J. Swain, V. Finkelstein, S. French and M. Oliver (eds), *Disabling Barriers – Enabling Environments*. London: SAGE, in association with the Open University. pp 49–60.

Scott, J. and Larcher, J. (2002) 'Advocacy for people with communication difficulties', in B. Gray and R. Jackson (eds), *Advocacy and Learning Disability*. London: Jessica Kingsley. pp. 170–87.

Stevens, S. (2002) 'Where did the disability movement go?', *Community Living*, 16 (1): 18–19.

Wetherell, M. and Maybin, J. (1997) 'The distributed self: a social constructionist perspective', in R. Stevens (ed.), *Understanding the Self*. London: SAGE, in association with the Open University. pp. 220–64.

6

Reflections on Doing Emancipatory Disability Research

Colin Barnes

In 1992, Mike Oliver coined the phrase 'emancipatory disability research' to refer to a new approach to researching disablement. It is rooted in a general dissatisfaction with conventional social research strategies amongst other socially oppressed groups that emerged in the 1970s and 1980s. Therefore, it has links with 'new paradigm' approaches such as feminist, 'Black' and education research. Its primary aim is to challenge and transform the social relations of research production (DHS, 1992). Since its inception, it has spawned a range of variants dealing with specific sections of the disabled population with broadly similar principles and goals. These include 'inclusive' research for people with 'learning difficulties' (Walmsley and Johnson, 2003) and 'survivor' research (Sweeney et al., 2009) for 'mental health systems users and survivors'.

This chapter provides a personal reflection on some key issues arising from this development. It is divided into three main sections. The first provides a brief introduction to the notion of emancipatory disability research. The second focuses on issues arising from this perspective. The concluding section argues that although there has been notable progress in transforming particular practices within disability research, further development is unlikely due to reactionary forces within the research establishment.

Emancipatory disability research?

Social scientists and sociologists in particular have been doing 'disability' research since at least the 1950s. There are studies dealing with 'doctor–patient' relations, stigma, institutional living, and large-scale surveys chronicling the numbers of disabled people in the general population. All of these have provided important insights into current thinking on disability and related issues (Barnes, 2009).

Yet the main problem with these and similar studies is that they are based on the orthodox view that impairments, whether physical, sensory or intellectual, are the main cause of disability and disadvantage. This began to change in the late 1960s and early 1970s with the emergence of the international disabled people's movement, the redefinition of disability by the UK's Union of the Physically Impaired Against Segregation (UPIAS), the emergence of the social model of disability, and an alternative approach to doing disability research known as 'emancipatory disability research'.

Hence during the 1980s, several, mostly disabled, researchers began to explore disabled people's individual and collective experiences to show how environmental and social forces influence disabled people's life chances. In 1989, the British Council of Organizations of Disabled People (BCODP) – then the UK's national umbrella for organisations controlled and run by disabled people – commissioned a large-scale study of discrimination encountered by disabled people in the UK to bolster their campaign for anti-discrimination legislation (Barnes, 1994). These developments led to the generation of an emancipatory disability research agenda.

In 1991, the Joseph Rowntree Foundation (JRF) initiated a series of seminars on researching disability that provided a forum for the development of this new approach. These events brought together disabled and non-disabled researchers from various organisations working on a range of disability issues. This resulted in a special issue of the international journal *Disability, Handicap and Society* (renamed *Disability & Society* in 1993) entitled 'Researching Disability'. The articles therein provided the basis for the development of the emancipatory disability research paradigm (DHS, 1992).

It is a radical research agenda that warrants a reversal of the conventional social relations of research production. In contrast to traditional 'top down' approaches whereby disability research is initiated and controlled by professional academics and researchers, researching disablement should be generated and controlled from the 'bottom up' by disabled people and their organisations. In the early 1990s, such ideas seemed utopian to say the least. Then most disability research was financed by large government agencies like the Department of Health (DoH). In many ways, these organisations were dominated by traditional medical and academic interests and conventional assumptions about disablement and disability-related research.

As the decade drew to a close, this began to change due to the politicisation of disability by disabled people and their organisations and a changing economy. Of note was the growing emphasis on market forces within universities and research agencies, the increased use and misuse of research data by politicians, policy makers and the media, and the inevitable widespread disillusionment with social research generally amongst the general public. Since the turn of the 1990s, most research projects focusing on disablement in the UK have been funded by charities and trusts, such as the JRF and National Lottery's Community Fund (now known as the Big Lottery's Research Programme). Both these organisations have prioritised user-led concerns over those of the academy and professional researchers (Barnes, 2009).

This resulted in the completion of several projects that, implicitly if not explicitly, conform to an emancipatory research agenda. Useful recent examples include: the BCODP's *Independent Futures: Creating User Led Disability Services in a Disabling Society* (Barnes and Mercer, 2006), Shaping Our Lives' *Transforming Social Care: Changing the Future Together* (Beresford and Hasler, 2009) and *Talking about Sex and Relationships: The Views of Young People with Learning Difficulties* (CHANGE, 2010). Additionally, there is a growing emphasis on user participation, if not control, within the research programmes of the various UK research councils and funding agencies (DoH, 2005: Frankham, 2009; NHS Involve, undated). Whilst these changes might not go as far as some might wish, and certainly their impact has yet to be comprehensively evaluated, they do mark something of a shift in the right direction.

Key issues in emancipatory disability research

Since 1992, there have been several attempts to identify the core characteristics of the emancipatory disability research model. These can be addressed under the following headings: accountability, the social model of disability, data collection and empowerment.

Accountability

Accountability is a key feature of all research. Professional researchers are usually accountable to either academic peers or the project's commissioning and funding body or both. An emanicpatory framework requires researchers to be accountable to their 'research subjects': disabled people and their organisations. But to be answerable to all disabled people is impossible. The label 'disabled' can be applied to almost anyone with ascribed impairment regardless of cause, severity, age or ethnicity. Hence, the potential disabled population is vast.

To address this problem, researchers must become regularly involved with disability organisations. They can then become familiar with organisational structures, their goals, their controlling bodies and procedures for accountability to members. This will enable them to work with those agencies and groups that are controlled and run by disabled people themselves, and/or those that are committed to and working for the empowerment of the disabled population generally. This does not mean that to do emancipatory disability research someone must have an impairment, although there is an acute shortage of disabled researchers. But it does mean researchers must learn how to put their knowledge and skills at the disposal of disabled people and their organisations.

This entails ensuring appropriate mechanisms are in place to enable the effective exchange of information for everyone involved in the research process. Meeting rooms and communication systems must be accessible to all so that the research aims, objectives, methods and outcomes are clearly understood by all participants. Appropriate feedback and reporting strategies should be established at each stage of the project to ensure participants are kept fully informed of progress and developments. Further, all those involved in the research process, including consultants and participants, should be properly rewarded for their involvement. In sum, making research fully accountable has important resource implications in terms of time and money.

Inevitably, such a strategy poses problems for researchers working within a market-led environment where funding is short and career prospects are determined by the ability to secure lucrative and long-term research contracts. Most organisations controlled by disabled people are local, hand-to-mouth operations with very limited resources. Consequently, money for research is often given a low priority. Also, when needed, the demand is usually for small-scale locally based projects that are relatively short-term in character.

The social model of disability

In 1981, Mike Oliver adopted the phrase 'the social model of disability' to reflect the growing demand by disabled people for policies and practices that focused on the ways the physical and cultural environment imposed limitations on 'certain categories of people', rather than on the assumed limitations of individuals and groups (p. 28). Until the 1990s, research that adopted this approach was a rarity, but this is no longer the case. In some respects, the social model has become the new orthodoxy. Social model rhetoric is evident in research documents and policy statements from a diverse range of national and international organisations, including central and local governments, charities and voluntary agencies. Sadly, the rhetoric is not always matched by policy change. This has generated considerable concern amongst disability activists (Jolly, 2012).

Part of the problem relates to the mis-reading and re-interpretation of the social model by disabled writers and academics. To summarise, it is suggested that the social model does not address the reality of disabled people's experiences regarding the negative aspects of impairment, the psycho-emotional consequences of disablement and the diversity within the disabled population in terms of impairment groupings, gender, ethnicity, sexuality and class. This has prompted some to suggest that the social model is an outdated ideology, no longer relevant to the postmodern world of the twenty-first century (Shakespeare, 2006; Goodley, 2011; Watson, 2012).

These assertions follow the launch of the World Health Organization's revised definition of disablement, the International Classification of Functioning, Disability and Health (ICF). Intended to replace its much criticised predecessor, the International Classification of Impairment, Disabilities and Handicaps (ICIDH), the ICF claims to bring together the medical and social models of disability into one unitary 'scientific' and expressly apolitical framework for policy analysts and researchers (WHO, 2002). Although an improvement on the ICIDH as it recognises that impairment, activity and participation are all subject to environmental forces, impairment is still the primary focus of analysis and a 'significant variation from the statistical norm'. This of course ignores the fact that the identification and labelling of impairment as socially deviant is subject to ideological, political and cultural forces; but more on this later.

All of this raises important questions about the role of experience in the context of social model research. It can be argued that including information about disabled people's experiences in research is empowering for isolated disabled individuals and that the inclusion of participants' narratives is necessary to illustrate the impact of oppression. It is important to remember though that social scientists have documented the experiences of powerless groups, including many who could be defined as disabled, for most of the last century. There is also the danger that experiential accounts may be interpreted as 'sentimental biography' or as being 'preoccupied with the medical and practical details of a particular affliction' (Hunt, 1966: ix).

Additionally, there is the problem of selection and representation. Researchers have yet to devise ways of collectivising experience, and experiential research has yet to yield any meaningful political or social policy outcomes. It is important, therefore, that within an emancipatory research framework any discussions of disabled people's individual and collective experiences are couched firmly within the context of disabling environments and cultures.

Data collection

Emancipatory disability research is often associated with qualitative rather than quantitative methodologies. This is attributable to the claim that large-scale surveys and quantitative analyses cannot capture the extent and complexity of human experience. Also, such studies are favoured by advocates of objectivity and value freedom and therefore are subject to political manipulation. Yet the notion of objectivity is a hotly contested issue in the social sciences and science generally. Philosophers, scientists and politicians since the Enlightenment have repeated the claim that 'scientists' of whatever persuasion can interpret data without reference to personal values or interests. But *all* information, whatever its source and format, can be interpreted in different ways, and those charged with the responsibility of interpreting it are influenced by various forces: economic, political and cultural.

Consequently, it is increasingly recognised that judgements are coloured by personal experience and that all propositions are limited by the meanings, implicit or explicit, in the language used in their formulation. Furthermore, all theories are produced and supported by particular social groups and all observations are theory-laden. Traditionally, medical and academic interests have dominated disability research. Until recently, these were viewed as objective and value-free. Alternatives, such as social model accounts, were seen as politically biased and/or subjective.

Notwithstanding, there is also common ground between the emancipatory research model and other contemporary social research methodologies, including positivism and post-positivism. Early positivism is founded on a 'realist ontology': the assertion that there is a 'reality out there' driven by natural laws. Social science is about uncovering the true nature of that reality in order to predict and control it. Moreover, post-positivism acknowledges important differences between the 'natural' and 'social' worlds in that the rules that govern the former are viewed as universal. Conversely, social realities are variable across time, place, culture and context. Proponents also recognise that subjective values may enter the research process at any point from conceptualisation to conclusion. They also accept that the outcomes of social research may also influence future behaviour and attitudes (Barnes, 2009).

Researchers adopting a social model perspective, regardless of their theoretical leanings – whether materialist, feminist or postmodernist – all assert that there is a 'reality' out there. The social oppression of disabled people, that is historically, environmentally and culturally variable, is influenced by subjective values and interests, and is politically and socially influential. The crucial difference between advocates of post-positivism and supporters of an emancipatory research model lies in their claims to political neutrality. For the former, although recognised as sometimes unattainable, objectivity and value freedom are the stated aims; for the latter, political commitment and empowerment are the unequivocal goals.

Inevitably, this leads to accusations that politically committed researchers reveal only their allegiance to a particular world view and therefore deny the significance of other perspectives, actions and beliefs. But similar criticisms can be made of all social research. In response, researchers adopting an emancipatory framework must make their standpoint clear at the outset, and ensure that choices of research methodology and data collection strategies are logical, rigorous and open to scrutiny, and commensurate with the goals of the sponsoring organisation and research participants. Finally, all data collection strategies have their strengths and weaknesses. It is not the research methods themselves that are the problem – it is the uses to which they are put.

Empowerment

To be truly emancipatory, disability research must be empowering. It must generate accessible data that have meaningful and practical outcomes for disabled people. Unfortunately, in common with social research generally, much disability research is written for academic rather than lay audiences and therefore has little relevance to the empowerment of disabled people and their organisations.

But empowerment is not something that can be given – it is something that people must do for themselves. The important point here is ownership. Within an emancipatory framework, it is organisations controlled by disabled people that devise and control the research agenda and, equally important, to whom and with whom the research findings are disseminated. Even so, research outcomes in themselves cannot bring about meaningful political and social transformation, though they can reinforce and stimulate the demand for change. Thus, the main targets for emancipatory disability research are disabled people and their allies.

Indeed, there is now a significant body of work produced by organisations controlled by disabled people and service users across the UK and Europe that adheres to emancipatory research principles. This includes large- and small-scale studies using both quantitative and qualitative methodologies. It is also apparent that these studies have had a significant impact on policy development both nationally and internationally. But this is not to suggest that user-controlled projects in themselves are responsible for these outcomes; they are not, but they can play an invaluable part in the struggle for a fairer and more just society.

Conclusion: So far but no further?

Certainly, much has changed over the last ten or so years in the field of disability research. There can be little doubt that the arrival of the social model of disability and the emancipatory research paradigm has had an important impact on many researchers engaged in disability research. But their impact on the social relations of research production has been only marginal and what progress has been made is now under threat. Over the last decade, they have been increasingly rejected by reactionary forces within the academy in favour of traditional scientific individualising strategies such as the ICF and critical realist research to explore both the experience of impairment and that of disablement (Shakespeare, 2006; Watson, 2012).

Apart from blurring the crucial conceptual distinction between impairment and disability and reifying personal tragedy theory, these approaches lend themselves to 'people fixing' rather than 'structural change' (Bickenbach, 2009: 120). Moreover, although the ICF is presented as apolitical, in the UK it is sponsored by insurance companies, 'healthcare' agencies and the Department of Work and Pensions to measure impairments in order to reduce welfare payments to disabled individuals (Jolly, 2012).

Given the enormity of the ongoing global economic crises and the ensuing attacks on disabled people's lifestyles in all countries, both rich and poor, now more than ever disability researchers should be focusing on the structural forces – economic, political and cultural – that create disablement, not shying away from them.

References

Barnes, C. (1994) 'Forward to the second impression', in *Disabled People in Britain and Discrimination: A Case for Anti-discrimination Legislation*. London: Hurst. pp. ix–xv.

Barnes, C. (2009) 'An ethical agenda in disability research: rhetoric and reality', in D.M. Mertens and P.E. Ginsberg (eds), *The Handbook of Social Research Ethics*. London: SAGE. pp. 458–73.

Barnes, C. and Mercer, G. (2006) *Independent Futures: Creating User-Led Disability Services in a Disabling Society*. Bristol: Policy Press.

Beresford, P. and Hasler, F. (2009) *Transforming Social Care: Changing the Future Together*. London: Shaping Our Lives.

Bickenbach, J.E. (2009) 'Disability, non-talent, and distributive justice', in K. Kristiansen, S. Velmas and T. Shakespeare (eds), *Arguing About Disability: Philosophical Perspectives*. London: Routledge. pp. 105–23.

CHANGE (2010) *Talking about Sex and Relationships: The Views of Young People with Learning Difficulties*. Leeds: CHANGE.

Department of Health (DoH) (2005) *Research Governance Framework for Health and Social Care*. London: Department of Health.

Department of Health and Security (DHS) (1992) 'Special Issue: Researching Disability', *Disability, Handicap and Society*, 7 (2): 99–203.

Frankham, J. (2009) *Partnership Research: A Review of Approaches and Challenges in Conducting Research in Partnership with Service Users*. Southampton: ESRC (Economic and Research Council) National Centre for Research Methods.

Goodley, D. (2011) *Disability Studies: An Interdisciplinary Introduction*. London: SAGE.

Hunt, P. (ed.) (1966) *Stigma: The Experience of Disability*. London: Geoffrey Chapman.

Jolly, D. (2012) A Tale of Two Models: Disabled People Vs. Unum, Atos, Government and Disability Charities, Disabled People Against Cuts. Available at: www.dpac.uk.net/2012/04/a-tale-of-two-models-disabled-people-vs-unum-atos-government-and-disability-charities-debbie-jolly/ [accessed 17/07/12].

NHS Involve (undated) Involve: Supporting Public Involvement in NHS Public Health and Social Care Research. Available at: www.invo.org.uk/ [accessed 6/07/12].

Oliver, M. (1981) 'A new model in the social work role in relation to disability', in J. Campling (ed.), *The Handicapped Person: A New Perspective for Social Workers*. London: RADAR. pp. 19–32. Available on the Disability Archive UK at http://disability-studies.leeds.ac.uk/files/library/Campling-handicapped.pdf [accessed 12/06/12].

Shakespeare, T.W. (2006) *Disability Rights and Wrongs*. London: Routledge.

Sweeney, A., Beresford, P., Faulkner, A., Nettle, M. and Rose, S. (eds) (2009) *This is Survivor Research*. Ross-on-Wye: PCCS Books.

Walmsley, J. and Johnson, K. (2003) *Inclusive Research with People with Learning Disabilities: Past, Present and Future*. London: Jessica Kingsley.

Watson, N. (2012) 'Searching disablement', in N. Watson, A. Roulstone and C. Thomas (eds), *The Routledge Handbook of Disability Studies*. London: Routledge. pp. 93–105.

World Health Organization (WHO) (2002) *International Classification of Functioning, Disability and Health*. Geneva: WHO.

7
International Perspectives on Disability

John Swain and Sally French

Introduction

The process of globalisation is controversial and contested and can be viewed in both positive and negative terms. The substantial and growing literature addresses questions of the how, why, extent and what of global social change. In relation to culture, Cree summarises both sides of a major debate:

> For many countries globalisation has been experienced as a kind of colonisation of local cultures and customs; a 'Westernisation' or even 'Americanisation'. Yet globalisation has also opened up so-called marginalised and peripheral communities throughout the world bringing the potential for greater awareness of diverse cultures that may challenge the hegemony of Western ideas. (2002: 299)

In relation to social and economic change, it has been noted by many writers and researchers that globalisation is strongly correlated with poverty and increasing inequalities both within and between countries, although the process is geographically uneven. Poverty and inequality do not just concern monetary wealth but include education, health, housing, communication, knowledge and information (Cree, 2002; Cochrane and Pain, 2004; Mackay, 2004; United Nations, 2005; Barnes and Sheldon, 2010; Shah, 2011).

In relation to disability, perhaps it is not surprising that, as Goodley points out, disability studies have developed 'right across the globe' (2011: 18), and he provides 32 references to literature to reflect this. Our aim in this chapter is to provide a necessarily brief overview, concentrating on the global causes of disability and impairment and the possibilities for positive global developments.

International experience

In all countries of the world, disabled people are markedly over-represented amongst the poorest stratum of society. This is not just in terms of money but also education, employment, housing, health, transport, leisure, family life and social relationships (Barnes and Sheldon, 2010). For instance, it was estimated by UNESCO in 2007 that only 10 per cent of disabled children in the majority world go to school. Disabled girls and women are particularly badly affected in all respects.

Maart et al. (2007), in their study of 475 disabled people in South Africa with a range of impairments, found that they faced a large number of barriers including inaccessible buildings, low educational and employment prospects, and prejudicial and discriminatory attitudes. Those from urban areas were more likely to be faced with environmental barriers, whilst those in rural areas were more likely to experience attitudinal barriers which were often reinforced by traditional beliefs and superstitions about disabled people and impairment.

Wehbi and El-Lahib (2007) investigated the employment situation of disabled people in the Lebanon: 50 per cent of their 200 participants were illiterate and many had spent years in institutions; 67 per cent were unemployed and most of those who worked were self-employed. They faced numerous barriers to employment, including physical inaccessibility of buildings and transport, low levels of educational attainment, discriminatory attitudes, poor health, lack of personal connections and an influx of foreign labour. Women who lived in rural areas were often prevented from working by their families. Those who were employed frequently earned less than the minimum wage, even when working for long hours, and their employment was often temporary. As Wehbi and El-Lahib state: 'The overall picture is of a workforce that is overworked, underpaid and has a very low income and little job security' (2007: 380).

Braathen and Kvam (2008) investigated the experiences of 23 disabled women in Malawi with visual, hearing and physical impairments and learning difficulties. They found that the women faced many barriers in terms of education and employment as schools and workplaces were not accessible to them. They also faced negative attitudes based on superstition and lack of understanding of disability and impairment. For instance, a common belief in Malawi is that impairment is contagious or associated with witchcraft. A woman who had had polio said:

> My parents could not believe it so they took me to a witch doctor who said that I had stepped on something that was put there by a certain woman who was not happy with me. He said I had been bewitched ... Other people regard my disability as witchcraft. They say that I fell from a witchcraft airplane at night while going to bewitch other people. (2008: 465)

Other women had problems within their families and with their acceptability for marriage. One woman said: 'Men were always saying that none of them could propose marriage to me. They said that I would bring bad luck to the family' (2008: 467).

Dhungama (2006) interviewed 30 disabled women in Nepal, 13 of whom were illiterate. As Dhungama explains:

being one of the poorest countries, access to health, education and work opportunities [in Nepal] is extremely limited for the entire population. People with disabilities and their families face additional barriers to accessing services due to the restriction of their own disabilities, poverty, the mountainous terrain and social stigma. (2006: 133)

Less than 3 per cent of disabled people in Nepal receive any kind of rehabilitation and 70 per cent receive no education. The environment is inaccessible in terms of buildings and transport and there is virtually no statutory provision. One disabled woman who managed to find a job had to leave because there was no accessible toilet. Furthermore, 24 of the 30 women experienced humiliation, in the form of taunting and teasing, on the streets.

There is a belief in Nepalese society that disabled women bring bad luck to families and 80 per cent remain unmarried even though marriage is the social norm. If married women become disabled, they often experience a lack of support and abuse from family members and are denied contact with other families, leading to isolation. The law in Nepal allows men to divorce their wives if they become disabled. According to Dhungama: 'The marital life of disabled women is even worse. Their husbands and parents-in-law do not accept their disabilities and often their husbands beat them ... they are regarded as misfortunes for the family' (2006: 145).

Disabled women are often reliant on institutions which can become a lifeline to them. One woman, for instance, expressed her fear about the possible closure of a Cheshire Home (a residential home for disabled people):

I do not know what will happen in coming days. Here ... I have had amenities for the last couple of years to survive ... I have been passing my days with full care. But the lack of sustainability of this organisation shocked me, makes me vulnerable to my condition. (2006: 137)

As Dhungama states:

The majority of disabled women in the study were not only unable to satisfy their basic needs but were confronted with the problem of actual survival: almost all households did not have basic facilities such as electricity, water or a toilet. (2006: 142)

Kassah (2008) interviewed eight disabled wheelchair users, seven men and one woman, who made their living from begging in Ghana. Kassah explains that disabled people in Ghana receive little education or medical care and even have difficulty finding the resources to feed themselves. Impairment in Ghana is often viewed as a punishment or curse and most disabled people fail to find a marriage partner or may be divorced if they become disabled. Thus, for many disabled people begging becomes a means of survival, even though it is stigmatised by the government who have tried to eliminate it. All eight respondents referred to begging as work which they pursued in order to buy essential equipment, such as wheelchairs, and to help maintain their families.

The social and economic causes of impairment

The social model of disability separates disability from impairment. Disability is socially and economically caused, as the experiences of disabled people summarised above clearly demonstrate. It is eradicated by the removal of social and economic barriers to inclusion and participation. Understanding the causes of impairment, however, is left under the umbrella of medicine and the medical model. Impairment is caused physically, genetically, by disease or injury. It is thus eradicated medically, including the abortion of possibly impaired foetuses, and surgery. From a global perspective, this overall understanding can be challenged and seen as simplistic. At heart, the causes of impairment are the same as those of disability. Impairment is demonstrably socially and economically caused. Poverty, and the consequences of poverty, cause impairment as they cause disability.

This discussion takes us towards evidence which basically lies within the minefield of statistics. How many people are impaired through social and economic causes as compared to genetic causes? There are gross statistics that are regularly referred to. For instance, the Department for International Development (DFID) (2000) reproduces the figures provided by the UN (UNESCO, 2007) – malnutrition: 20%, accident/trauma/war: 16%, infectious diseases: 11%, non-infectious diseases: 20%, congenital diseases: 20%, and other (including ageing): 13%. Poverty underlies or is closely associated with most causes of impairment, including poor nutrition, dangerous working and living conditions, limited access to vaccination programmes, and to health and maternity care, poor hygiene and bad sanitation.

Though the precise meaning of the available statistics is not easy to pin-point, they clearly paint a bleak picture. It is estimated that chronic food deficits affect about 792 million people in the world (FAO, 2000), including 20 per cent of the population in the majority world countries. Malnutrition affects all age groups, but it is especially common among the poor and those with inadequate access to health education and to clean water and good sanitation. More than 70 per cent of children with protein-energy malnutrition live in Asia, 26 per cent live in Africa, and 4 per cent in Latin America and the Caribbean (WHO, 2000) (see www.who.int/water_sanitation_health/diseases/malnutrition/en/). The WHO states that, globally, 2.4 billion people, most of them in majority world countries, do not have access to improved sanitation facilities. Perhaps most telling, the WHO state that the 'data collected over ten years show that little progress has been made in reducing this number' (see www.who.int/ceh/risks/cehwater/en/). The statistics summarised by Barnes and Mercer (2010), using sources such as WHO (2001) and Stone (1999), provide further grim details: over 100 million people have acquired impairments through chronic malnutrition; 250,000 children lose their sight each year through lack of Vitamin A; and towards 800 million people have acquired a cognitive impairment due to a lack of iodine in their diet.

It is not possible to provide even an estimate of the number of people who have been impaired through recent conflicts and wars. Bilmes (2011), in a discussion of the economic consequences, states that over 90,000 US veterans of the Iraq and Afghanistan wars required medical evacuation from the conflicts. This, of course, does not include the numerous survivors of these conflicts who develop mental health issues after returning to the USA. The figures are, of course, serious, but can give only an indication of the possible number of people from Iraq and Afghanistan who were impaired during these conflicts. Since the Second World War, 41 million people have been killed in wars or 'by human decision' (Leitenberg, 2006). All that can be said is that the number of survivors impaired in these conflicts is inestimable.

Natural disasters, such as floods, tornadoes, hurricanes, earthquakes, droughts and disease epidemics, including AIDS, cause impairments as well as the more often headlined numbers of deaths. They are also not as random or haphazard as the term 'natural' might imply. Typically, the poor around the world are the worst hit and lack the resources and services to minimise the human effects. There are causes too which affect only women. The DFID (2000) reports that 20 million women a year are impaired as a result of pregnancy and childbirth, and 100 million girls and women have become impaired as a result of female genital mutilation.

Even hereditary causes cannot be divorced from the social and economic. Hagrass (2005) states that in Egypt hereditary factors are associated with endogamous marriage. People marry cousins for social, economic and cultural reasons and thus increase the incidence of many different types of impairment. Whatever the validity of the specific statistics above, it is clear that looking globally the prevention of impairment lies substantially in the eradication of poverty which requires social and economic action rather than medical interventions such as prenatal detection. The roots of impairment and disability are ultimately closely aligned: social and economic. It can be argued that this global perspective unites not only disabled people but all who would fight social and economic injustice and inequality. It is this fight which we turn to next.

A universal movement and rights-based perspective

At the centre of possibilities for positive repercussions of globalisation for disabled people lies the international voice of disabled people. The most significant development has been the growth of the organisation Disabled People's International (DPI). The global significance of the DPI was emphasised in 1998 by Kalle Konkkola (then the chairperson of the DPI) as follows:

As chairperson I have felt that DPI's meaning is more important in the Southern, Eastern and developing countries than in the Western countries especially when we look at the level of commitment. Of course the organisations in Western Europe have a commitment of working together but it appears as if the expectations on DPI are greater outside of Europe than in Europe. (cited in Priestley, 2001: 6)

As recognised by the DPI, the main political imperative in relation to globalisation is poverty:

A major goal of Disabled People's International is the full participation of all disabled people in the mainstream of life, particularly those in developing countries, who form the vast majority of the world's 500 million disabled people. DPI recognizes that poverty not only leads to disability, but also allows for few concessions for the needs and aspirations of disabled people. (www.dpi. org/en/about_us/)

However, detailed reports of the achievements of the disabled people's movement in countries in the majority world are rather mixed. Dube et al. (2006), for instance, provide examples of successful initiatives in South Africa, including the establishment of the Office on the Status of People with Disabilities, a parliamentary presence and representation on key statutory bodies. Disability policy, though, as in many majority world countries, 'has tended to be stuck on the page, rather than being used to improve the lives of disabled people' (p. 131). Hurst (2005) writes of 'the silencing of DPI through lack of funding' (p. 77).

It has been common for some years for the universal establishment of human rights to be identified as the single most important political development (Bickenbach, 2001). Bickenbach (2001) argues that human rights embody values of the respect for differences, equality of opportunity and full participation in all aspects of social life. The human rights approach is the main international thrust for social change emanating from the social model of disability and the global challenge to the oppression of disabled people. There are much-cited positive examples such as the United Nations' *Standard Rules on the Equalization of Opportunities for People with Disabilities* (UN General Assembly, 1993). However, only a third of countries have anti-discrimination legislation and the laws in many of those that do are of questionable effectiveness (UN Department of Public Information, 2008).

Conclusion

A chapter which attempts to address the lives of disabled people within the global context can only begin to recognise the complexities, controversies and inadequacies of any predictions for the future. Nevertheless, there are fundamental realities which reverberate around the globe. Any analysis begins with the realisation that disabled people are the poorest of the poor. Poverty and all its manifestations define the lives of disabled people around the globe, underpin causes of disability and underpin, too, the multiplicity of causes of impairment. It is clear that the benefits of globalisation do reach some disabled people of the majority world but they tend to be among the better educated and the least poor. For instance, in a study of 122 disabled Internet users in China, it was found that they had high levels of educational attainment and received the necessary equipment from family members if their wages were low or if they were unemployed (Guo et al., 2005). We are living in a shrinking political, economic and cultural world and disability remains in the rear.

References

Barnes, C. and Mercer, G. (2010) *Exploring Disability* (2nd edn). Cambridge: Polity.

Barnes, C. and Sheldon, A. (2010) 'Disability politics and poverty in a majority world context', *Disability & Society*, 25 (7): 771–82.

Bickenbach, J.E. (2001) 'Disability human rights, law, and policy', in G.L. Albrecht, K.D. Seelman and M. Bury (eds), *Handbook of Disability Studies*. Thousand Oaks, CA: SAGE. pp. 565–84.

Bilmes, L.J. (2011) Current and Projected Future Costs of Caring for Veterans of the Iraq and Afghanistan Wars. Available at: www.costsofwar.org/sites/default/files/articles/52/attachments/Bilmes Veterans Costs.pdf

Braathen, S.H. and Kvam, M.H. (2008) 'Can anything come out of this mouth? Female experiences of disability in Malawi', *Disability & Society*, 23 (5): 461–74.

Cochrane, A. and Pain, K. (2004) 'A globalising society', in D. Held (ed.), *A Globalising World? Culture, Economics, Politics*. London: Routledge. pp. 5–46.

Cree, V.E. (2002) 'Social work and society', in M. Davies (ed.), *The Blackwell Companion to Social Work*. Oxford: Blackwell. pp. 289–303.

Department for International Development (DFID) (2000) Disability, Poverty and Development. London: DFID. Available at: www.handicap-international.fr/bibliographie-handicap/4PolitiqueHandicap/hand_pauvrete/DFID_disability.pdfwww.handicap-international.fr/bibliographie-handicap/4PolitiqueHandicap/hand_pauvrete/DFID_disability.pdf

Dhungama, B.M. (2006) 'The lives of disabled women in Nepal: vulnerability without support', *Disability & Society*, 21 (2): 133–46.

Dube, T., Hurst, R., Light, R. and Malinga, J. (2006) 'Promoting inclusion? Disabled people, legislation and public policy', in B. Albert (ed.), *In or Out of the Mainstream: Lessons from Research on Disability and Development Cooperation*. Leeds: The Disablity Press. pp. 104–18.

FAO (2000) *The State of Food Insecurity in the World*. Rome: FAO.

Goodley, D. (2011) *Disability Studies: An Interdisciplinary Introduction*. London: SAGE.

Guo, B., Bricout, J.C. and Huang, J. (2005) 'A common open space or a digital divide? A social model perspective on the online disability community in China', *Disability & Society*, 20 (1): 49–56.

Hagrass, H. (2005) 'Definitions of disability and disability policy in Egypt', in C. Barnes and G. Mercer (eds), *The Social Model of Disability: Europe and the Majority World*. Leeds: The Disability Press. pp. 148–62.

Hurst, R. (2005) 'Disabled People's International: Europe and the social model of disability', in C. Barnes and G. Mercer (eds), *The Social Model of Disability: Europe and the Majority World*. Leeds: The Disability Press.

Kassah, A.K. (2008) 'Begging as work: a study of people with mobility disabilities in Accra, Ghana', *Disability & Society*, 23 (2): 163–70.

Leitenberg, M. (2006) *Deaths in Wars and Conflicts in the 20th Century* (3rd edn), Occasional Paper No. 29, Cornell University Peace Studies Program. Ithaca, NY: Cornell.

Maart, S., Eide, H., Jelsman, J., Loeb, M.E. and Ka Toni, M. (2007) 'Environmental barriers experienced by urban and rural disabled people in South Africa', *Disability & Society*, 22 (4): 357–69.

Mackay, H. (2004) 'The globalisation of culture', in D. Held (ed.), *A Globalising World? Culture, Economics, Politics*. London: Routledge. pp. 47–84.

Priestley, M. (ed.) (2001) *Disability and the Life Course: Global Perspectives*. Cambridge: Cambridge University Press.

Shah, A. (2011) Causes of Poverty. Available at: www.globalissues.org [accessed 31/03/12].

Stone, E. (1999) 'Disability and development in the majority world', in E. Stone (ed.), *Disability and Development: Learning from Action and Research on Disability in the Majority World*. Leeds: The Disability Press. pp. 1–20.

UNESCO (2007) *EFA Global Monitoring Report 2007 – Strong Foundation: Early Childhood Care and Education*. Paris: UNESCO.

United Nations (UN) (2005) *Report on the World Situation 2005: The Inequality Predicament*. New York: United Nations.

United Nations (UN) Department of Public Information (2008) Backgrounder: Disability Treaty Closes a Gap in Protecting Human Rights. Available at: www.un.org/disabilities/default.asp?id=476

UN General Assembly (1993) Resolution 48/96. Standard Rules on the Equalization of Opportunities for Persons with Disabilities (A/RES/48/96). 48th Session, 20 December. Available at: www.un.org/esa/socdev/enable/dissre00.htm

Wehbi, S. and El-Lahib, Y. (2007) 'The employment situation of people with disabilities in Lebanon', *Disability & Society*, 22 (4): 371–82.

World Health Organization (WHO) (2000) *Turning the Tide of Malnutrition: Responding to the Challenge of the 21st Century*. Geneva: WHO.

World Health Organization (WHO) (2001) *Rethinking Care from the Perspective of Disabled People*. Geneva: WHO.

Part 2

In Our Own Image

8

Disability and the Body

Bill Hughes

Introduction

In describing the principles of what was to become the social model of disability, UPIAS (1976) made a clear distinction between impairment and disability. Disability was defined as social oppression and impairment as biological deficit. This distinction 'crippled' the medical model but removed impairment and the body from radical disability discourse. This new perspective made it clear that disability was a problem of social organisation (Oliver, 1990). The solution to the problem of disability, therefore, did not lie in the efforts of rehabilitation science but in systematic social change. Though disability was made into a social and political category, impaired bodies were consigned to nature.

Over the last 20 years, there has been some considerable effort made in disability studies literature to politicise disabled embodiment (Morris, 1991; Hughes and Paterson, 1997; Shakespeare and Watson, 1997; Hughes, 2002; Goodley, 2011), with the culturally oriented humanities tradition in North America playing a significant role (Garland Thomson, 1997, 2009; Davis, 2002; McRuer, 2006; Snyder and Mitchell, 2006). More importantly, embodied differences within the disability movement that were grounded in the different experiences of impairment indicated that disability identity could not be conceived of as a homogeneous package. Identity so conceived signalled the marginalisation of, for example, people with cognitive disabilities (Goodley, 2001) and raised question marks in the minds of Deaf activists as to whether the disabled people's movement is hospitable enough for their political purposes (Scully, 2012). If the celebration of difference was to be used as a mantra to counter the politics of exclusion, then it had to be applied to relations among disabled people as well as to relations between disabled and non-disabled people. The debate about impairment and the body was partly a challenge to the process by which disability identity was dominated by the interests of people with mobility impairments. The fact that questions of physical access to public space had come to dominate disability politics was manifest most explicitly in the adoption of the figure of the wheelchair user as the universal symbol for disability. These debates signified that the bodies of disabled people were political; and could not be reduced to biology or conceded to the medical profession. Impairment, like disability, was social and historical:

> Scholars have only recently discovered that the human body itself has a history. Not only has it been perceived, interpreted and represented differently in different epochs, but it has also been lived differently, brought into being within widely dissimilar material cultures, subjected to various technology and means of control and incorporated into different rhythms of production and consumption, pleasure and pain. (Gallacher and Laqueur, 1987: vii)

In practice, disabled people began to take pride in their lives and their bodies. Bodies that had been excluded from the labour market by the epic transformation of industrial capitalism (Oliver, 1990) and invalidated by the normalising proclivities of modern medicine began to discover that the physical and mental 'defects and deficits' by which they had been known for the last 150 years were a matter of social construction rather than biological fact. The social model made adjustments to incorporate impairment because 'all disabled people have impairments' (Oliver et al., 2012: 30). This concession to the obvious was, in part, a response to noisy theoreticians but it was mostly a result of the affirmative strategies (Swain and French, 2000) of disabled people who began to trade in the stigma of shameful imperfection for the audible voice of the independent agent. The discourse that impairment is opposed to physical, cognitive and social integrity was exposed as a lie. The pathologisers had got it wrong and the social model adjusted itself to contend with the dynamic of a politics of pride and the arrival of new waves of social theory.

Thinking impairment

The social model has focused on the claim that disabled people are and have been excluded from participation in social life, but it has been much more reticent to examine the processes by which disabled people's bodies have been represented as inferior, blighted or in deficit. Disabled people are second-class citizens but they have also had their bodies invalidated and demeaned by a variety of cultural systems of meaning. Thinking about the social aspects of impaired bodies has been inspired, mostly, by three theoretical traditions: feminism, poststructualism and phenomenology. I will briefly review the contribution that these traditions have made to the understanding of disabled embodiment.

Feminism

Disabled feminists were first to argue that impairment could not be conceived of in politically neutral terms (Morris, 1991; Wendell, 1996; Garland Thomson, 1997; Thomas, 1999, 2001; Fawcett, 2000). Originally, the social model had contended that whilst disability was a collective issue, impairment was a personal problem. Feminists, however, lived by the slogan that the 'personal was the political'. Logic suggested that if one's corporeal status was personal, then to consign it to political neutrality and make medicine its natural mentor was a mistake. If one lives with both impairment and disability, then both contribute to the experience of disability at a personal level. Feminists charged the social model with failing to take into consideration the whole realm of the 'personal and the experiential' (Thomas, 2001: 48), including what Jenny Morris (1991: 10) called 'the experience of our own bodies'. Disabled feminists prefer to admit that some impairments involve pain and suffering and that it is politically honest and valuable to speak about such issues rather than take the *malestream* view that politics can be reduced to the elimination of barriers. Besides, oppression is not simply something that is manifest in the discriminatory constitution of social organisation. It is also something that is 'felt' – as anger, frustration or even pain – as a consequence of experiencing the 'ableism' of culture (Campbell, 2009).

Feminists also faced up to the difficult question of whether or not impairment can be regarded as a cause of disability. The social model was unequivocal that this could not be the case and that disability could be traced, causally, to forms of social organisation. However, Sally French (1993: 17) argued that, whilst she supports the 'basic tenets of the social model', she is compelled to argue – from her experience of visual impairment – that 'some of the most profound problems experienced by people with certain impairments are difficult, if not impossible, to solve by social manipulation'. In order to address this problem of causality, Carol Thomas (1999: 43) has proposed the concept of 'impairment effects' by which she means 'restrictions of activity which are associated with being impaired but which are not disabilities', in so far as they have nothing to do with the unequal power relations between disabled and non-disabled people. She also makes it clear that impairment effects 'should not be naturalized, or dealt with as pre-social "biological" phenomena'.

Poststructuralism

Feminism is a broad church and a number of feminists who have contributed significantly to disability studies can be described as postmodernists or poststructuralists (Corker and French, 1999; Shildrick, 2002; Tremain, 2005). Poststructuralists and postmodernists deconstruct the dualistic thinking that separates the world into binaries like body and society, private and public, and impairment and disability. This, they argue, represents the modernist tradition of thinking and its day is done. The terms we use – like impairment and disability – are linguistic signs that only have an arbitrary and conventional connection with the things that they are supposed to give meaning to. If language is to be reduced to its effects, as poststructuralists argue, then the body is primarily a cultural or discursive product. From this point of view – strongly influenced by the work of Michel Foucault – impairment is fully cultural. Put another way, the impaired body is a historically contingent product of power and, therefore, not – as the medical profession would have it – a set of universal biological characteristics amenable to and objectively defined by diagnostic practices.

Whilst some feminist writers, like Susan Wendell (1996), think that there are real biological differences between disabled and non-disabled bodies, poststructuralists reject such claims on the grounds that they are essentialist, and argue that the body is produced by meaning and interpretation and is, therefore, best understood in terms of discourse or cultural representation. Perhaps the best way to understand this 'anti-essentialist' argument is, ironically, to think about non-disabled bodies. The non-disabled body is usually described as 'normal'. But what do we mean by 'normal'? Clearly, it is not a precise term, more of a statistical average. In other words, in reality, the normal or non-disabled body does not exist. What does exist is the linguistic convention or discourse of normality that conveys something to us about bodies and helps us to make some sense of them. If the non-disabled body does not exist in any essential sense, then the same applies to impairment. It is a metaphor, a cultural representation that, in modern times, has become located in a negative language of defect and deficit.

Phenomenology

Phenomenology starts with experience or the perception of the subject. The impaired body is not so much a biological datum as a fundamental point of reference for whosoever experiences it (Hughes and Paterson, 1997; Paterson and Hughes, 1999). The body is the material basis of everybody's experience. It is 'our point of view on the world'. It is the 'place' in which we live and by which we are recognised, but it is also an object upon which we can reflect. In all these incarnations, it is social. It is the where, why and when of our daily activities and experiences. The body is the existential foundation of self and culture. Given this social repertoire associated with our physicality, it is fair to claim that impairment is social and disability, embodied. Ableism makes the world alien to impaired bodies and, therefore, simultaneously produces impairment as a particular sort of experience – one that is frequently exclusionary, restrictive, discriminatory and oppressive.

We live in a world that is characterised by a carnal hierarchy. The non-impaired body is privileged and advantaged. The impaired body is judged as incompetent, and such an evaluation (of worth) is often carried, as a core assumption, by non-disabled persons into their everyday encounters with disabled people (Titchkosky, 2007). This kind of argument locates the oppression of disabled people not in its structural origins in objective barriers but in the concrete world of lived experience and the everyday world of mundane social relationships. Impairment cannot be siphoned out from the mosaic of dimensions that make everyday encounters into unsatisfactory experiences for disabled people. Such encounters compel disabled people to reflect upon their bodies and on the way in which they are perceived as 'alien'. As Kevin Paterson put it:

> In the context of a social environment saturated with disablist images, attitudes and behaviour and devoid of carnal information that reflects my corporeal

status, I am perpetually reminded of my body. These incidents can be major or minor – depending on how I feel or their frequency that day. They may range from being stared at or side-stepped in the street, treated as a young child, considered drunk when I am not, to being called disablist names. (Paterson and Hughes, 1999: 605)

The social and physical world has been made in the image and likeness of non-disabled people. It is a home for *their* bodies. Even the norms and codes of movement and timing which structure everyday communication are informed by and devised in an idiom that is based on the carnal and emotional needs of non-disabled people.

The three theoretical positions described above are different in many ways but what they all have in common is that they do not treat impairment simply as biology or nature. This transforms the meaning of impairment from an individual medical problem into a site of social and political debate. The social model, in its infancy, did exactly this for the concept of disability and it is important to keep impairment sociologically alive, primarily because disability itself should be understood in terms of the invalidating responses to impairment that have developed historically in the non-disabled imaginary (Hughes, 2012) or mindset.

Conclusion

The debate about impairment has been central to the development of a revisionist view in disability studies, most clearly associated with the work of Tom Shakespeare (2006). Yet, if the legitimacy of the social model is to be sustained, it must be inclusive of and support the aspirations of all disabled people. Disabled people have much in common and while it is unity that makes disability politics possible, impairment is a significant dimension of the experience of disability and of the differences in experience. It is important to keep the debate about impairment alive and well. 'It should be possible to understand the "impaired body" as simultaneously biological, material and social – in short as bio-social in character' (Thomas, 2007: 135). It is also politically desirable.

It is to impairment that non-disabled people react – emotionally violently, with hatred, through exclusion, segregation, marginalisation, sterilisation, genocide, and so on – and it is the non-disabled imaginary or mindset that needs to be named and shamed by the disabled people's movement and deconstructed by critical disability studies. The idea of critical disability studies has emerged out of the theoretical flux described above and from the intention embedded in these perspectives to treat impairment and the body as socially and politically meaningful (Goodley et al., 2012; Shildrick, 2012). The fact that the body is variously culturally and historically interpreted and understood, should be put to use in the endeavour of disability emancipation because it is through such interpretations that disabled people are invalidated and demeaned; transformed from manifestations of 'human variation' (Siebers, 2008: 25) into sub-human 'objects' of pity, fear and disgust (Hughes, 2012).

References

Campbell, F.K. (2009) *Contours of Ableism*. Basingstoke: Palgrave Macmillan.
Corker, M. and French, S. (eds) (1999) *Disability Discourse*. Buckingham: Open University Press.
Davis, L. (2002) *Bending over Backwards: Disability, Dismodernism and Other Difficult Positions*. New York: New York University Press.
Fawcett, B. (2000) *Feminist Perspectives on Disability*. London: Prentice Hall.
French, S. (1993) 'Disability, impairment or something in between', in J. Swain, V. Finkelstein, S. French and M. Oliver (eds), *Disabling Barriers – Enabling Environments*. London: SAGE, in association with the Open University. pp. 17–25.
Gallacher, C. and Laqueur, T. (eds) (1987) *The Making of the Modern Body*. Berkeley: University of California Press.
Garland Thomson, R. (1997) *Extraordinary Bodies: Figuring Physical Disability in American Culture and Literature*. New York: Columbia University Press.
Garland Thomson, R. (2009) *Staring: How We Look*. Oxford: Oxford University Press.
Goodley, D. (2001) 'Learning difficulties, the social model of disability and impairment: challenging epistemologies', *Disability & Society*, 16 (2): 207–31.
Goodley, D. (2011) *Disability Studies: An Interdisciplinary Introduction*. London: SAGE.
Goodley, D., Hughes, B. and Davis, L. (eds) (2012) *Social Theories of Disability: New Developments*. Basingstoke: Palgrave.
Hughes, B. (2002) 'Disability and the body', in C. Barnes, L. Barton and M. Oliver (eds), *Disability Studies Today*. Cambridge: Polity. pp. 58–76
Hughes, B. (2012) 'Fear, pity and disgust: emotions and the non-disabled imaginary', in N. Watson, A. Roulstone and C. Thomas (eds), *Routledge Handbook of Disability Studies*. London: Routledge. pp. 68–78.
Hughes, B. and Paterson, K. (1997) 'The social model of disability and the disappearing body: towards a sociology of impairment', *Disability & Society*, 12 (3): 325–40.
McRuer, R. (2006) *Crip Theory: Cultural Signs of Queerness and Disability*. New York: New York University Press.
Morris, J. (1991) *Pride against Prejudice: Transforming Attitudes to Disability*. London: The Women's Press.
Oliver, M. (1990) *The Politics of Disablement*. London: Macmillan.
Oliver, M., Sapey, B. and Thomas, P. (2012) *Social Work with Disabled People* (4th edn). Basingstoke: Palgrave.
Paterson, K. and Hughes, B. (1999) 'Disability studies and phenomenology: the carnal politics of everyday life', *Disability & Society*, 14 (5): 597–610.
Scully, J.L. (2012) 'Deaf identities in disability studies', in N. Watson, A. Roulstone and C. Thomas (eds), *Routledge Handbook of Disability Studies*. London: Routledge. pp. 109–21.
Shakespeare, T. (2006) *Disability Rights and Wrongs*. London: Routledge.
Shakespeare, T. and Watson, N. (1997) 'Defending the social model', *Disability & Society*, 12 (2): 293–300.
Shildrick, M. (2002) *Embodying the Monster*. London: SAGE.
Shildrick, M. (2012) 'Critical disability studies', in N. Watson, A. Roulstone and C. Thomas (eds), *Routledge Handbook of Disability Studies*. London: Routledge. pp. 30–41.
Siebers, T. (2008) *Disability Theory*. Ann Arbor: University of Michigan Press.
Snyder, S. and Mitchell, D. (2006) *Cultural Locations of Disability*. Chicago and London: University of Chicago Press.

Swain, J. and French, S. (2000) 'Towards an affirmation model of disability', *Disability &
Society*, 15 (4): 569–82.

Thomas, C. (1999) *Female Forms: Experiencing and Understanding Disability*. Milton
Keynes: Open University Press.

Thomas, C. (2001) 'Feminism and disability: the theoretical and political significance of the
personal and the experiential', in C. Barton (ed.), *Disability Politics and the Struggle for
Change*. London: David Fulton. pp. 48–58.

Thomas, C. (2007) *Sociologies of Disability and Illness*. London: Palgrave Macmillan.

Titchkosky, T. (2007) *Reading and Writing Disability Differently: The Textured Life of
Bodiment*. Toronto: Toronto University Press.

Tremain, S. (2005) *Foucault and the Government of Disability*. Ann Arbor: University of
Michigan Press.

UPIAS (1976) *Fundamental Principles of Disability*. London: UPIAS.

Wendell, S. (1996) *The Rejected Body: Feminist Philosophical Reflections on Disability*. New
York: Routledge.

9

Disability and Psychology

Dan Goodley

Introduction

Can we bring together psychological and disability studies theory in ways that help us make sense of the external conditions and relational experiences of disablism? What is the psychological impact of living with impairment in a disabling society? How are we to understand and confront non-disabled individuals' reactions to disability? This chapter seeks to address these questions. First, we will trace some of the ways in which the psychological has been attended to in the disability studies literature. Second, we will examine a number of analytical moments when disability and psychology have interconnected. Third, we will draw on the theory of emotional labour and the concept of demanding publics to probe disabled people's relational and subjective engagements with their wider environments and the non-disabled people that populate them.

Psychology *in* disability studies

We should acknowledge but not detail tensions between disability studies and psychology (for more developed accounts, see contributions to Goodley and Lawthom, 2005, 2008; Goodley, 2012). Instead, we will begin by pulling out some examples from British disability studies that have engaged with psychology. Disabled people's organisations have responded to the psychological impact of living in a disabling society through politicisation (Campbell and Oliver, 1996), the provision of peer counselling (Priestley, 1999) and the promotion of disability arts as powerful forms of catharsis (Hevey, 1992). The self-advocacy movement of people with the label of intellectual disabilities has established safe spaces for the sharing of aspirations

* Parts of Chapter 6 of Goodley (2011) *Disability Studies: An Interdisciplinary Introduction* (London: SAGE ©) have been reproduced with all permissions received.

(Goodley, 2000), mental health activists have subverted normative understandings of sanity (Chamberlin, 1990) and 'queer crips' have celebrated their transgression (McRuer, 2003). Accordingly, disability studies has addressed the psychology of disablism, defined by Thomas (2007: 73) 'as a form of social oppression involving the social imposition of restrictions of activity on people with impairments and the socially engendered undermining of their psycho-emotional well being'. Fanon (1993: 12–13) describes this as a process of socio-diagnosis: of waging war on both levels of the socio-economic and psychological. Disablism, like racism, can seriously threaten psychological life.

It is possible to trace a strong psychological thread of thinking from the early to the contemporary days of British disability studies. Oliver et al.'s (1988) text was one of the first to work with a clear politicised understanding of disability while representing the subjective experiences of living with an acquired impairment. Similarly, in the first edition of this volume, Swain et al. (1993) included a number of psychological accounts of disability. Amongst them was the pioneering chapter by Finkelstein and French (1993) that called for a psychology of disability that was in tune with the conditions of disabling society and the subjective lives of disabled people. The feminist collection by Morris (1996) offered clear expositions of the subjective experiences of impairment and disability. Many feminists view the socio-political as present in the interstices and intimacies of day-to-day private life, as they do in public domains (Thomas, 2002: 49). The significance of the personal is highlighted by Stramondo (2009), who observes that a recurring anxiety alluded to by those advocating for assisted suicide is the question of whether or not 'you would want someone to wipe your ass'. Intimate relationships are an important part of our social and political lives. Theorising the relational and subjective qualities of self and other, individual and society would appear to be a growing concern for disability studies. But what kinds of psychological entanglements would be most beneficial to disability studies? We move now to contemplate how we might borrow from psychology to service the needs of disability studies. What we should have in mind is a recasting of psychology as 'a discipline of and for the (disabled) community that helps us challenge disabling conditions of everyday psychological and cultural life' (Goodley, 2012: 310).

Psychology *for* disability studies

A review of the literature would suggest that there have been a number of attempts to politicise the emotional and psychological registers through the lens of disability studies (see contributions to Goodley and Lawthom, 2005; see also Olkin and Pledger, 2003). The concept of *psycho-emotional disablism* encapsulates the psychological consequences of in/direct forms of discrimination, recognising that disablism is felt within as well as outside (Thomas, 2002, 2007; Reeve, 2008). *Distributed competence* acknowledges the extent to which psychological competence is enabled or stifled through the networks of support one has in one's life. Intelligence and capacity are understood in terms of the quality of relational networks of support rather than the disposition of an individual (Booth and Booth, 1994; Tobbell and Lawthom, 2005). *The corporeal or embodied* experience of disability and impairment has been theorised as contributing to the subjective status of the individual, dependent not only on essentialist characteristics of embodiment but also on the body's social and relational engagements with its environment (Hughes and Paterson, 1997; Paterson and Hughes, 1999).

The *metaphorical* manufacturing of the disabled self can be found in dominant forms of cultural production, where disability is used as a metaphor for psychological, social and cultural discourses of 'lack', 'tragedy' and 'flawed' (Davis, 1995; Mitchell and Snyder, 1997, 2006). Such disabling subjective and objective encounters bring with it the risk of *internalised oppression* and the psychological consequences of the material exclusion of disabled people from mainstream life including false consciousness (Oliver, 1996: Chapter 13). Hence, the dynamic interplay of biology, psychology and the environment has led some to argue for a *relational* understanding of disability (Wendell, 1996; Shakespeare, 2006). *Discursive* analyses interrogate the constitution of self, body and social world through the practices and discourses of societal institutions and cultural narratives (Corker, 1998; Tremain, 2005). Recent engagements with *social psychoanalytic* theory unpick the dynamic relational and inseparable nature of the psychological and social life in the constitution of disabled and non-disabled subjectivities (Marks, 1999; Goodley, 2011). Meanwhile, *queer and postcolonial* interventions have blurred the binaries of self/other; nature/society; private/public; psychological/material through an analysis of heteronormative, occidental and patriarchal societies, in which the psychology of disability is both oppositional to normative society and viewed as positively disruptive (McRuer, 2003; Ghai, 2006). *Existential* and *phenomenological* writings have understood emotions as being directly related to how close our expectations, hopes and desires come to being met (Shuttleworth, 2000; Michalko, 2002; Titchkosky, 2003).

All these analytical encounters render the emotional and the intimate legitimate subjects of social scientific analysis (Thomas, 2004). Each contemplates the person's interiority and their relationship with the exteriority of others. Or, as Ghai (2006: 26) puts it, they attend to alterity: how the disabled self is made in the image of others. These developments have addressed what Finkelstein and French (1993) describe as the need for a psychology of disability, 'which focuses on the psychological anxieties and distresses caused by the social relations of disability' (Reeve, 2008: 53). Each, to varying extents, shifts attention from the psychology of impairment, to a psychology of dis/ability and disablism.

Psychology *for* disability studies contests the individualisation of disability and seeks to expose psychological elements of living with an impairment in a disabling world. Psychology *for* disability engages in what Hook (2004: 115) defines as psycho-politics: the explicit politicisation of the psychological, which occurs through the placing of a series of ostensibly psychological concerns and concepts within the register of the political. For the remainder of this chapter, we will subject an ostensibly psychological idea – the reaction of others to the self – to political and theoretical interrogation. As Michalko (2002) puts it, the problem of disability is rarely the problem for disabled people. Instead, the ways in which non-disabled others respond to the presence of disability creates problems for disabled people. The self–other dichotomy is a key relationship in psychology. As Hollway (2007: 128) has argued, 'if we are seen in ways that make us feel we exist, that confirm us, then we are free to go on looking, and our sense of self is enlarged as we internalise the other and their sense of us'. For disabled people, this potential for enlargement of the self risks being stifled because engagements with the other take place in a context of disablism. It is therefore crucial that we interrogate the politics of these psychological relations.

Psychology *of* disablism: Emotional labour and demanding publics

A feature of psychological and emotional disablism relates to the kinds of perfor-mances expected of disabled people. We know that disabled people are expected to emotionally labour in response to a demanding non-disabled public (Goodley, 2012: 318). Liddiard (2012) reminds us that even during the most intimate of encounters with others – personal care, assistance and sexual activities – disabled people are expected to manage their selves in relations with others. A theoretical route for mak-ing sense of these encounters is provided by Williams's (2003) discussion of *emo-tional labour*, a term coined by Hochschild (1983). Williams provided a study of air hostesses in which she acknowledges the huge emotional and physical pressures placed on these workers by the passengers they serve. Disabled people also serve the public in a number of ways: existing as convenient emotional objects and recipients of pity, fascination, curiosity – a point not lost on disabled feminists (Malec, 1993; Wendell, 1996). The concept of emotional labour seeks to account for the assault on the self that occurs in response to demanding publics. Emotions are corporeal thoughts, embodied processes, imbricated with social values and frequently involved in preserving social bonds, social rules and displays of behaviour (Williams, 2003: 519–20). Hochschild's (1983) concept of emotional labour refers to those times when the self has to act in ways that fit the expectations of others. Disabled people learn biographical responses to the expectations of non-disabled culture – the demanding public – which might range from acting as the passive disabled bystander, the grateful recipient of others' support, the non-problematic receiver of others' disabling attitudes. Maintaining this emotional labour can be psychologically test-ing. Williams (2003) discusses the notion of 'corpsing' where the social actor fails to maintain the management of their emotional labour and the illusion of stability. They freeze. Corpsing can occur when publics demand too much. Following Fanon (1993: 33), these demands may reside in 'the stigmata of a dereliction' in non-disabled people's relationships with disabled others. Here are a few examples that I have collected:

> Your child's the naughty boy in my child's class, isn't he? (A parent's question to the mother of a child with the label of ADHD)

I never think of you as disabled. (A common 'positive' comment from friends of the disabled writer Michalko, 2002)

At least he's not *too* disabled. (A health visitor's comments to the mother of a newborn baby)

Did you read on the web that 52% of the American public would prefer to be dead than disabled? (Bar chat on a November night)

You are just so brave, I don't know how you cope. (A mother's comment to another mother of a disabled child in the playground)

I don't know how you can work with those people … It must be so rewarding to work with those people. (Contradictory comments from a friend to a key worker for people with learning difficulties)

I've had coins dropped in my lap by strangers in the street. (Hewitt, 2004)

Don't worry about paying, love; we don't charge for retards. (Comment from a fairground assistant to the mother of a disabled child, cited in Goodley, 2011)

The other mothers asked that I did not bring my Autistic sons on the school trip because they were worried that my boys might attack their children. (Anonymous story handed to me after a seminar, April 2009)

When the public demands so much emotional labour from disabled people, then it is hardly surprising the latter would corpse. People deal with corpsing in different ways. Some are productive (embracing disability activism; challenging the public; joking about it; kicking the cat), whilst others are potentially destructive (avoiding social settings where such questions may arise; internalising these comments as indicators of psychological flaws; feeling powerless). Whatever the reaction, the response is energy-sapping: 'many disabled people are tired of being symbols to the able bodied' (Wendell, 1996: 252). Williams's (2003) analysis presumes that the (non-disabled) public is already demanding. This rings true for many disabled people. Non-disabled people appear, at times, to expect responses to the most inappropriate of questions; assume that it is perfectly acceptable to share their own curiosities around impairment with disabled people; demand quick responses to hurtful and thoughtless commentaries. Williams (2003) refers to these as 'strong scripts' of individuals in culturally powerful positions who feel authorised to make such demands. This might explain why disabled people find it easier to identify themselves as disabled to themselves (and other disabled people) than they do to other (non-disabled) people (Wendell, 1996).

Clearly, the emotional lives of disabled people risk being policed by these publics. Olkin (2002) describes the experience of affect regulation: that is the prescription of certain affects/emotions (such as cheerfulness and gratefulness) alongside the pro- hibition of other affects (including anger and resentment). When disabled people display the latter types of emotion, they are often dismissed by demanding publics as being arrogant, unreasonable, ungrateful and having a chip on their shoulders.

Just as black people are expected to be, in the words of Fanon (1993: 34), 'good niggers' *[sic]*, disabled people are supposed to be 'good cripples'; 'eternal victims of an essence, of an appearance, for which they are not responsible' (Fanon, 1993: 34). The psychological and emotional experience of disablism is one subjected to every-day, mundane and relentless examples of cultural and relational violence.

Conclusion

In this chapter, we have considered the place and value of psychological concepts, theories and appropriations to the development of disability studies. One key area of analysis that requires highlighting and challenging relates to the demands expected of disabled people by the non-disabled public. This is not to suggest that all non-disabled people are equally as demanding, nor that all disabled people are subjected to the same kinds of demands. As Reeve (2012) has observed, different impairment categories, variegated life opportunities and the kinds of spaces we occupy bring with them varying forms of psycho-emotional disablism. Nevertheless, the non-disabled register remains a troubling space requiring understanding and politicisation. Perhaps one way in which disability studies and psychology can work together by turning the gaze from disabled people onto non-disabled, disabling and ableist culture is to ask: what is the psychological impact of trying to live up to the ideals of being cognitively and physically 'able' when ableist standards are so impossible to achieve? How do disabled people challenge and queer the demands of ableist societies? How can we theorise and contest this precarious phenomenon of the 'able-bodied'? In answering these questions, a psycho-politics may be developed that learns from the expertise of disabled people, their politics and their everyday encounters with society.

References

Booth, T. and Booth, W. (1994) *Parenting under Pressure: Mothers and Fathers with Learning Difficulties*. Buckingham: Open University Press.

Campbell, J. and Oliver, M. (1996) *Disability Politics: Understanding Our Past, Changing Our Future*. London: Routledge.

Chamberlin, J. (1990) 'The ex-patients movement: where we've been and where we are going', *Journal of Mind and Behaviour*, 11 (3): 323–36.

Corker M. (1998) *Deaf and Disabled or Deafness Disabled*. Buckingham: Open University Press.

Davis, L.J. (1995) *Enforcing Normalcy: Disability, Deafness, and the Body*. New York: Verso.

Fanon, F. (1993) *Black Skins, White Masks* (3rd edn). London: Pluto Press.

Finkelstein, V. and French, S. (1993) 'Towards a psychology of disability', in J. Swain, V. Finkelstein, S. French and M. Oliver (eds), *Disabling Barriers – Enabling Environments*. London: SAGE, in association with the Open University. pp. 26–33.

Ghai, A. (2006) *(Dis)embodied Form: Issues of Disabled Women*. Delhi: Shakti Books.

Goodley, D. (2000) *Self-advocacy in the Lives of People with Learning Difficulties: The Politics of Resilience*. Buckingham: Open University Press.

Goodley, D. (2011) 'Social psychoanalytic disability studies', *Disability & Society*, 26 (6): 715–28.

Goodley, D. (2012) 'The psychology of disability', in N. Watson, C. Thomas and A. Roulstone (eds), *Routledge Companion to Disability Studies*. London: Routledge, pp. 310–23.

Goodley, D. and Lawthom, R. (eds) (2005) *Disability and Psychology: Critical Introductions and Reflections*. London: Palgrave.

Goodley, D. and Lawthom, R. (2008) 'Disability studies and psychology: emancipatory opportunities', in S. Gabel and S. Danforth (eds), *Disability and the Politics of Education: A Reader*. New York: Peter Lang. pp. 477–98.

Hewitt, S. (2004) 'Sticks and stones in a boy', in B. Guter and J. Killacky (eds), *Queer Crips: Disabled Gay Men and Their Stories*. New York: Haworth Press. pp. 117–20.

Hevey, D. (1992) *The Creatures Time Forgot: Photography and Disability Imagery*. London: Routledge.

Hochschild, A.R. (1983) *The Managed Heart: Commercialisation of Human Feeling*. Berkeley: University of California Press.

Hollway, W. (2007) 'Self', in W. Hollway, H. Lucy and A. Phoenix (eds), *Social Psychology Matters*. Maidenhead: Open University Press. pp. 33–64.

Hook, D. (2004) 'Fanon and the psychoanalysis of racism', in D. Hook (ed.), *Critical Psychology*. Lansdowne, South Africa: Juta Academic Publishing. pp. 114–37.

Hughes, B. and Paterson, K. (1997) 'The social model of disability and the disappearing body: towards a sociology of "impairment"', *Disability & Society*, 12 (3): 325–40.

Liddiard, K. (2012) (S)exploring Disability: Sexualities, Intimacies, and Disabilities. Unpublished PhD thesis, Warwick University.

McRuer, R. (2003) 'As good as it gets: queer theory and critical disability', *GLQ: A Journal of Lesbian and Gay Studies*, 9 (1–2): 79–105.

Malec, C. (1993) 'The double objectification of disability and gender', *Canadian Woman Studies*, 13 (4): 22–3.

Marks, D. (1999) *Disability: Controversial Debates and Psychosocial Perspectives*. London: Routledge.

Michalko, R. (2002) *The Difference That Disability Makes*. Philadelphia, PA: Temple University Press.

Mitchell, D. and Snyder, S. (eds) (1997) *The Body and Physical Difference: Discourse of Disability*. New York: Verso.

Mitchell, D. and Snyder, S. (2006) 'Narrative prosthesis and the materiality of metaphor', in L. Davis (ed.), *The Disability Studies Reader* (2nd edn). New York: Routledge. pp. 1650–2000.

Morris, J. (ed.) (1996) *Encounters with Strangers: Feminism and Disability*. London: The Women's Press.

Oliver, M. (1996) *Understanding Disability: From Theory to Practice*. London: Macmillan.

Oliver, M., Zarb, G., Silver, M., Moore, M. and Salisbury, V. (1988) *Walking into Darkness: The Experience of Spinal Cord Injury*. Tavistock: Macmillan.

Olkin, R. (2002) 'Could you hold the door for me? Including disability in diversity', *Cultural Diversity & Ethnic Minority Psychology*, 8 (2): 130–7.

Olkin, R. and Pledger, C. (2003) 'Can disability studies and psychology join hands?', *American Psychologist*, 58 (4): 296–304.

Paterson, K. and Hughes, B. (1999) 'Disability studies and phenomenology: the carnal politics of everyday life', *Disability & Society*, 14 (5): 597–610.

Priestley, M. (1999) *Disability Politics and Community Care*. London: Jessica Kingsley.

Reeve, D. (2008) Negotiating Disability in Everyday Life: The Experience of Psycho-emotional Disablism. Unpublished PhD thesis, Lancaster University.

Reeve, D. (2012) 'Psycho-emotional disablism: the missing link', in N. Watson, C. Thomas and A. Roulstone (eds), *Routledge Companion to Disability Studies*. London: Routledge, pp. 78–93.

Shakespeare, T. (2006) *Disability Rights and Wrongs*. London: Routledge.

Shuttleworth, R. (2000) 'The search for sexual intimacy for men with cerebral palsy', *Sexuality and Disability*, 18 (4): 263–82.

Swain, J., Finkelstein, V., French, S. and Oliver, M. (eds) (1993) *Disabling Barriers – Enabling Environments*. London: SAGE, in association with the Open University.

Stramondo, J. (2009) Fear, Anxiety, and Authentic Understanding of Disability: A Heideggerian Examination. Paper presented to the Society for Disability Studies conference, Tucson, AZ, 17–20 June.

Thomas, C. (2002) 'The "disabled" body', in M. Evans and E. Lee (eds), *Real Bodies*. Basingstoke: Palgrave. pp. 64–78.

Thomas, C. (2004) 'How is disability understood? An examination of sociological approaches', *Disability & Society*, 19 (6): 569–83.

Thomas, C. (2007) *Sociologies of Disability, 'Impairment', and Chronic Illness: Ideas in Disability Studies and Medical Sociology*. London: Palgrave.

Titchkosky, T. (2003) *Disability, Self and Society*. Toronto: University of Toronto Press.

Tobbell, J. and Lawthom, R. (2005) 'Dispensing with labels: enabling children and professionals to share a community of practice', *Educational and Child Psychology*, 22 (3): 89–97.

Tremain, S. (2005) (ed.) *Foucault and the Government of Disability*. Ann Arbor: University of Michigan Press.

Wendell, S. (1996) *The Rejected Body: Feminist Philosophical Reflections on Disability*. New York: Routledge.

Williams, C. (2003) 'Sky service: the demands on emotional labor in the airline industry', *Gender, Work and Organisation*, 10 (5): 513–51.

10

Women and Disability

Alison Sheldon

Disability – the restriction imposed on top of our impairments by the way our society is organised – is a form of social oppression to which *all* disabled people are subject. The disabled population is not, however, a homogeneous one. It consists of people with a wide variety of impairments, and is intercut by a number of other forms of structural disadvantage. The majority of those affected by disability are women. Subject to both disablism and sexism, disabled women find themselves disadvantaged in countless aspects of their existence, yet often feel their concerns are overlooked. This chapter does not set out to create hierarchies by singling out individual disabled people as more or less oppressed than others. It recognises, though, that disablism cannot be confronted in isolation. Any consideration of disablism, or indeed sexism, inevitably exposes unpalatable truths about society, the same society which disadvantages all oppressed people. It is impossible then 'to confront one type of oppression without confronting them all' (Barnes, cited in Campbell and Oliver, 1996: xii). This point is crucial for our understanding of disability and gender. For disabled women to achieve collective emancipation, disability, sexism and all other dimensions of oppression must be challenged head-on. In reality, however, these oppressions are generally considered in isolation one from another, thus weakening any meaningful challenge to the system and marginalising those, like disabled women, who are subject to more than one form of oppression.

Calls for a greater focus on 'difference' within feminist writings have been embraced by many women who experience disability, anxious that their specific experiences of oppression are neglected by the identity-based movements of which they are part – the women's movement and the disabled people's movement. The marginalisation of disabled women has thus prompted the development of a significant body of work within disability studies highlighting their plight (e.g. Fawcett, 2000; Hall, 2012; Hans and Patri, 2003; Thomas, 1999). Much of this work has borrowed heavily from feminist scholarship, in its insistence on the primacy of personal experience. How much such writings move disabled women towards what must be their ultimate goal – an end to oppression – is, however, debatable.

This chapter will consider similarities between the struggles of disabled men and women before examining the specific nature of disabled women's oppression and their lack of unity with their non-disabled sisters. Key areas of conflict arising from this lack of unity will then be discussed. Finally, a plea will be made for a more productive way forward for disabled women.

Oppression and disabled women

While having differing manifestations depending on which devalued social group or groups are involved, oppression is a unitary phenomenon of which disabled people's oppression and women's oppression are just specific examples. Disabled people and women have much in common, then, with both groups adversely affected by society's oppressive structures.

Since individuals do not fall into singular social groupings, there has been much debate about the importance of studying the interactions between different dimensions of oppression. How, for example, does disability affect women who are also subject to sexist oppression? Some regard such questions as vitally important, and are concerned about the exact nature of these interactions (Vernon, 1999). In contrast, others are concerned that: 'characterising people's experiences in terms of multiple jeopardies may only serve to marginalise their experiences even further and divert attention from common concerns and issues' (Zarb, 1993: 194).

This anxiety is not unfounded. There is little recognition from those who experience disability oppression and those who experience sexist oppression that their concerns are similar (Sheldon, 1999). Disabled women are said to fall between two stools – peripheral as women in the disabled people's movement, invisible as disabled people in the women's movement (Lloyd, 2001). Thus, the gendered nature of disability is not given a high priority, giving rise to some specific concerns for disabled women.

The specific concerns of disabled women

Disabled women's concerns are in many ways identical to those of disabled men and non-disabled women. They have, however, identified various areas in which they are at a unique social disadvantage, and which are peripheral issues for the movements purporting to represent their interests. For example:

> Disabled women are concerned to explore questions of sexuality and sexual identity, to challenge stereotypical images and oppressive mores relating to child-bearing and motherhood, and to identify dominant imperatives around physical and social aspects of self-presentation critically. (Lloyd, 2001: 716)

It could be argued that these are, to a great extent, concerns for *all* women. Why then is mainstream feminism disinterested in these issues as they pertain to disabled women? Whilst we live in a disablist society, perhaps it is inevitable that non-disabled feminists should share society's negative attitudes towards disabled people.

Alternatively, it could be argued that feminists have special reasons for wanting to distance themselves from us. Feminism's historical support for eugenics is well-documented (Davis, 1982; Lamp and Cleigh, 2012), and early feminists were both anxious to separate women from the inferior category of 'defectives', and reluctant to challenge the production of the category itself. Thus, disability became 'central to feminism as a negative trope' (Lamp and Cleigh, 2012: 176), with a preoccupation with autonomy and independence identified as 'one of the most pervasive feminist assumptions that undermines ... disabled women's struggle' (Thompson, 1997: 286). Hence, it is proposed that: 'Perceiving disabled women as childlike, helpless, and victimized, non-disabled feminists have severed them from the sisterhood in an effort to advance more powerful, competent, and appealing female icons' (Fine and Asch, 1988: 4).

The 'personal is political' has been the rallying call of feminism for many years. Ironically, this approach can also be blamed for mainstream feminism's neglect of disability. It is often thought sufficient to examine only the personal experiences of privileged, white, non-disabled, heterosexual women. Those on the margins are over-looked. It is crucial then that mainstream feminists go beyond simply understanding their own immediate experiences, and incorporate the concerns of a more diverse group of women.

Feminism has fought long and hard to challenge society's rigid gender roles, but this struggle may not mean much to disabled women. Disabled women are perceived to be needy, dependent and passive – stereotypical feminine qualities. At the same time, they are deemed incapable of aspiring to other 'feminine' roles, especially those relating to appearance, partnering and motherhood. It is posited, then, that disabled women 'have not been "trapped" by many of the social expectations feminists have challenged' (Fine and Asch, 1988: 29). This may make it difficult for disabled women to identify with the struggles of feminism. It is further suggested that the desire to be like other women may even create a tolerance of sexism in disabled women, who 'will never fight such sexism until they are enabled to discover their commonalities with non-disabled women' (1988: 29).

Whilst disabled women are oppressed in much the same way as non-disabled women, it seems that there may be little recognition of this commonality from either group. Hence, there are tensions between the two groups' agendas for change. Two such areas of tension will now be briefly considered – reproductive freedom and 'care'.

Disabled and non-disabled women: Irreconcilable differences?

Whilst feminism insists that the right to reproductive freedom must be a cornerstone of women's liberation, the early twentieth-century movement for birth control was championed primarily by white, middle-class, non-disabled westerners. For less privileged women, the movement advocated the eugenic strategy of population control, 'not the individual right to *birth control*' (Davis, 1982: 215). The twentieth century saw the widespread 'sterilisation abuse' of thousands of disabled women, a violation of human rights that still continues today (Human Rights Watch, 2011). Now though, disabled women are often discouraged from becoming mothers in more subtle ways. They are persuaded that their own health might suffer as a consequence of motherhood, that their baby might inherit their 'problem', or that their own impairment(s) will make them incapable of mothering (Thomas, 1997). Reproductive freedom must not be seen, then, solely as the right *not* to bear children; it must include the right for women to *bear* children should they wish – otherwise it can become a demand which implicitly condones eugenics.

Abortion, too, is a crucial issue for both the disabled people's movement and the women's movement. Disabled people have been highly critical of prenatal screening and selective abortion, seeing them as a new strategy of eugenics (Shakespeare, 1998). Non-disabled feminists, however, have largely welcomed prenatal testing, seeing it as 'another means through which women can gain control over their own reproduction' (Bailey, 1996: 143). There seems, then, to be a conflict between this feminist perspective on abortion and the perspective of the disabled people's movement. Some argue that the two positions are irreconcilable (Sharp and Earle, 2002), but there *are* non-disabled feminists who recognise the costs of prenatal screening, both for disabled people and for women generally (Hubbard, 1997). Perhaps these women will enter into discussions with the disabled people's movement and the geneticists to forge a new way forward. Alternatively, it may be that this dilemma cannot be solved amicably without radical changes in society. I would suggest that this is where disabled people, feminists and other oppressed people should be focusing their attention.

A key concern for the emergent British disabled people's movement was the disadvantaged position of disabled residents in institutions (Campbell and Oliver, 1996). In recent years, there has been a gradual move away from 'institutional care' in favour of community-based services. Whilst problems with 'community care' policies have been voiced by disabled and older people, they have largely been seen as an important step forward. These policies have, however, done little to improve the lives of younger non-disabled women. Since women are still responsible for the bulk of the 'caring' work that now takes place outside of institutions, 'community care' has perpetuated their dependent role in the family by putting yet more unpaid labour their way (Finch, 1984). The CBR (Community Based Rehabilitation) programmes supported by international agencies such as the World Health Organization (2010) have exported such practices to non-western contexts, placing a further burden on poor women in low-income countries (Erevelles, 2012). Rather than advocating changes to the patriarchal structures that support this oppressive division of domestic labour, many non-disabled feminists have come out in support of residential 'care', claiming, for example, that it is the only route that 'will offer us a way out of the impasse of caring' (Finch, 1984: 16). This assumption that a split exists between women who 'care' and 'dependent' people (gender irrelevant) both denies the reality that most people being 'cared for' are women, and obscures the fact that many people who need help with daily living tasks are also looking after others.

Even recent attempts to describe a 'feminist ethics of care' are still largely grounded in western concepts of autonomy, with the 'care recipient' implicitly constructed as non-autonomous (Erevelles, 2011: 180).

Both the debates around birth control and selective abortion, and those around 'care', demonstrate how the continuing oppression of disabled people and women has created situations where it seems sides must be taken – where disabled people's best interests are seen to be at odds with those of women. It is important for all of us, and especially for disabled women, to recognise where the blame lies for these situations: not with feminism or the disabled people's movement, but with a society which both movements must seek to change.

The way forward for disabled women: Personal or political?

Disabled women have been instrumental in applying feminist analyses to the understanding of disability, and an innovative body of work is growing as a result. There is, however, no one feminist means of analysis, so different writers have used different feminist approaches to support their arguments. Here, I will briefly assess the merits of just two of these approaches for furthering disabled women's ultimate cause.

Much feminist work within disability studies has been critical of the 'malestream' focus on social barriers, claiming that it pays insufficient attention to *differences* among disabled people (Fawcett, 2000), and effectively denies our personal experience of disability and indeed impairment (Crow, 1996; French, 1993). This individualistic approach, often equated with a feminist disability politics, is not, however, without its critics (Sheldon, 1999). Whilst experience is a 'necessary starting point', it should not be viewed as 'an end in itself' (Kelly et al., 1994: 29). There are concerns from both disabled people and feminists that the limited use of 'the personal is political' as the only analytical tool can be counterproductive. As one feminist has argued, the slogan:

> became a means of encouraging women to think that the experience of discrimination, exploitation or oppression automatically corresponded with an understanding of the ideological and institutional apparatus shaping one's social status ... When women internalized the idea that describing their own woes was synonymous with developing a political consciousness, the progress of feminist movement was stalled. (hooks, 1984: 24–5)

Likewise, it is said that those who demand more inclusion of personal experience are hampering the development of the disabled people's movement (Finkelstein, 1996). As a solution to similar tensions within feminism, an approach is suggested that examines 'the personal that is political, the politics of society as a whole, and global revolutionary politics' (hooks, 1984: 25). Perhaps this would be a useful way forward for the disabled people's movement.

In disability studies, though, a feminist analysis is often assumed to preclude any reference to revolutionary politics, or indeed economic structures. However, many feminists have adopted such an approach to explain their oppression. It is argued that progress for disabled people will not be achieved through a stress solely on equality of opportunity, but can best be achieved by borrowing from socialist feminists 'who call for societal transformations in addition to equality of opportunity within existing arrangements' (Fine and Asch, 1988: 27). It is not enough for women from oppressed groups to simply argue for equal rights with men, since 'knowing that men in their groups do not have social, political, and economic power, they would not deem it liberatory to share their social status' (hooks, 1984: 18). Disabled women also need to challenge the structures that create and perpetuate disability, sexism and other forms of oppression.

Through the work of early disabled activists, this materialist approach became the dominant way of conceptualising disability in the UK. In a similar vein, materialist feminists have argued that the current form of women's oppression has its roots in the capitalist system, and its particular division of labour (Delphy, 1984). Some kind of gender division of labour is apparent in most known societies, and where these divisions are found, women are always less valued than men. It is suggested, however, that prior to the industrial revolution, women were able to contribute to the process of production. As men began to operate in the economy outside of the home, women filled the gap they left behind – the private space of the home. Excluded from productive work, they became economically dependent on male wage-earners. Hence, with industrialisation both women and disabled people became further excluded.

A materialist analysis then seems to provide an invaluable way of theorising the interaction between disability and sexism. It highlights the fact that disabled people and women need to fight for a new kind of society; and it shows us that there is enormous scope for coalitions between the disabled people's movement, like-minded feminists and other oppressed groups. Such an analysis must be put centre-stage if we are ever to achieve a truly effective feminist disability studies (Erevelles, 2012).

Conclusion

However we experience disability and sexism as individuals, the lives of *all* disabled women are shaped by these oppressive structures. In order to eliminate all kinds of oppression, we need to transform society. Different oppressed groups may come to this realisation through the politicisation of very different personal experiences, yet in a way we are all engaged in a similar struggle. Perhaps when we all begin to challenge the same structures and institutions, significant changes will occur. We must then hold on to what we have in common. The key to all our liberation is unity among oppressed people. Rather than 'competing for "our" piece of a reduced pie ... what we need to do is demand a transformation that delivers a different pie – one big enough for all of us' (Russell, 1998: 231). Disabled women, consistently denied their piece of the pie, may be in an ideal position to forge such a collective agenda for an improved society.

76

In Our Own Image

References

Bailey, R. (1996) 'Prenatal testing and the prevention of impairment: a woman's right to choose?', in J. Morris (ed.), *Encounters with Strangers: Feminism and Disability*. London: The Women's Press. pp. 143–67.

Campbell, J. and Oliver, M. (1996) *Disability Politics: Understanding Our Past, Changing Our Future*. London: Routledge.

Crow, L. (1996) 'Including all of our lives: renewing the social model of disability', in J. Morris (ed.), *Encounters with Strangers: Feminism and Disability*. London: The Women's Press. pp. 55–72.

Davis, A. (1982) *Women, Race and Class*. London: The Women's Press.

Delphy, C. (1984) *Close to Home: A Materialist Analysis of Women's Oppression*. London: Hutchinson.

Erevelles, N. (2011) *Disability and Difference in Global Contexts: Enabling a Transformative Body Politic*. London: Palgrave Macmillan.

Erevelles, N. (2012) 'The color of violence: reflecting on gender, race and disability in wartime', in K.Q. Hall (ed.), *Feminist Disability Studies*. Bloomington: Indiana University Press, pp. 117–35.

Fawcett, B. (2000) *Feminist Perspectives on Disability*. Harlow: Prentice Hall.

Finch, J. (1984) 'Community care: developing non-sexist alternatives', *Critical Social Policy*, 3 (9): 6–18.

Fine, M. and Asch, A. (eds) (1988) *Women with Disabilities: Essays in Psychology, Culture and Politics*. Philadelphia, PA: Temple University Press.

Finkelstein, V. (1996) 'Outside, "inside out"', *Coalition*, April, 30–6.

French, S. (1993) 'Disability, impairment or something in between?', in J. Swain, V. Finkelstein, S. French and M. Oliver (eds), *Disabling Barriers – Enabling Environments*. London: SAGE, in association with the Open University. pp. 17–25.

Hall, K.Q. (ed.) (2012) *Feminist Disability Studies*. Bloomington: Indiana University Press.

Hans, A. and Patri, A. (eds) (2003) *Women, Disability and Identity*. New Delhi: SAGE.

hooks, b. (1984) *Feminist Theory: From Margin to Center*. Boston, MA: South End.

Hubbard, R. (1997) 'Abortion and disability: who should and should not inhabit the world?', in L. Davis (ed.), *The Disability Studies Reader*. London: Routledge. pp. 187–200.

Human Rights Watch (2011) Sterilization of Women and Girls with Disabilities. A briefing paper. New York: Human Rights Watch. Available at: www.hrw.org/news/2011/11/10/sterilization-women-and-girls-disabilities [accessed 29/10/12].

Kelly, L., Burton, S. and Regan, L. (1994) 'Researching women's lives or studying women's oppression? Reflections on what constitutes feminist research', in M. Maynard and J. Purvis (eds), *Researching Women's Lives from a Feminist Perspective*. London: Taylor and Francis. pp. 27–48.

Lamp, S. and Cleigh, W.C. (2012) 'A heritage of ableist rhetoric in American feminism from the eugenics period', in K.Q. Hall (ed.), *Feminist Disability Studies*. Bloomington: Indiana University Press, pp. 175–90.

Lloyd, M. (2001) 'The politics of disability and feminism: discord or synthesis', *Sociology*, 35 (3): 715–28.

Russell, M. (1998) *Beyond Ramps: Disability at the End of the Social Contract*. Monroe, ME: Common Courage.

Shakespeare, T. (1998) 'Choices and rights: eugenics, genetics and disability equality', *Disability & Society*, 13 (5): 665–81.

Sharp, K. and Earle, S. (2002) 'Feminism, abortion and disability: irreconcilable differences?', *Disability & Society*, 17 (2): 137–45.

Sheldon, A. (1999) 'Personal and perplexing: feminist disability politics evaluated', *Disability & Society*, 14 (5): 645–59.

Thomas, C. (1997) 'The baby and the bathwater: disabled women and motherhood in social context', *Sociology of Health and Illness*, 19 (5): 622–43.

Thomas, C. (1999) *Female Forms: Experiencing and Understanding Disability*. Buckingham: Open University Press.

Thompson, R.G. (1997) 'Feminist theory, the body and the disabled figure', in L. Davis (ed.), *The Disability Studies Reader*. London: Routledge. pp. 279–92.

Vernon, A. (1999) 'The dialectics of multiple identities and the disabled people's movement', *Disability & Society*, 14 (3): 385–98.

World Health Organization (WHO) (2010) Community-based Rehabilitation Guidelines. Geneva: WHO. Available at: www.who.int/disabilities/cbr/guidelines/en/index.html [accessed 29/10/12].

Zarb, G. (1993) 'The dual experience of ageing with a disability', in J. Swain, V. Finkelstein, S. French and M. Oliver (eds), *Disabling Barriers – Enabling Environments*. London: SAGE, in association with the Open University. pp. 186–95.

11

Men, Masculinities and Disability

Steve Robertson and Brett Smith

The aim of this chapter is to consider the main issues relating to the intersections of men, masculinities and disabilities. Drawing on and integrating empirical and theoretical work from both the Critical Studies of Men and Disability Studies fields, we begin by briefly reviewing the emergence of interest in men and disability before considering more recent key literature in the field that moves beyond homogenising views of masculinity and disability. Finally, we conclude by suggesting important points to consider in future research on men and disability.

From whence it came

Since the 1980s, work by feminists has highlighted how much disability research has been 'gender blind' [sic]; that is, gender has been invisible and the experience of disabled men has been taken as representative of disabled experience in general (Morris, 1993). Yet around the same time, key disability studies writers were also pointing out that little research existed which specifically explored the experiences of disabled men (Shakespeare, 1996, 1999). This apparent contradiction, that men's experiences are representative of all persons' experiences yet men's actual experiences are rarely researched, is paralleled in social science generally. Within the Critical Studies of Men field, Hearn and Morgan (1990) addressed this apparent contradiction. They suggested that this 'invisibility' occurs because men are too much in the foreground, so whilst men may frequently constitute the research subject, the research is rarely 'about men in a more complex, more problematised, sociological sense' (p. 7).

Shakespeare (1996) further suggests that within disability studies, in general, women working in predominantly feminist contexts tended to explore more personal aspects of sexuality, relationships and identity, whilst men concentrated on employment, housing and other material social issues. This, he says, reproduced the public (realm of the male)/private (realm of the female) split and led to an under-representation of disabled men's experiences. Such invisibility of men as gendered beings in research may not be accidental. It may, in fact, 'serve men's interests, keeping their activities apart from critical scrutiny, by other men as well as by women' (Hearn and Morgan, 1990: 7).

However, during the 1980s and 1990s, accounts of men's personal experiences of impairment and links to 'masculinity' were emerging. Issues of 'gendered identity' became key, and autoethnographic accounts of the impact of impairment on one's sense of masculinity (Kriegel, 1991, 1998; Murphy, 1987; Zola, 1982) were supplemented by empirical research theorising the nature of masculinities and disability (Gerschick, 1998; Gerschick and Miller, 1995; Oliver et al., 1988). Building on the premise that traditional (hegemonic) masculinity is predicated on strength, rationality, self-reliance, potency and action, and that 'True masculinity is almost always thought to proceed from men's bodies' (Connell, 1995: 44), these personal accounts highlighted the difficulties some men had in negotiating their gendered identity, usually following acquired physical impairment. These accounts tended to describe an 'embattled identity'; a struggle men had to meet society's (and their own) conflicting expectations of what it is to be male: 'Paralytic disability constitutes emasculation of a more direct and total nature. For the male, the weakening and atrophy of the body threaten all the cultural values of masculinity' (Murphy, 1987: 94).

Yet these personal accounts also showed that (hegemonic) masculinity could assist with helping survive the experience of becoming impaired. As Kriegel states:

> Be a man! An old battered idea that has not fared well. Like all clichés, it embarrasses. Yet clichés spring from the cultures that give them life, and to the idea of what it meant to be a man in 1944 I owe my survival. (1998: 5)

Being a man – strong, determined, not willing to show weakness or give up – Kriegel feels helped him through to his present sense of (male) self.

Such work was important in highlighting how 'disability' is a gendered issue for men. However, it risks reproducing an overly individualised focus on how men 'handle' the experience of impairment. Critical questions lay dormant regarding cultural representations of 'disability' and 'masculinity', the structural embedding of these representations, and how this structural embedding is responsible for contributing to and generating such identity conflict.

Oliver et al.'s (1988) research into the experiences of men following spinal cord injury (SCI) moved away from an individualised, personal tragedy model of disability. A social adjustment model was proposed that saw social context, including the social meanings attached to impairment, as crucial to understanding the consequences and experiences of impairment. This work developed links between men's experience and the wider social context, showing how structural (material) issues were significant in shaping such experience. However, it failed to fully consider 'gendered identity' as part of the socially integrated meanings that impact on the experience of impairment for these men. This is important because, as Shakespeare (1994) highlights, masculinity is wrapped up with notions of bodily invincibility (and therefore bodily fragmentation) through concerns with potency, supremacy and domination.

The empirical work of Gerschick and Miller (1995) drew on interview data to develop more nuanced approaches to theorising masculinities and disability in ways that explored individual experience in relation to the wider gender order; that is, it linked the interpersonal and the institutional. They suggested that disabled men developed three main coping strategies in the (re)negotiation of gendered identity: *reliance*, where great effort is made to continue to try and fulfil traditional/hegemonic ideals; *reformulation*, where hegemonic ideals were redefined in new ways; and *rejection*, where hegemonic ideals are renounced and one's own ideas about what constitutes 'masculinity' are inverted or its importance in life is downplayed. These three strategies were not seen as fixed. Rather, disabled men move into and out of different strategies at different places and times. Gerschick (1998) later shifted the emphasis slightly by opting for a model with two strategies: compliance with, or resistance to, societal norms of hegemonic masculinity. In both models, rejection/ resistance – the construction of 'counter-hegemonic alternatives' (1998: 208) – is seen as the approach that provides men with impairments the best opportunity for escaping what he terms 'gender domination'.

Diverging paths

Since the previous version of this chapter (Robertson, 2004), work has developed that recognises the importance of understanding the plurality of 'masculinities' and their intersections with diverse 'disabilities'. Influenced by wider discussions from within postmodernism and poststructuralism, by the late 1990s and early 2000s significant debate was taking place within disability studies about the limitations of both individualised, personal experiential approaches to disability and the social model of disability. The former was often seen as running the risk of slippage into biomedical 'personal tragedy' models, whilst many (pro-)feminist disability scholars (Corker, 1998; Morris, 1996; Shakespeare, 1994; Shakespeare and Watson, 1995; Thomas, 1999) and activists were highlighting the limitations of the social model in exploring the socially integrated nature of the personal effects that impairment might have for an individual.[1] One of the significant outcomes of these debates was a desire to extend the social model of disability into questions of culture, representation and meaning, and this has relevance for understanding how these personal 'impairment effects' (Thomas, 1999) differ, both quantitatively and qualitatively, not only between disabled men and women but between different groups of disabled men. As Shuttleworth et al. (2012) highlight, early work on masculinities and disability often presented 'disability' as an almost generic category. It focused less on understanding how masculinities intersect differently with varying types of impairment.

An area very rarely considered in terms of its gendered nature is that of learning impairment. Work by Wilson and colleagues (Wilson, 2009; Wilson et al., 2011, 2012) suggests the notion of *conditionally masculine* to help elucidate the intersection of sexual health, masculinity, gendered care-giving and intellectual disability. This work links ideas about malleable embodied notions of masculinity with maintaining the importance of cognition: the greater the cognitive impairment, the less gendered sociocultural scripts shape these men's masculinities. Furthermore, the greater the cognitive impairment, the greater influence support staff will have in shaping these men's gendered identities. Following earlier calls to 'bring the body back in' to the disability debate (Williams, 1999), Wilson's work provides a good example of the importance of biopsychosocial approaches in helping fully capture the links between issues of gendered representation and materiality, and between issues of structure and agency within the context of learning impairment.

Men with acquired impairment, notably SCI, have featured much in research. Building on their early work (Sparkes and Smith, 2002), Sparkes and Smith (2009) focused on the bio-social character of the body with men who acquired an SCI through playing rugby and their experiences of pain. They found that, despite potential costs to their health, these men initially hid their pain from others whilst in rehabilitation as speaking about pain was considered a threat to the men's masculine self-identity. More recently, Smith (2013) drew on Connell's (1995) relational theory of gender and Thomas's (2007) relational theory of disability to examine disabled men's understanding of health several years after acquiring an SCI. In this study, men felt they *should* care about health and this was partly a result of the materiality of impaired bodies that require daily health work. However, such concern about one's health can put masculinities at risk as health is often constructed as a feminine domain. Thus, these men also stated that whilst they cared about their health, they did not care too much (see also Robertson, 2007). This narrative addition, Smith argues, works for the disabled men by enabling each to accrue masculine capital (de Visser et al., 2009) and uphold masculinities.

Moreover, Smith (2013) proposes that the men upheld gendered identities by performing resilience. Resilience is about the ability to positively adapt to adversity or risk. Resilience was, for these men, a health resource, helping them recover quickly if illness or health problems arose. But resilience was also a resource for gaining masculine capital and upholding masculinities. For example, the men stated that they did not need to care too much about their health because they had the strength, courage, power and control to positively adapt if a health problem arose. Thus, by drawing on masculine signifiers – like strength and control – resilience became a resource for legitimating not caring about health too much, and therefore a way of 'doing' masculinity.

The work of Gibson et al. (2007) on men with Duchenne Muscular Dystrophy (DMD) is also illustrative of how masculinities intersect differently with different types of impairment. Drawing on Bourdieu's critical social theory, Gibson and colleagues revealed that in certain social microcosms (i.e. fields) men with DMD adapted masculine signifiers such as strength, intelligence, leadership and autonomy, and expressed them in non-traditional ways. For example, in the field of the family, masculinities were established through observable behaviours, beliefs, strategies, thoughts, attitudes and tastes (i.e. practices) in which the men provided emotional, physical or financial support for family and pets. However, in different fields, and through more traditional gendered practices, the men with DMD reproduced hegemonic forms of masculinity. For instance, when talking about education, some participants recalled intimidating younger, emotionally or cognitively weaker (but physically stronger) boys through physical violence or verbal aggression. In this field, such acts were a key source of 'positive' gendered capital, in that they helped sustain a dominant position amongst other disabled persons. Moreover, with regard to dating, some men suggested that to be regarded as 'fully male' males should have successful, lucrative careers and be able to sexually satisfy a woman in narrowly defined ways. Within such fields, and through such practices, the men thus both reproduced what constitutes masculine capital and also engaged in practices that contributed to transforming these meanings.

Yet, as Gibson et al. (2007) also suggest, the men with DMD rarely openly questioned dominant masculinities or consciously attempted to create spaces for alternate forms of masculinity. They noted that whilst they claimed power in some fields and thrived with varying degrees of success within the context of their lives, within the larger social space, and across most fields, they were profoundly marginalised. For instance, they were marginalised through the inaccessibility of the built environment and the various ways that their visible bodily differences were negatively marked across social space. Importantly, this marginalisation was embodied, being part of their habitus (the set of socially learned dispositions, skills and ways of acting that are taken for granted), acquired and internalised through the fields and practices of everyday life. One result of this was that marginalisation was experienced as troubling, but also as 'normal': marginalisation was 'an embodied reality for men with DMD whereby they come to "believe" that the margin is (more or less, and with some exceptions in particular fields) where they belong' (2007: 514).

Conclusion: Pointing a way forward

Having considered where work on men, masculinities and disabilities has come from and what recent thinking has offered, it remains important here to consider what the most salient points are as we continue to take research in this area forward. To us there seems to be three major opportunities in this regard.

First, mentioned briefly above, is recent work in Critical Men's Studies which suggests that men not only accrue 'masculine capital' but, importantly, act to trade certain types of 'masculine capital' for others (de Visser et al., 2009). Yet, following de Visser et al.'s argument, it is vitally important to also recognise that the capacity to trade such capital is limited because different masculine and non-masculine behaviours have different values and, we would add, because varied impairments are structurally disabling, enabling and constraining in differing ways. Considering how and where forms of masculine capital are developed and traded as masculinities intersect with different impairments will therefore help facilitate more nuanced (rather than simplistic) ways of understanding these intersections.

Second, whilst the debate about social and individual models of disability remains (Hughes, 2009), we believe that continuing to expand the social model to incorporate aspects of 'impairment effects' provides a sensible and practical way to understand the complexity of disability and its intersection with gender/masculinities. Utilising sociological work on embodiment, particularly that based within critical realist frameworks (Williams, 1999), presents us with the opportunity to explore important issues of structure and agency in ways that avoid both a disembodied and an overly somaticised view of disability (for empirical examples, see Gibson et al., 2007; Robertson, 2006; Robertson et al., 2010).

Finally, we believe it important to link revised approaches to understanding masculinities as configurations of practice embedded within sets of gender relations

(Connell and Messerschmidt, 2005) with a relational theory of disability (Thomas, 2007). Using a social relational framework allows full consideration of the issues of structure and agency and helps highlight the role and movement of power within sets of relations. 'Disability'/'masculinities' can then be explored in ways that simultaneously appreciate: (a) the fluidity of individual subject positions; (b) how specific (hegemonic) practices become embedded in and reproduced through social institutions (structures); and (c) ways that facilitate and constrain individual actions (agency). In short, it helps us consider the gendered nature of disabled men's varied social interactions, how these are shaped and also how they themselves act to shape and (re)form social structures and institutions.

Note

1 These authors were by no means suggesting an abandonment of the social model, rather a return to and expansion of the theoretical framework from which it emerged – see Shakespeare and Watson (1995) and Thomas (2004, 2007).

References

Connell, R.W. (1995) *Masculinities*. Cambridge: Polity.

Connell, R.W. and Messerschmidt, J.W. (2005) 'Hegemonic masculinity: rethinking the concept', *Gender & Society*, 19 (6): 829–59.

Corker, M. (1998) *Deaf and Disabled, or Deafness Disabled?* Buckingham: Open University Press.

de Visser, R., Smith, J.A. and McDonnell, E.J. (2009) '"That's not masculine": masculine capital and health-related behaviour', *Journal of Health Psychology*, 14 (7): 1047–58.

Gerschick, T.J. (1998) 'Sisyphus in a wheelchair: men with physical disabilities confront gender domination', in J. O'Brien and J. Howard (eds), *Everyday Inequalities: Critical Inquiries*. Malden, MA: Blackwell. pp. 189–211.

Gerschick, T.J. and Miller, A.S. (1995) 'Coming to terms: masculinity and physical disability', in D. Sabo and D.F. Gordon (eds), *Men's Health and Illness: Gender, Power and the Body*. London: SAGE. pp. 183–204.

Gibson, B.E., Young, N.L., Upshur, R.E.G. and McKeever, P. (2007) 'Men on the margin: a Bourdieusian examination of living into adulthood with muscular dystrophy', *Social Science & Medicine*, 65: 505–17.

Hearn, J. and Morgan, D.H.J. (1990) 'Men, masculinities and social theory', in J. Hearn and D.H.J. Morgan (eds), *Men, Masculinities and Social Theory*. London: Unwin Hyman. pp. 1–18.

Hughes, B. (2009) 'Disability activisms: social model stalwarts and biological citizens', *Disability & Society*, 24 (6): 677–88.

Kriegel, L. (1991) *Falling into Life: Essays*. San Francisco, CA: North Point Press.

Kriegel, L. (1998) *Flying Solo: Reimagining Manhood, Courage and Loss*. Boston, MA: Beacon Press.

Morris, J. (1993) 'Gender and disability', in J. Swain, V. Finkelstein, S. French and M. Oliver (eds), *Disabling Barriers – Enabling Environments*. London: SAGE, in association with the Open University. pp. 85–92.

Morris, J. (1996) *Encounters with Strangers: Feminism and Disability*. London: The Women's Press.

Murphy, R. (1987) *The Body Silent*. London: Phoenix House.

Oliver, M., Zarb, G., Silver, J., Moore, M. and Salisbury, V. (1988) *Walking into Darkness: The Experience of Spinal Cord Injury*. London: Macmillan.

Robertson, S. (2004) 'Men and disability', in J. Swain, S. French, C. Barnes and C. Thomas (eds), *Disabling Barriers – Enabling Environments* (2nd edn). London: SAGE. pp. 75–80.

Robertson, S. (2006) '"I've been like a coiled spring this last week": embodied masculinity and health', *Sociology of Health & Illness*, 28 (4): 433–56.

Robertson, S. (2007) *Understanding Men and Health: Masculinities, Identity and Wellbeing*. Buckingham: Open University Press.

Robertson, S., Sheikh, K. and Moore, A. (2010) 'Embodied masculinities in the context of cardiac rehabilitation', *Sociology of Health & Illness*, 32 (5): 695–710.

Shakespeare, T. (1994) 'Cultural representations of disabled people: dustbins for disavowal', *Disability & Society*, 9 (3): 283–301.

Shakespeare, T. (1996) 'Power and prejudice: issues of gender, sexuality and disability', in L. Barton (ed.), *Disability and Society: Emerging Issues and Insights*. Harlow: Longman. pp. 191–214.

Shakespeare, T. (1999) 'When is a man not a man? When he's disabled', in J. Wild (ed.), *Working with Men for Change*. London: UCL Press. pp. 47–58.

Shakespeare, T. and Watson, N. (1995) 'Defending the social model', *Disability & Society*, 12 (2): 293–300.

Shuttleworth, R., Wedgewood, N. and Wilson, N.J. (2012) 'The dilemma of disabled masculinity', *Men & Masculinities*, 15 (2): 174–94.

Smith, B. (2013) 'Disability, sport, and men's narratives of health: a qualitative study', *Health Psychology*, 32 (1): 110–19.

Sparkes, A. and Smith, B. (2002) 'Sport, spinal cord injuries, embodied masculinities, and narrative identity dilemmas', *Men and Masculinities*, 4 (3): 258–85.

Sparkes, A. and Smith, B. (2009) 'Men, spinal cord injury, memories, and the narrative performance of pain', *Disability & Society*, 23 (7): 679–90.

Thomas, C. (1999) *Female Forms: Experiencing and Understanding Disability*. Milton Keynes: Open University Press.

Thomas, C. (2004) 'How is disability understood? An examination of sociological approaches', *Disability & Society*, 19 (6): 569–83.

Thomas, C. (2007) *Sociologies of Disability and Illness: Contested Ideas in Disability Studies and Medical Sociology*. Basingstoke: Palgrave Macmillan.

Williams, S.J. (1999) 'Is anybody there? Critical realism, chronic illness and the disability debate', *Sociology of Health & Illness*, 21 (6): 797–819.

Wilson, N.J. (2009) Conditionally Sexual: Constructing the Sexual Health Needs of Men and Teenage Boys with a Moderate to Profound Intellectual Disability. Unpublished PhD thesis, University of Sydney.

Wilson, N.J., Parmenter, T.R., Stancliffe, R.J. and Shuttleworth, R.P. (2011) 'Conditionally sexual: men and teenage boys with moderate to profound intellectual disability', *Sexuality & Disability*, 29 (3): 275–89.

Wilson, N.J., Shuttleworth, R.P., Stancliffe, R.J. and Parmenter, T.R. (2012) 'Masculinity theory in applied research with men and boys with intellectual disability', *Intellectual & Developmental Disabilities*, 50 (3): 261–72.

Zola, I. (1982) *Missing Pieces: A Chronicle of Living with a Disability*. Philadelphia, PA: Temple University Press.

12

Lying Down Anyhow: Disability and the Rebel Body

Liz Crow

In this chapter, I begin with a short autobiographical piece about lying down in public places. This is followed by an exploration of the influences involved in the process of *Lying Down Anyhow*.

We sip from glasses of orange juice and half-pint lagers on a cool afternoon in autumn, a gentle rise and fall of conversation, and I nudge off my shoes to lie upon the cushioned window seat. From behind the bar, the landlord hurls himself towards me, his face as livid as the velvet beneath me: 'Get up, get up, get out. This is a *respectable* establishment.'

– – –

When I lie down, it is clean mountain air, cool water in blistering summer, soft rains of release. Sit up, and I am fragile as ice, a light breeze might shatter me. Sitting up, I am beyond my body; lying down, cradled by gravity, I creep back in to occupy my self.

In the privacy of home, I move from bed to sofa, sofa to floor, pillow, rugs and hardwood boards. I lie down wherever I happen to be, with the ease of twenty years' practice, freely.

But in the world outside, I am censored. I seek out-of-the-way spaces: corridors and empty classrooms, fields and first aid rooms and once, even, a graveyard. I wait to be alone, tuck myself from sight and then, only then, as though it is a thing of shame, I recline.

To be a part of the social world, I must sit: brace myself, block body from mind, steel will. To lie down is to absent myself from ordinary spaces. I wonder how many of us there are skulking in the in-between spaces. And I wonder at how such an everyday action, a simple thing born of necessity, became a thing to conceal. What taught us our shame?

– – –

'Lie down on the job' and we purposely neglect our work. 'Let something lie' and we decline to take action. A 'layabout' slacks and skives and shirks. The English language tells me my shame. Is that why, when I look around, I see lying down in public places only in the merest snatches and swatches of life, as though those of us who lie down have been written out?

Work hard enough, and I may recline, guiltless, in the green of summer parks or bake on sun-kissed beaches. With degrees of censure, young enough, slim enough, pretty enough, I can enter a young love's tryst, entwined on grassy banks. I can child's play Sleeping Lions and make angels in the snow, or pose as death on a yoga mat until body and self dissolve.

Ill enough, and I can lie down on doctor's couch or in hospital bed, a properly licensed space. In extremis – grand mal and hypo, knife attack and heart attack – I can make the street my bed; although, mistaken for drunk or overly-dramatic, my saviour might just 'let it lie' and cross over the road.

Human beings do not, apparently, much lie down and, if they must, then they tempt accelerated demise. In the annals of research, lying down is all let-this-be-a-warning treatises on the dangers of bedrest, of bone demineralisation and blood clots. Yet for me, lying down is my holding together; far from demise, this is my way to life.

In well-earned leisure, in pleasure, play and extremes, we may lie down in public places. In carefully controlled circumstances, we will not be judged for idleness and sloth. But why is it, as adults, to lie down amongst others, we must either be productive or chasing death? It is as though, in permitting ourselves to lie down in carefully sanctioned spaces, we have become convinced of our autonomy, when all we have proved is the strength of its prohibition.

Out in the urban jungle, edgy young designers create street furniture to dissuade the populace from lying down: benches divided by armrests, rails for perching, seats which revolve to prevent extended idling.[1] New laws in multiple cities around the world make it an offence to lie down in public places. If Westminster Council prevails, lying down could cost me £500;[2] in San Bruno it could earn me six months in jail.[3] This is not, you understand, a bid to address the social costs of homelessness, just to move on, design out, that which does not conform. Lying down in public spaces is no longer merely invisible; it is to be *disappeared*.

It seems it will take a brave woman to undertake public lying down. I intend to be her. I will not be disappeared.

I vowed to write lightly because I am writing of something so simple: of stretching out my legs, reclining my body, resting my head, amongst people. Lying down, for me, *is* lightness. But this is not light. To lie down, in social spaces, is not a simple act of physiology; it is a statement. In the midst of codes that say *you do not do this*, to lie down in public is confrontation.

Perhaps if it did not matter so much, it would be easy.

Still, I worry about the small things.

To lie down in front of others feels so *exposed*. The bed exists in private space; it is sleep and sex, intimacy and guard let down. In public, reclined, I have *so much body*; it unfolds and unravels on the horizontal plane, taking up more than its share of space. It flaunts itself, 'look at me', and eclipses face and mind. I watch myself through the eyes and ideas, the anxieties and judgements of others; danger lurks in being misread. And I wonder: shall I keep my boots on or tuck them neatly to one side? There is no guidebook.

Lying down in public places demands portion control, dress sense and, in summer months, attention to the calluses on my feet. If I am to become a poster girl for the disappeared, I'd like to look my best.

The absence of a guidebook could yet become my freedom. If the rules cannot be kept, then they are there for the breaking. And so I shall search for better ways.

– – –

Tying my bootlaces by the front door, I glance up and see anew a picture that has hung so long it had blended to invisibility. A black-and-white engraving from the 1893 *Graphic* celebrates the fashionable seaside resort of Brighton where wealthy society brought ailments for salt-water cures. A gentleman, pale-faced in bowler hat and waxed moustache, reclines upon a bath chair. His arm rests languidly upon the furs that swathe him and his fingers grip tight upon a cigarette. Well-wishers smile and hang upon his every word: a lady admirer takes him by the hand, a gentleman rests an arm tenderly on the hood of the chaise, and a large dog stands sentinel. He is, the title tells us, *An Interesting Invalid*, and, though the chair's canopy frames him like a halo, he better describes a more fabulous, dissipated, dolce vita of invalidism. Perhaps this is a disposition to aspire to.

Closer to nirvana, the Reclining Buddha rests his head upon a lotus flower. He lies feet together, long toes aligned, adorned in offerings of oranges and marigolds. In Thailand, the Buddha lies vast in stone, wrapped Christo-like in saffron folds,[4] which billow in the breeze. There are four 'respect-inspiring forms'[5] in Buddhism, and the fourth of these is lying down. A lighter expression of being, it shifts us 'out of the way of the Way',[6] so that we may more readily find the path to an authentic self. Is there revelation in this for me? Lie down and I am freed from the distraction of physicality to reoccupy my self; transcending the tethers of the social world, I find there are other ways to be.

The reclining figures of Henry Moore survey the landscape with a gaze that is far-seeing. Rooted in this earth, organic, monumental, they cast aside the myth of beauty to embrace the energy, barely contained, of the static form. His figures rise from stone so embodied, so absolutely *present*, they almost breathe. I read of the themes of the sculptor's work – truth to the material, form-knowledge,[7] resurrection[8] – and I smile. I respond to my own materiality, shaping myself to its truth and find, for me, that lying down is life restored. And, just as the figures echo the contours of the Yorkshire in which they belong, when I lie down, I come home.

Moore would 'give everything'[9] to chisel figures 'more alive than a real person',[10] though few could outdo the *cojones* of Frida Kahlo. All passion and flesh, she painted her very *self*. From her bed, reflecting her gaze in a ceiling-mounted mirror, she described the play of gravity on the contours of a body lying down. I see her now, muddying the bed sheets with oil and turpentine, lust and rebellion hand-in-hand. Always one for the grand entrance, she is photographed lying in state at the opening of a solo show, the paintings hastily rearranged to accommodate her bed,[11] until Frida herself became a work of art. No fears holding her back. Even after she had left the room, her bed remained.

When he was ill, Christopher Newell would have his bed wheeled to the front of the tiered lecture theatre in Hobart Hospital, from where he would address future-doctors on the ethics of their profession, urging his audiences to 'dare to encounter the muckiness of everyday ethical decision making'.[12] As associate professor, he lay down with authority, and he lay down knowingly. He unfolded and unravelled his body amongst people in a bid to move his students from 'other to us',[13] to bring them to a point of knowing deep down the humanity of those they would meet in their later professional lives. He lay down for both his comfort and his campaign.

— — —

In the sand dunes of Kijkduin, on the North Sea coast of the Netherlands, lies a crater, 30 metres across, entered through an underground passage.[14] At its core lies a bench of stone built for lying down, in sculpture that can only ever be appreciated prone. Supporting the whole of the body, it tips the head back until your gaze is cast upwards, beyond the circle of the crater's rim, from where you fall up up up into a canopy of sky. We believe we know the sky, arched above us in the everyday, but Turrell's sculpture of light wraps it, traces its edges, and the world looks different from here.

I vowed to write lightly because lying down, for me, *is* lightness and Turrell's *Celestial Vault* begins to uncover a lighter way. When I gaze up, does his sky fall in upon me, or does it fall away? Does it threaten to come hurtling down, or can I reach up to touch it? When I lie down, transgressing my society's norms, should I brace myself for disapproval or shall I lean towards it in curiosity and embodied exploration? Is lying down an act, or is it a process of discovering the people who surround me? There are many ways to be in the world.

And now I remember. I lay down another time in public. In Covent Garden, cobbles unyielding, I dragged a large foam cushion behind me. Oh, this time it was *good*. We were a festival of artists with rebel bodies and an outsider view. For that day, we occupied the space, discovering who we might be in a world that was ours. I lay down amongst people and it felt just fine.

So here is my choice: I can absent myself from the social world, or I can lie down anyhow. If there is no guidebook, I shall write one for myself. I will not 'take this lying down'.

My guide is not about managing shame or the troubled body. My guide is about seizing some small courage and breaking rules that cry out to be broken. It is about laughing with the results and going back for more. And it's about realising that, when I push the boundaries, others find their courage too: that time, that conference, where I sat on the floor and, two days later, amidst sighs and wry smiles, at least half the people there had made themselves more comfortable too.

My guide shows me that lying down is not a simple act of physiology but my marking out a place in the world. Sitting up is about my body, but lying down is a declaration of liberty, the soft rain of release.

And so, I see it now; here is my freedom: I shall be fabulous in my dissipation, delight in the earth-mother voluptuousness of a Henry Moore, get out of the way of the Way in my drapes of gold and protest from the very heart of body and soul. I shall be Frida Kahlo, has she no shame, brazen hussy, wearing her wounds with pride. And my boots I shall tuck neatly to one side.

And every time I venture out and lie down, it will be a fanfare for the disappeared, a toast to the rebel body, and I will say, *we are here and we are here and we are here*.

Lying Down Anyhow begins in the physicality of the body, the freedom that is, for me, the act of lying down. Yet, when I ask why lying down in public is so very hard to do, it transforms into a story about external codes and constraints, those emotional, social, political and cultural influences that shape the body's way of being. *Lying Down Anyhow* is less the story of a troubled body than of its interface with the language, values and physical structures that limit the possibilities of lying down in public places.

Those codes and constraints permeate my internal world, shaping my thinking and behaviour. Internalising external sanctions and their attendant shame, I censor myself, believing that lying down in public places cannot be done. But, when I question their validity, I find there are other ways to respond. *Lying Down Anyhow* extends from a story of why it is so difficult to lie down in public to a decision that the constraints cannot be allowed to limit my life or the life of others; it is a decision not to be 'disappeared'.

In changing my response, I shift to the role of activist. Since there is no guidebook, I write my own, producing a counter-narrative to say beyond doubt that 'we are here'. I find myself in a process of freeing the imagination to new ways of being in the world. Setting out to make sense of my own world, I find I am also drafting a map for others to follow. My response is an antidote to the constraints and, even as they continue to hold me back, I begin to reform them in return.

I tell a story of lying down despite the constraints, to spite the constraints. And whilst such prohibitions become apparent only in collision with bodies which do not, or cannot, conform, I realise that theirs is an influence exerted upon us all. *Lying Down Anyhow* begins with my body but is, more truthfully, a tale for every body in a social world.

I begin to question whether this is a story of disability at all. In writing *Lying Down Anyhow*, increasingly I find the difficulty of lying down in public to be a symbol of the universal constraints that impact upon us all. It is a symbol of the collective need to find courage to break those myriad rules that cry out to be broken. *Lying Down Anyhow* becomes a story of the larger human condition and our need for better ways of being in the world.

In passing the text onwards, I ponder what it might set in motion. I hope there will be readers who recognise their own experience in mine and, in doing so, find 'some small courage' too. Perhaps they will not lie down in public, but find from inside themselves the capacity to confront other constraints that hold them back. In questioning who we are and how we want to be, *Lying Down Anyhow* opens up possibilities for celebrating the rebel body and finding a more curious way of living.

Notes

1 Lockton, D. (2008) Anti-Homeless 'Stools': Design with Intent Blog. Available at: http://architectures.danlockton.co.uk/category/benches/ [accessed 26/05/12].
2 Bullivant, S. (2011) Sweeping the Homeless – and Charity – from Westminster's Streets, *The Guardian Online*. Available at: www.guardian.co.uk/commentisfree/belief/2011/mar/04/homeless-victoria-london-westminster-bylaw (paragraph 4) [accessed 04/03/12].
3 San Bruno, California (2011) Title 5 Public Peace, Morals and Welfare; Chapter 6.12 Trespassing and Loitering; 6.12.060 Sitting or lying down in designated zones prohibited, San Bruno Municipal Code, Quality Code Publishing. Available at: http://qcode.us/codes/sanbruno/view.php?topic=6-6_12-6_12_060&frames=on [accessed 26/05/12].
4 Visbeek, B. (2009) A Sign of Enlightenment and Beauty (photograph). Available at: www.flickr.com/photos/visbeek/4002506546/ [accessed 26/05/12].
5 Tophoff, M. (2006) 'Mindfulness-Training: Exploring Personal Change Through Sensory Awareness', *Internet Journal for Cultural Studies* (Internet-ZeitschriftfürKulturwissenschaften, in translation). Available at: www.inst.at/trans/16Nr/09_2/tophoff16.html (paragraph 5) [accessed 26/05/12].
6 Vassi, M. (1984) *Lying Down: The Horizontal Worldview*. Santa Barbara, CA: Capra Press. p. 14.
7 Wilkinson, A. (ed.) (2002) *Henry Moore: Writings and Conversations*. Berkeley and Los Angeles: University of California Press.
8 Wright, F.S. (1947) 'Henry Moore: reclining figure', *Journal of Aesthetics and Art Criticism*, 6 (2): 95–105.
9 Wilkinson, A. (ed.) (2002) *Henry Moore: Writings and Conversations*. Berkeley and Los Angeles: University of California Press. p. 200.

10 Wilkinson, A. (ed.) (2002) *Henry Moore: Writings and Conversations*. Berkeley and Los Angeles: University of California Press.

11 Herrera, H. (1983) *Frida: A Biography of Frida Kahlo*. New York: Perennial Library/ Harper & Row. p. 406.

12 Newell, C. (2002) cited in Goggin, G. (2008) 'Bioethics, disability and the good life: remembering Christopher Newell: 1964–2008', *Bioethical Inquiry*, 5: 235–8.

13 Newell, C. (2006) 'Moving disability from other to us', in P. O'Brien and M. Sullivan (eds), *Allies in Emancipation: Shifting from Providing Service to Being of Support*. Melbourne: Thomson/Dunmore. pp. ix–xi.

14 Frank, T. (2011) Untitled, Nothing into Something: A Blog About Light, 6 July. Available at: www.nothingintosomething.com/blog/james-turrell-celestial-vault [accessed 26/05/12].

13

Psycho-emotional Disablism and Internalised Oppression

Donna Reeve

The original UPIAS definition of disability (1976) which underpins the social model of disability states a clear social relational approach whereby disability arises from the social barriers imposed on people with impairments. Using this UPIAS document as her starting point, Carol Thomas has produced an extended social relational definition of disablism: 'Disablism is a form of social oppression involving the social imposition of restrictions of activity on people with impairments and the socially engendered undermining of their psycho-emotional well-being' (Thomas, 2007: 73).

This definition of disablism recognises the importance of both *structural* and *psycho-emotional* disablism (also 'psycho-emotional dimensions of disability', in Thomas, 1999), differentiating forms of oppression that operate at an outside/public level from those that are found at an inner/private level. Locating the cause of psycho-emotional disablism in oppressive social relationships rather than individual psychopathology means that the solution is to be found in changes at the social and cultural level rather than through individual therapy (see also Chapter 33). Thomas has advocated a move to using the term 'disablism' rather than 'disability' in order to align the oppression faced by people with impairments firmly in the realm of the social relational along with hetero/sexism, racism and ageism which people are more familiar with (see Chapter 3).

Whilst the social model of disability has never specifically excluded a discussion of the barriers which disabled people face that operate at the psycho-emotional level, nonetheless when most people think of disabling barriers, they tend to concentrate on *structural* barriers such as inaccessible buildings, exclusion from the workplace or lack of sign-language provision for Deaf people. Forty years ago, there needed to be a focus on removing structural and institutional barriers which physically excluded disabled people from society, but it is now time to examine the impact of these more private experiences of oppression, which can exclude someone from society as effectively as structural barriers. This chapter will discuss examples of *indirect* and *direct* psycho-emotional disablism and show how the latter relates to the existing concept of 'internalised oppression'.

Indirect psycho-emotional disablism

In addition to differentiating between structural and psycho-emotional disablism, it is also possible to separate out two sources of this latter kind of disablism (Reeve, 2008). *Indirect* psycho-emotional disablism is associated with the experience of structural disablism, recognising the psycho-emotional consequences of exclusion and discrimination. When a disabled person is faced with a structural barrier such as an inaccessible bus or broken hearing loop, the act of exclusion can operate at both a material and psycho-emotional level because this barrier to physical inclusion also serves to remind the disabled person that '"you are out of place", "you are different"' (Kitchin, 1998: 351), in addition to emotional reactions such as anger/ hurt at being excluded.

It could also be argued that some of the 'reasonable adjustments' made to meet the requirements of the Equality Act 2010 can result in indirect psycho-emotional disablism for those disabled people forced to use them. For example, a public building may require disabled people (and those with pushchairs) to use a back entrance, whereas everyone else can enter via the front entrance. The 'reasonable adjustments' clause in the law legalises these forms of spatial apartheid, which can result in the user of the back entrance feeling like a second-class citizen; ironically, the removal of the spatial structural barrier has created a psycho-emotional barrier. Needless to say, those 'reasonable adjustments' which are too humiliating to use will mean that the disabled person remains excluded from that public place/activity.

Direct psycho-emotional disablism

The rest of this chapter will focus on *direct* psycho-emotional disablism, which arises from the relationships that a disabled person has with other people or themselves and is the most important form of psycho-emotional disablism. These 'acts of invalidation' can be found in looks, words or actions that occur in relationships with family members, friends, strangers or professionals, both disabled and non-disabled people. So a common experience for disabled people with visible impairments is that of being *stared at* by others when away from the home because they look or behave differently to 'normal' people. It may be understandable to attract a glance because of this difference, but it is at the point at which the casual glance turns into a hardened stare that this gaze becomes pathologising and an act of invalidation (Hughes, 1999). Another related example is that of having the gaze deliberately withdrawn when others avoid interacting with a disabled person, or engage in the 'Does he take sugar?' conversation with someone pushing the wheelchair.

Psycho-emotional disablism can also arise from the thoughtless *words* of others; for example, comments shouted out in the street such as 'I'd rather be dead than be in one of those [wheelchair]' (Laura in Reeve, 2008: 146) reveal more about the speaker's fears of frailty, vulnerability and death (Hughes, 2007) than the ways in which Laura feels about her own life as a disabled person. Nonetheless, these prejudiced comments can still be upsetting for the recipient of such an outburst. Invasive questions can be difficult to handle; the 'What is *wrong* with you?' question asked by a stranger can be deeply unsettling because it serves to underscore impairment as negative/bad/wrong.

As well as emerging from looks and words, another source of direct psycho-emotional disablism arises from what people *do* when interacting with a disabled person, and this area is particularly pertinent to professional practice. The way that a professional treats the disabled person they are working with can impact on emotional well-being; for example, if two carers talk to each other rather than the disabled person they are helping to get up in the morning, then this can be experienced as infantilising and exclusionary (Reeve, 2008). Whilst this is not a deliberate act of disablism per se by the two carers, nonetheless the consequences of the failure to consider how the person they are helping might feel when talked over in this way still impacts on the psycho-emotional well-being of the disabled person. Psycho-emotional disablism can also result from the cost-cutting measures of local authorities, particularly when services are cut which a disabled person needs in order to retain their dignity around toileting, for example, such as being forced to use incontinence pads at night instead of having support to use a commode (*The Guardian*, 2011).

Finally, it could be argued that there are important interconnections between psycho-emotional disablism and disablist hate crime – acts such as hate speech have resonances with the comments from strangers discussed earlier. Disablist hate crime covers a range of actions from intimidation and vandalism/graffiti, to kidnap, rape, torture and murder (Quarmby, 2008). The same roots which feed psycho-emotional disablism also fuel disablist hate crime – prejudice and contempt for disabled people 'rooted in the view that disabled people are inferior; in some cases less than human' (Quarmby, 2008: 8).

One of the difficulties of psycho-emotional disablism is its unpredictability; whilst someone may know from experience that they will find it difficult to physically access a particular restaurant, they cannot predict how strangers will react to them in the street on any given day. So on a 'bad' day, they may decide to stay at home rather than run the gauntlet of negative reactions, consequently remaining as excluded from participating in society as by structural barriers such as steps. Whilst people with invisible impairments may be able to avoid many of the examples of psycho-emotional disablism described previously, nonetheless there is always the risk that their disability status will be revealed and this fear forms the basis for 'the negative psycho-emotional aspects of concealment' (Thomas, 1999: 55). This is particularly true for people living with pain and fatigue, impairments which are often fluctuating and invisible.

In part, these kinds of social interactions between disabled people and others – staring, avoidance, comments and questions which assume the tragedy of impairment and disability – come about because there is a lack of agreed rules of cultural engagement about social interactions between disabled people and others (Keith, 1996: 72). Therefore, whilst it is usually considered rude in UK society to stare or comment that one is fat, there is often no such restraint shown when the other person is disabled. One of the consequences of the lack of 'rules' means that often disabled people will undertake considerable 'emotion work' to ease the social inter-action, facilitating inclusion rather than exclusion (Reeve, 2008).

Internalised oppression

All of the previous section refers to direct psycho-emotional disablism arising from the relationships that a disabled person has with other people. In contrast, direct psycho-emotional disablism present in the relationship that a disabled person has with *themselves* relates to the existing phenomenon of *internalised oppression*. Internalised oppression is not unique to disabled people – it is a common experience for any subordinated group in society (Young, 1990). The recognition of the impact of internalised oppression within disability studies is not new: 'We harbour inside ourselves the pain and the memories, the fears and the confusions, the negative self-images and the low expectations, turning them into weapons with which to re-injure ourselves, every day of our lives' (Mason, 1992: 27).

Internalised oppression operates at a psychic level and is often largely uncon-scious, which makes it insidious and difficult to challenge (Marks, 1999). Internal-ised oppression is a powerful example of psycho-emotional disablism because it has a direct impact on who disabled people can *be* (Thomas, 2007); for example, a disabled person may decide not to be a parent because they have internalised the prejudice that people 'like them' do not have children.

One approach to unpacking this form of oppression is found in the work of Fiona Kumari Campbell (2009), who draws on the concept of internalised racism from crit-ical race theory to discuss what she terms 'internalised ableism'. Campbell discusses the harm that is done by living in a culture where disability is relentlessly and inher-ently negative; consequently 'the processes of ableism, like those of racism, induce an internalisation or self-loathing which devalues disablement' (Campbell, 2009: 20).

Campbell suggests that internalised oppression is the driver behind the distancing of disabled people from each other (dispersal) and the ways in which disabled people adopt ableist norms (emulation). Dispersal can be seen at work within hierarchies of impairment whereby disabled people position themselves relative to other disabled people (Deal, 2003). Emulation can be seen in the phenomenon of 'passing' which can happen in two ways. At its most benign, this could be someone hiding their impairment in order to avoid having to deal with the reactions of others, as discussed earlier. Another example would be that of the 'supercrip', a disabled person who overachieves in order to prove that they are better than normal, thus widening the gap between that which is loathed (disability) and that which is desired (non-disability). However, a disabled person who is struggling to emulate the ableist norm, is manu-facturing an identity as non-disabled; this takes emotional energy, is forever at risk of fracture and exposure, and denies access to alternate ways of being in which dis-ability is associated with diversity, as a site of potential resistance and possibility.

Internalised oppression is difficult for someone to challenge because disability, unlike ethnicity for example, is not usually common to other family members. This is particularly problematic for disabled children because their less powerful position means they are more vulnerable to the views of society and their parents may be unwitting oppressors in the process, because their beliefs and expectations will be shaped by the professionals they defer to (French, 1994). Finally, people who acquire impairments in adult life and who now find themselves members of this devalued social group, can struggle to make sense of this new identity which clashes with how they see themselves (Young, 1990). Therefore, it is clear that access to positive images of disability and contact with other disabled people could help someone resolve these conflicting aspects of their new life, helping to identify and remove their own internalised oppression.

Conclusion

In this chapter, I have discussed the different forms that psycho-emotional disablism can take and have related internalised oppression to a particular form of direct psycho-emotional disablism arising from the relationship a disabled person has with themselves. Because of the way that psycho-emotional disablism can impact so negatively on self-esteem and self-respect, it has much in common with the experience of emotional abuse; hence psycho-emotional disablism is cumulative and often past experiences can exacerbate current psycho-emotional disablism (Reeve, 2008). However, it should be pointed out that psycho-emotional disablism is not experienced by all disabled people – many disabled people are able to shrug off the thoughtless reactions of others while others actively resist. A good example of this resistance is the statue of Alison Lapper Pregnant (Milmo, 2004), whereby the archetypal image of beauty personified by the Venus de Milo is reflected by a statue of a pregnant disabled woman. Additionally, the form that psycho-emotional disablism takes will be influenced by the type and visibility of impairment (Reeve, 2012), as well as by the cultural messages about disability in that particular society. Therefore, it would be expected that psycho-emotional disablism might take different forms in countries in the majority world, compared to minority world countries such as the UK.

   Although Thomas first introduced the concept of psycho-emotional disablism in 1999, disability studies has been slow to engage with this particular form of disablism. This is not because psycho-emotional disablism is slowly being eradicated in the UK – the rise in disablist hate crime in recent years has been in part fuelled by media representations of disabled people on benefits as workshy scroungers (Scope, 2011). In addition, I have shown how some of the implementations of the Equality Act to include people can *create* indirect psycho-emotional disablism, even if the original structural barriers are removed.

   The psychic processes which underpin the experience of psycho-emotional disablism are complex – in real life, different examples of direct/indirect psycho-emotional disablism are difficult to untangle completely from the experiences of impairment and structural disablism, as well as gender, age, ethnicity, sexuality, time, place, etc. For example, a wheelchair user who finds themselves having to act out the 'grateful disabled person' role, in order to get someone to help them access an inaccessible shop, could be juggling anger at being excluded, dealing with thoughtless comments from strangers, as well as internalised oppression from acting out a stereotype. Whilst the sociological concept of psycho-emotional disablism has achieved much by *naming* these inner forms of disablism, this work needs to be extended by drawing on fields outside disability studies, such as critical psychoanalysis, if a 'politically engaged, contextual psychology of disability' (Watermeyer, 2012: 161) is to be achieved.

References

Campbell, F.K. (2009) *Contours of Ableism: The Production of Disability and Abledness*. Basingstoke: Palgrave Macmillan.

Deal, M. (2003) 'Disabled people's attitudes toward other impairment groups: a hierarchy of impairments', *Disability & Society*, 18 (7): 897–910.

French, S. (1994) 'The disabled role', in S. French (ed.), *On Equal Terms: Working with Disabled People*. Oxford: Butterworth-Heinemann. pp. 47–60.

Hughes, B. (1999) 'The constitution of impairment: modernity and the aesthetic of oppression', *Disability & Society*, 14 (2): 155–72.

Hughes, B. (2007) 'Being disabled: towards a critical social ontology for disability studies', *Disability & Society*, 22 (7): 673–84.

Keith, L. (1996) 'Encounters with strangers: the public's responses to disabled women and how this affects our sense of self', in J. Morris (ed.), *Encounters With Strangers: Feminism and Disability*. London: The Women's Press. pp. 69–88.

Kitchin, R. (1998) '"Out of place", "knowing one's place": space, power and the exclusion of disabled people', *Disability & Society*, 13 (3): 343–56.

Marks, D. (1999) *Disability: Controversial Debates and Psychosocial Perspectives*. London: Routledge.

Mason, M. (1992) 'Internalised oppression', in R. Rieser and M. Mason (eds), *Disability Equality in the Classroom: A Human Rights Issue* (2nd edn). London: Disability Equality in Education, pp. 27–8.

Milmo, C. (2004) 'The woman on the plinth: the story of Alison Lapper', *Independent News*. Available at: http://news.independent.co.uk/uk/this_britain/story.jsp?story=501958 [accessed 22/03/04].

Quarmby, K. (2008) *Getting Away With Murder: Disabled People's Experiences of Hate Crime in the UK*. London: Scope.

Reeve, D. (2008) Negotiating Disability in Everyday Life: The Experience of Psycho-emotional Disablism. Unpublished PhD thesis, Lancaster University.

Reeve, D. (2012) 'Psycho-emotional disablism: the missing link?', in N. Watson, A. Roulstone and C. Thomas (eds), *Routledge Handbook of Disability Studies*. London: Routledge. pp. 78–92.

Scope (2011) Deteriorating Attitudes Towards Disabled People. Available at: www.scope.org.uk/news/attitudes-towards-disabled-people-survey [accessed 17/05/11].

The Guardian (2011) 'Carer battle over as ex-ballerina loses Supreme Court fight', *The Guardian*, 6 July. Available at: www.guardian.co.uk/society/2011/jul/06/care-battle-ballerina-supreme-court [accessed 11/07/11].

Thomas, C. (1999) *Female Forms: Experiencing and Understanding Disability*. Buckingham: Open University Press.

Thomas, C. (2007) *Sociologies of Disability and Illness: Contested Ideas in Disability Studies and Medical Sociology*. Basingstoke: Palgrave Macmillan.

UPIAS (1976) *Fundamental Principles of Disability*. London: UPIAS and The Disability Alliance.

Watermeyer, B. (2012) 'Is it possible to create a politically engaged, contextual psychology of disability?', *Disability & Society*, 27 (2): 161–74.

Young, I.M. (1990) *Justice and the Politics of Difference*. Princeton, NJ: Princeton University Press.

14

Generating Debates: Why We Need a Life-Course Approach to Disability Issues

Mark Priestley

This chapter argues that we should include issues of generation and the life course when thinking about disability in modern societies. This perspective is important because it highlights how disabling societies affect people of different generations in different ways (for example, disabled children, young people, adults or older people). It helps us to avoid an over-simplification of disabled people's collective experiences and redresses the marginalisation of under-represented groups (especially disabled children and older people).

Generation as difference

Disability studies has tended to emphasise the collective experiences of disabled people, as an oppressed group in society, and this has been a very productive approach. However, there are dangers in over-simplifying the collective experience when we know that disabling societies affect different people in different ways. For example, there have been long-standing claims that the disability experience is markedly different for women and men, for people with different kinds of impairment, for people from different ethnic backgrounds, and in different cultural contexts. In this context, a life course approach suggests that disability also carries a different significance for people of different ages and at different stages of life.

Just as gender theorists have shown how much can be gained by distinguishing between the experiences of disabled women and disabled men, so a life course approach suggests that we can gain a great deal by thinking more carefully about the generational experiences of 'disabled children', 'disabled adults' or 'disabled elders', for example. When we look at the way disability is produced and regulated within modern societies, there are some very important generational dimensions. Thinking about disability in terms of generation helps us to understand more clearly how disability and impairment are produced, how they are socially constructed, and how they are regulated in significantly different ways across the life course.

Generation, in this sense, is about more than just age. It involves thinking about the ways that important generational categories (like childhood, youth, adulthood or old age) are constructed, and how transitions between them are governed through social institutions. A good example here is the enduring lack of critical debate about disability issues in old age, despite the fact that the likelihood of impairment increases with age and, in western industrialised societies, the majority of disabled people are over retirement age. Yet, older people are rarely considered 'disabled' in quite the same way that younger adults and children with impairments are (even within activist debates on disability rights). Understanding these anomalies is only possible if we consider the relationship between disability and generation.

To summarise, adopting a life course approach involves thinking about the way in which life course transitions are organised at a collective level within societies and about the generational significance of disability issues as they affect people of different ages. It adds a new dimension to our understanding of disability and offers new ways of thinking about a wide range of debates (in a similar way to the introduction of a gendered analysis). The following sections suggest some of these themes in relation to the body, identity, culture and structure. These arguments are developed in more detail in three books: *Disability and the Life Course: Global Perspectives* (Priestley, 2001), *Disability: A Life Course Approach* (Priestley, 2003) and *Disability and Social Change: Private Lives and Public Policies* (Shah and Priestley, 2011).

Generating bodies

The development of critical disability theory has seen a shift from historical concerns with the impaired body towards a more social and political view of disability. This shift of focus from embodied impairment to society was critical in the development of a social model of disability. However, it has also attracted some criticism from those who take a more social view of the body (e.g. Hughes and Paterson, 1997; Hughes, 2009). Thinking about the body in its social and cultural sense is less problematic for disability studies than traditional medical views of the body and has much relevance for the relationship between disability, generation and the life course.

For example, we might note that bodily impairment characteristics appear to carry a much greater social significance for disabled children and young people than they do in later life. In this sense, social concerns with bodily imperfection seem to play more heavily on disabled children and the unborn than on older people. Although social theorists have suggested an increasing tolerance towards bodily diversity in postmodern consumer societies (Featherstone, 1991, 2010), there is little evidence of such developments in relation to tolerance about the birth of disabled children. The pressures on parents and doctors to produce 'normal' children certainly appear to have less in common with celebrations of diversity than with pursuing uniformity and the normalisation of the body.

Thinking about youth and adulthood also highlights the generational significance of the body in disability debates. Idealised constructions of youthfulness play heavily on the pursuit of bodily perfection in consumer societies, while constructions of independent adulthood emphasise autonomy in physical and cognitive function. These bodily ideals contribute to disability in two ways. First, they provide cultural scripts for decoding the body's potency as an object of beauty or sexual desire – leading to the aesthetic oppression of those whose bodily characteristics are not read in this way (e.g. Hughes, 2000). Second, there is the underlying assumption that young adult bodies should be fit for production and reproduction in the interests of capital, patriarchy and the state.

The significance of a generational account of the body is also underlined in the case of old age. The impaired body has figured prominently in constructions of old age, yet rarely has this been articulated as a disability debate. Indeed, embodied experiences of impairment have been viewed as less 'disruptive' in old age than in childhood or young adulthood (e.g. Williams, 2000; Larsson and Grassman, 2012). It is tempting to conclude that the biographical normality of the impaired body in old age may explain why older people with impairments are rarely seen as disabled in the way that younger adults are.

Disability studies and disability activism have posed some significant challenges to the normalisation of the body, such as resistance to the 'myth of bodily perfection' (Stone, 1995). There has also been active resistance to the elimination of diversity through genetic technologies and eugenic practices. Similarly, disability culture has offered new representations of the body that place greater value on difference and diversity in constructions of physical beauty or sexual attractiveness (Shakespeare, 2000). However, it is also evident that such claims remain rooted in associations between beauty and youth, thereby failing to challenge the power relationships of a generational system that devalues bodies in later life.

Generating identities

Just as a consideration of the body throws up a number of generational issues, thinking about identity is also a useful approach. Encounters with disabling barriers and practices have a considerable impact on disabled people's identity (Shah and Priestley, 2011). For example, the construction of disabled births as 'wrongful lives' and attempts to eradicate impairment characteristics devalue the perceived worth of disabled people in society. Similarly, the normalisation of child development, and the segregation of children with impairments, reinforces negative associations with 'developmental delay' and abnormality. Barriers to participation in the socially val-ued areas of paid employment and parenting have denied many disabled people access to the social networks and citizenship rights upon which adult identities are premised.

Institutional responses to disability have relied on definitions that tend to group disabled people together according to impairment labels or the convenience of ser-vice bureaucracies. This has been reflected in the denial of more nuanced and situated identities. For example, disabled children and young people have often been ascribed relatively static identities that privilege their impairment status above attributes of gender, class, ethnicity or sexuality. Here, age and generation are also important, since generational identities and cultures (especially youth cultures) are a significant aspect of personal biography and identity.

For example, limited access to peer networks and youth cultures may create con-flicts of identity management for young disabled people, forcing them to choose between their disability identity and their youth identity. By contrast, it has been suggested that identity management in old age may be less affected by impairment or by disabling barriers. That is not to say that older people with impairments are not discriminated against as disabled people – far from it. Rather, the assertion is that impairment and disability in old age might be construed as less disruptive to normal identities of ageing than say impairment in younger adulthood (because disability is more widely anticipated in old age).

The development of disability culture and disability politics has been important in promoting more positive identities. However, these new identity resources are very adult-focused. Disabled children, young people and elders remain conspicuous by their absence from disability culture. For both younger and older people then, choos-ing positive disability identities within the movement may mean losing contact with important generational networks and identities. If disability culture is to maintain the inclusiveness of a shared disability identity, it must also resist the temptation to accept the kind of power relationships that place adult interests first.

Generating cultural representations

Cultural analyses also show how disability is constructed in different ways at dif-ferent points in the life course. There is also a certain cultural similarity in the way that disability, childhood and old age have been constructed as 'non-adult' social categories (both marginal to and dependent upon adults). Such constructions have been important in the governance of disability through social institutions. For example, the cultural construction of disabled people as childlike (as innocent, asexual or untamed) has been reproduced in the legitimation of adult power rela-tionships based on custodial care and surveillance. Similarly, the infantilisation and social death of older people in institutional settings has much in common with that experienced by both children and disabled adults, impacting on rights (Hockey and James, 1993; Mégret, 2011).

Culturally, life course expectations in modern societies continue to be defined in relation to idealised notions of modern adulthood. Such constructions have been highly gendered, with a traditional emphasis on distinctive male and female adult roles centred on participation in productive or reproductive labour respectively (specifically, employment and parenting). By contrast, children, young people, elders and disabled people of all ages have been constructed as lacking the kind of adult attributes upon which full personhood and citizenship are premised.

However, there have been significant cultural challenges to this adult-centred construction of the life course. The recognition of generational conflict and power relationships has been mirrored in a new generational politics, in which non-adult minority groups have made new claims to adult rights and responsibilities. The emergence of movements for the rights of children and older people place an increasing strain on traditional constructions of citizenship as a uniquely adult-centred concept. Social claims from the disabled people's movement have raised similar challenges, emphasising self-determination, reflexivity and interdependence over the cultural ideals of autonomous functioning.

Generating social structures

The development of social models of disability was underpinned by a structural analysis, demonstrating how people with perceived impairments become disabled through processes of social transformation (Oliver, 1990; Oliver and Barnes, 2012). In particular, materialist accounts pointed to historic changes in the social relations of production and reproduction within western capitalist economies as a driving force for the creation of disability as a social and administrative category. Here, the changing demands of industrialisation, competitive labour markets, new technologies and the patriarchal nation-state have all been important.

Structural analyses also help to explain the emergence of the generational system. For example, it could equally be argued that similar processes of social change created the categories of childhood and youth. Thus, the increasing demands of industrialisation and individuation in knowledge societies have led to an extension of the training required before young people can participate effectively in productive adult labour (Irwin, 1995; MacDonald, 2011). In this sense, the regulation of childhood and youth as dependent non-adult states has been driven by economic developments and the changing structure of adult labour markets. At the same time, increased longevity and the exemption of older workers from those same labour markets (through retirement) created a parallel category of old age. Clearly, there are considerable parallels between these processes and those that have produced the structural dependency of disabled people in modern societies.

So, a structural analysis of disability makes little sense as a 'special case', in isolation from the production of the generational system. In particular, it is important to understand the centrality of adult work and employment in producing both disability and generational boundaries. This may help to explain why the political focus of disability debates still falls so heavily on adult-centred issues (particularly on issues of employment and parenting). While disability in youth and old age can be partially accommodated within an existing generational system of dependency, disability in adulthood stands out as a greater structural challenge. In this sense, social responses to disabled children have had much to do with structural concerns about their potential for participation in future adulthood. Conversely, the distinct lack of institutional or policy focus on disability in old age reflects the fact that older people are often already structurally exempt from productive or caring adult labour.

These structural analyses of both disability and the generational system have been premised on a particular view of the social relations of production in modern societies. As the life course scholar, Meyer (1988: 57) concluded:

> The life course in modern societies is itself a construct with deep cultural supports. It is not simply the aggregate product of a series of individual choices, nor is it the accidental construction of institutions organized around other cultural purposes. To a substantial extent, the life course is a conscious and purposive cultural product of the modern system.

Given that much contemporary social theory is concerned with explaining transitions from modern societies towards late modern or postmodern forms of social organisation, it is important to question how this affects our understanding of disability and the generational system for the future. Two themes seem important here. First, processes of individuation have undermined the apparent predictability of our traditional life course pathways and expectations. As a consequence, the 'normal' life course has been increasingly redefined in terms of individually negotiated 'life projects' and risks (e.g. Giddens, 1991; Rustin, 2000; Mayer, 2009). As these traditional life expectations break down, it is perhaps unsurprising that the progress of disabled people's claims to full participation and equality have occurred at the same time as parallel claims from 'non-adult' generational minorities (particularly children and older people). Second, social status is becoming increasingly defined by our patterns of consumption rather than our contribution to production. Since our understanding of both disability and the generational system are premised on an analysis of the social relations of production, such changes pose an additional challenge.

Conclusion

As I hope this brief chapter shows, the concepts of generation and the life course add another dimension to our understanding of disabling barriers and disability debates. Adopting a life course approach also raises a number of important generational questions. Why, for example, have states gone to such lengths to limit or prevent the birth of disabled children? Why have disabled children been so often excluded from mainstream education? What is the significance of youth culture and youth transitions for *young* disabled people? How does the expectation of an 'independent' *adulthood* contribute to the production of disability in modern societies? Why are *older* people with impairments rarely seen as disabled in quite the same way that *younger* adults often are? Why are different moral standards applied to the death and dying of disabled and non-disabled people? Inserting age and generation into our questions about disability leads us to new insights and understandings of disability, of normalcy in the life course and its social organisation in contemporary societies.

References

Featherstone, M. (1991) 'The body in consumer culture', in M. Featherstone, M. Hepworth and B. Turner (eds), *The Body: Social Process and Cultural Theory*. London: SAGE. pp. 170–96.

Featherstone, M. (2010) 'Body, image and affect in consumer society', *Body & Society*, 16 (1): 193–221.

Giddens, A. (1991) *Modernity and Self Identity*. Cambridge: Polity.

Hockey, J. and James, A. (1993) *Growing Up and Growing Older: Ageing and Dependency in the Life Course*. London: SAGE.

Hughes, B. (2000) 'Medicine and the aesthetic invalidation of disabled people', *Disability & Society*, 15 (4): 555–68.

Hughes, B. (2009) 'Disability activisms: social model stalwarts and biological citizens', *Disability & Society*, 24 (6): 677–88.

Hughes, B. and Paterson, K. (1997) 'The social model of disability and the disappearing body: towards a sociology of impairment', *Disability & Society*, 12 (3): 325–40.

Irwin, S. (1995) *Rights of Passage: Social Change and the Transition from Youth to Adulthood*. London: UCL Press.

Larsson, A. and Grassman, E. (2012) 'Bodily changes among people living with physical impairments and chronic illnesses: biographical disruption or normal illness?', *Sociology of Health & Illness*, 34 (8): 1156–69.

MacDonald, R. (2011) 'Youth transitions, unemployment and underemployment: plus ça change, plus c'est la même chose?', *Journal of Sociology*, 47 (4): 427–44.

Mayer, K. (2009) 'New directions in life course research', *Annual Review of Sociology*, 35: 413–33.

Mégret, F. (2011) 'The human rights of older persons: a growing challenge', *Human Rights Law Review*, 11 (1): 37–66.

Meyer, J. (1988) 'Levels of analysis: the life course as a cultural construction', in M.W. Riley (ed.), *Social Structures and Human Lives*. Newbury Park, CA: SAGE pp. 46–92.

Oliver, M. (1990) *The Politics of Disablement*. Basingstoke: Macmillan.

Oliver, M. and Barnes, C. (2012) *The New Politics of Disablement*. Basingstoke: Palgrave Macmillan.

Priestley, M. (ed.) (2001) *Disability and the Life Course: Global Perspectives*. Cambridge: Cambridge University Press.

Priestley, M. (2003) *Disability: A Life Course Approach*. Cambridge: Polity.

Rustin, M. (2000) 'Reflections on the biographical turn in social sciences', in P. Chamberlayne, J. Bornat and T. Wengraf (eds), *The Turn to Biographical Methods in Social Science: Comparative Issues and Examples*. London: Routledge. pp. 53–70.

Shah, S. and Priestley, M. (2011) *Disability and Social Change: Private Lives and Public Policies*. Bristol: Policy Press.

Shakespeare, T. (2000) 'Disabled sexuality: toward rights and recognition', *Sexuality and Disability*, 18 (3): 159–66.

Stone, S.D. (1995) 'The myth of bodily perfection', *Disability & Society*, 10 (4): 413–24.

Williams, S. (2000) 'Chronic illness as biographical disruption or biographical disruption as chronic illness? Reflections on a core concept', *Sociology of Health & Illness*, 22 (1): 40–67.

15

The Representation of Disabled People in the News Media

Robert Williams-Findlay

Introduction

During an interview in 2009, Colin Cameron said, 'How do disabled people manage to feel good about who they are in a culture that keeps on telling us that we're shit – through charity, through the media, through the way services are organised and delivered, through countless everyday interactions with intrusive strangers, condescending professionals, family members who just don't get what it's about?' (Disability Arts Online, 2009: unpaginated). Cameron was discussing his exploration of the affirmative model which centres upon people with impairments' view of themselves and their lives (2008) (see Chapter 4). Existing cultural representations of disabled people do more than reinforce oppressive stereotypes, they construct 'stories' around who and what we are, and in so doing *explain away* disabled people's marginalised position within society.

Oliver (1996), through outlining the 'individual tragedy' approach towards disability, explains how disabled people are viewed as being unable to live worthwhile lives. If disabled people's lives are *made sense of* in terms of their lack of social worth and this in turn legitimates disabled people's lived experience of social exclusion and marginalisation within society, how has the news media addressed the growing social movements for change among disabled people? In 2009, I researched the reporting of disability-related matters in *The Times* and *The Guardian* by looking at language usage and representation over an eight-week period for the years 1988 and 2008. I was looking to see if the language and representation had radically altered or not. The aim was to contrast my findings with previous research conducted by Smith and Jordan (1991), Cooke et al. (2000) and Haller et al. (2006). This chapter builds upon questions that emerged from my study.

Before proceeding, let us clarify the notion of media representation. A basic understanding would be that representation refers to:

the construction in any medium (especially the *mass media*) of aspects of 'reality' ... Such representations may be in speech or writing as well as still or moving pictures. The term refers to the *processes* involved as well as to its *products*. (Chandler, 2012)

Representation therefore 'involves not only how identities are represented (or rather *constructed*) within the text but also how they are constructed in the processes of production and reception' (Chandler, 2012: unpaginated). My research required me to investigate the production of news within newsprint, however I believe similar processes exist within other forms of news production. The focus of this chapter is more on the processes involved in news production, but we begin with an introduction to research that has studied the relationship between disabled people and news production.

The story so far: Research on disability and the news industry

A considerable volume of material has been written on the representation of disabled people within the news industry. Research conducted by Smith and Jordan (1991) and Cooke et al. (2000) was UK-based and concerned language, imagery and the practice of the press. Cooke et al. argued that 'disabled people are, of course, the subject of news items and occasionally of features but these stories tend to be on disability from a non-disabled perspective' (p. 6). Hall (1973: 186) explains that 'ideological concepts embodied in photos and texts in a newspaper, then, do not produce new knowledge about the world. They produce recognitions of the world as we have already learned to appropriate it.' Cooke et al. (2000: 4) stated: 'many disabled people feel the press does not reflect the reality of their lives' and the 'types of subjects relating to disability are more likely ... to contain derogatory language'.

This links in with Cameron's views. Both the research undertaken by Cooke et al. (2000) and Williams-Findlay (2009) employed modified lists of words considered 'negative' by Smith and Jordan.

In the USA, similar types of research have been undertaken. Clogston (1990) offered a set of five categories or models which reveal dominant attitudes within what are called 'news frames'. The use of news frames will be discussed in a moment, but first I want to outline the categories that are thought to capture 'stories' about disabled people. The first three are called 'traditional' because they all correspond to the dominant ideologies which define disability as 'an individualised tragedy'. The first category is the 'medical model' which presents disability as illness or malfunction. This was very evident through my research. The second, the 'social pathology model', is where disabled people are viewed as disadvantaged and in need of care and support (charity or state intervention). The 'supercrip model' operates within the duality of 'tragic, but brave', where disabled individuals are portrayed as 'deviant' because they go 'beyond expectations' and do 'incredible feats'.

The next two categories are viewed as 'progressive' and whilst they were used in this study, the usage was less culturally based than the meanings offered by Clogston (1990). The 'minority/civil rights model' sees disabled people as part of a disabled community with legitimate civil rights grievances. The second 'progressive' category – 'cultural pluralism' – is where disabled people are considered to be multifaceted and there is not a focus on their impairments (Haller and Ralph, 2000). Haller (1995), following the passing of the Americans with Disabilities Act (ADA), introduced three further models which related to responses in society to the Act. In addition, Clogston analysed news items in terms of the extent to which disabled people could be regarded as being either 'active' or 'passive' within the texts. 'Active' refers to evidence of disabled people contributing to the item either as a source or authorship, and 'passive' means disabled people are reported or commented upon by a third party thereby having no influence on the text. These are the main research studies that underpinned my own research and subsequently influenced my thinking for this chapter.

Making the news

A crucial question to ask when talking about 'making the news' is: what makes something newsworthy? Park (1994: 13) addressed 'newsworthiness' in terms of impact upon the audience in these terms: 'dog biting man would probably not be newsworthy, whereas the opposite would ... it will be remembered and repeated'. What news is, the functions it plays within society, and the question of 'newsworthiness' cannot however be considered in isolation. How news is produced and the organisation behind it, are also important factors. White (1950) spoke about the 'gatekeepers' involved in selecting the news, suggesting they decide the style of stories best suited for their particular paper. Shoemaker (1991) argued that the processes were more complex. Hall et al. (1978), for example, state that 'Just as each paper ... has a particular organisational framework, sense of news and readership, so each will also develop a regular and characteristic *mode of address*.' The production of news for television has its own format, however – even with 24/7 news channels, news items and their style of presentation tend to fit 'the house style' in a similar pattern to newsprint.

Golding and Elliot (1979) expanded upon this by suggesting news is the transmission of an ideology belonging to specific social groups and arises from the production process and identified demands of the audience. Others consider this 'hypodermic' transmission model too simplistic. Within my study, there was evidence to suggest the language employed and subject areas covered reflected the differing media audiences. Hall et al. (1978: 59) suggest that certain social groups benefit through having special status. It is having institutional power, being seen as a representative voice or laying claim to expert knowledge that confers this status and sees the exercising of ideological power: 'The media, then, do not simply "create" the news; nor do they simply transmit the ideology of the "ruling class" in a conspiratorial fashion.'

Olien et al. (1989) suggest: 'Media reports social movements as a rule in the guise of watchdogs, while actually performing as "guard dogs" for the mainstream.' Hence, disabled people and their lives become framed by well-established stereotyped representations which are maintained because, as Hall et al. (1978: 56) point out, 'Events, as news ... are regularly interpreted within frameworks derived, in part, from this notion of *the consensus* as a basic feature of everyday life.' This links with the view that most stories about disabled people are from non-disabled people's perspectives. The relationship between journalists, sources and audiences is complex, however research acknowledges the location of the news media as agents in the social construction of reality, and by the same token the role it plays in the creation of a societal world view (Cohen and Young, 1982). It is necessary therefore to enquire as to the extent to which dominant ideologies associated with disabled people co-exist with 'common sense' ideologies within the construction of disability-related 'news frames'.

News frames, disability and stereotyping

Because of societal barriers, the general public gets much of its information about the disability community from media sources rather than through interpersonal contact (Haller, 1999; Makas, 1993). Haller cites Higgins (1992) who says we, as a society, 'make disability' through our language, media and other public and visible ways. There was a shared view among the writers that stereotypical assumptions about disabled people are 'inherent to our culture and persist partly because they are constantly reproduced through the communications media' (Barnes, 1992). This raises issues regarding the influences that impact upon journalists' writing about disabled people.

Gamson (1989: 161), speaking about the journalist and the audience, explains that they are likely to share the same culture, therefore enabling an exchange of meanings. He states: 'The frames for a given story are frequently drawn from shared cultural narratives and myths.' It is therefore argued that many journalists continue to represent disability as a medical problem or social deviance which denies disabled people's own perspectives. Media researchers have employed the notion of 'framing' to describe how a social phenomenon, such as disability, can be presented in ways which influence or shape readers' attitudes towards that phenomenon. A number of researchers argue that these news frames are created at an unconscious level by news workers who gravitate toward familiar understandings, rather than new or unique frames (Clogston, 1990). Journalistic routines and practices lead them to official or 'authoritative' sources, rather than those considered marginal or minority. This suggests newspapers are more likely to approach disability charities than disabled people's organisations. My study revealed that *The Times* has a close relationship with the

RNIB, and a search for key words within texts failed to register any national self-organised disability groups or high-profile campaigns led by the disabled people's movement.

Acknowledging the stereotypes employed within news framing, however, does not tell the whole story. Some research studies address stereotyping by suggesting the use of more 'positive' language and imagery (Smith and Jordan, 1991; Barnes, 1992). Hevey (1992), however, is critical of this argument. I would suggest that stereotypes often play the role of *confirming* what the audience believe they 'know'; however, the location of disabled people within news frames, how they are reported upon and even their absence from the news can play a role in establishing whether they are considered 'newsworthy' or not. On this note, our attention turns to where disabled people appear in the news.

How the news industry frames disabled people: The ambiguity of living disabled lives

The representation of disabled people within the news industry is determined by the type of language employed, the use of visual imagery and how they are 'framed' within specific stories (Figure 1.1). In relation to language deployment, evidence to suggest that since the 1980s there has been some change in the use of language, however, it is not consistent across the board. The newspapers, whilst cutting down on the traditional pejorative terms associated with disabled people, appeared less open to embracing language disabled people would prefer. Evidence also exists to suggest that within the last decade, especially in the UK, there has been an increase in the volume of disability-related news stories, however this is accompanied by an increased politicisation of media coverage, and with it comes a new language which assists in stereotyping and stigmatising people on benefits or receiving welfare support (Briant et al., 2011).

The role of language becomes clearer when contextualised in terms of 'news frames' and 'subject matter' vis-à-vis the interrogation of news items. My own study considered items in terms of being 'negative' or 'progressive' news frames (Clogston, 1990) and the extent to which disabled people were 'active', for example, drove the piece or 'passive', for example, silent and reported upon. The majority of the subject areas found within Smith and Jordan were repeated in mine with little change between 1988 and 2008, except for a slight increase in 'rights-based' stories.

Health – Medical research – Medical negligence – Benefits – Mainstream politics – Government policy – Campaigning/rights – Employment – Education – Services – Charity – Housing – Community care – Local authorities – Transport – Media/arts – Human interest – Sport – Legal/crime – Miscellaneous

Figure 1.1   How the news industry frames disabled people: the ambiguity of living disabled lives

The implications behind this are simple: the news industry only views disabled people as 'newsworthy' within certain bands of 'subject areas'. Similarly, the sources for these news items appear to be agencies which have traditionally been associated with controlling the lives of disabled people. Finally, within the items and subject areas disabled people were found to be more likely to be framed in 'negative' representations than 'progressive' ones; more 'passive' than 'active'. Cameron's assertion that disabled people find it difficult to feel good about themselves because of the external pressures coming from within dominant culture certainly applies to the news industry. Whether it is intentional or not, the reproduction of traditional news frames over more progressive ones simply helps maintain the status quo; however, this situation, I would argue, cannot be altered simply by changing the internal culture of the news industry.

The majority of representations of disabled people in the news media reflect the ways disabled people are viewed from dominant perspectives vis-à-vis what it means to live 'disabled lives'. This does not necessarily portray how disabled people see themselves or their lived experiences. Hevey (1992: 17) explains that: 'disability imagery can comprise multiple viewpoints or gazes, ranging from the impairment and the body to the disabling social environment, [and this] is not yet clear to many people concerned with this area'. Failure to address these viewpoints or gazes means 'the efforts of the media and the charitable organisations have been to turn the political discourse on disability imagery into, at best, a superficial debate on "positive" or "negative" imagery'. In other words, the social and political issues around what it means to be disabled people are rarely articulated or viewed in terms of *conforming* to 'normality'. Research shows little evidence of the news industry seeing disability represented as 'social oppression or restriction'. Within the global disabled people's movement and disability studies, debates rage around the question of 'disabled identities' – however, these debates largely by-pass the news industry.

The traditional representations of disabled people still hold sway because the news media, through its production, sources and the social influences upon its audiences, remains unwilling or unable to address the challenging issues raised by disabled people's struggles for self-determination.

References

Barnes, C. (1992) *Disabling Imagery and the Media: An Exploration of the Principles for Media Representations of Disabled People*. Halifax: British Council of Organisations of Disabled People and Ryburn Publishing. Available at: http://disabilitystudies.leeds.ac.uk/files/library/Barnes-disabling-imagery.pdf (accessed 15/07/13).

Briant, E., Philo, P. and Watson, N. (2011) *How the Newspapers are Reporting Disability*. Glasgow: Strathclyde Centre for Disability Research and Glasgow Media Unit, University of Glasgow.

Cameron, C. (2008) 'Further towards an affirmation model', in T. Campbell, F. Fontes, L. Hemingway, A. Soorenian and C. Till (eds), *Disability Studies: Emerging Insights and Perspectives*. Leeds: The Disability Press. pp. 14–30.

Chandler, D. (2012) Media Representation. Available at: www.aber.ac.uk/media/Modules/MC30820/represent.html (accessed 03/04/12).

Clogston, J.S. (1990) *Disability Coverage in 16 Newspapers*. Louisville, KY: Avocado Press.

Cohen, S. and Young, J. (1982) 'Models of presentation: the manufacture of news', in S. Cohen and J. Young (eds), *Social Problems, Deviance and the Mass Media*. London: Constable. pp. 157–68.

Cooke, C., Daone, L. and Morris, G. (2000) *Stop Press! How the Press Portrays Disabled People*. London: Scope.

Disability Arts Online (2009) Discussion: Colin Cameron – Further Towards an Affirmative Model of Disability. Available at: www.disabilityartsonline.org.uk/affirmative-model-of-disability (accessed 02/04/12).

Gamson, W.A. (1989) 'News as framing', *American Behavioral Scientist*, 33: 157–61.

Golding, P. and Elliot, P. (1979) *Making News*. Harlow: Addison Wesley Longman.

Hall, S. (1973) 'The determinations of news photographs', in S. Cohen and J. Young (eds), *The Manufacture of News: Social Problems and the Mass Media*. London: Constable.

Hall, S., Critcher, C., Jefferson, T., Clarke, J. and Roberts, P. (1978) *Policing the Crisis*. London: Macmillan.

Haller, B.A. (1995) Narrative Conflicts: News Media Coverage of the Americans with Disabilities Act at the National Communication Association annual meeting, San Antonio.

Haller, B.A. (1999) 'How the news frames disability: print media coverage of the americans with disabilities act', *Research in Social Science and Disability*. JAI Press, Vol. 1.

Haller, B.A. and Ralph, S.M. (2000) 'Content analysis methodology for studying news and disability: case studies from the United States and England', *Research in Social Science and Disability*, 2: 229–53.

Haller, B.A., Dorries, B. and Rahn, J. (2006) 'Media labelling *versus* the US disability community identity: a study of shifting cultural language', *Disability & Society*, 21(1): 61–75.

Hevey, D. (1992) *The Creatures that Time Forgot: Photography and Disability Imagery*. London and New York: Routledge.

Higgins, P.C. (1992) *Making Disability: Exploring the Social Transformation of Human Variation*. Springfield, IL: Charles C. Thomas.

Makas, E. (1993) 'Changing channels: the portrayal of people with disabilities on television', in G.L. Berry and J.K. Asamen (eds), *Children and Television*. Newbury Park, CA: SAGE. pp. 255–68.

Olien, C., Tichenor, P. and Donohue, G. (1989) 'Media and protest', in L. Grunig (ed.), *Monographs in Environmental Education and Environmental Studies*. Troy, OH: North American Association for Environmental Education.

Oliver, M. (1996) *Understanding Disability: From Theory to Practice*. Basingstoke: Macmillan.

Park, R.E. (1994) 'News as a form of knowledge: a chapter in the sociology of knowledge', *American Journal of Sociology*, 45: 669–86. [Reproduced in Schlesinger, P. and Tumber, H. (1994) *Reporting Crime: The Media Politics of Reporting Crime*. Oxford: Oxford University Press.]

Shoemaker, P.J. (1991) *Gatekeeping*. London: SAGE.

Smith, S. and Jordan, A. (1991) *What the Papers Say and Don't Say about Disability*. London: Spastics Society.

White, D.M. (1950) 'The gatekeeper: a case study in the selection of news', *Journalism Quarterly*, Vol. 27.

Williams-Findlay, R. (2009) Is there Evidence to Support the View that the Language and Subject Matter Selected by *The Times* and the *Guardian* in Relation to Disabled People has Changed over the Last Twenty Years? Unpublished MA thesis, University of Leeds.

16

Disability Culture: The Story So Far

Alison Wilde

Raymond Williams called culture 'one of the two or three most complicated words in the English language' (Williams, 1983: 87). Its meaning is not clear and unambiguous, and it is used in different ways and by and in different disciplines. Even within cultural studies, there have been long and complex debates on this topic (see, for example, Barker, 2011; Peters, 2000; Storey, 2012 for a discussion of cultural theory in relation to disability).

Given this, it might be better to avoid the term altogether. But despite the inherent ambiguities, it is still a term with potential for explanatory power, and it does (however imperfectly) reflect a fundamental aspect of the world, having a particular significance for disabled people.

I will be considering two aspects or types of culture: as artefacts of performance, as creative communicative practices in a specific domain – art, theatre, cinema, TV, and so on; and as something more down-to-earth, the practices and knowledges of living or being, the substance of 'ways of life', shaping our membership of social groups, feelings of belonging and our identities.

Similarly, disability culture can be conceptualised in two main ways. First, as an expressive and demonstrative force, disability arts has played a leading role in highlighting some of the realities of disabled people's lives, challenging the hegemony of non-disabled cultural norms, and inspiring and galvanising other disabled people. Although disability culture cannot be reduced to disability art, it is clearly seen by many to be a vital part of disability culture (see, for example, Sutherland, 1997; Vasey, 2004).

Disability art has played a crucial part in the development of new disability aesthetics, making important contributions to disability politics which has informed us in our struggles for social and cultural inclusion. Notwithstanding ongoing disagreements on what disability art is, has been or should be (Darke, 2003), disability art as 'art by disabled people with a commitment to (some form of) disability politics' has burgeoned. Defined so loosely, it concerns itself with many things: impairment experiences, disabling barriers, critiques of 'normality', sexuality, gender, medicine, ethnicity, psycho-emotional issues, empowerment, disempowerment, joy, desperation and much more. And it does so in a wide variety of forms including film, visual arts, poetry, literature, theatre, live art, comedy, dance, music and cabaret/burlesque. It is also significant that, with a few notable (but sadly visible) exceptions, disability arts (in its many guises, so widely defined) is predominantly authored and practised by disabled people.

As such, it has provided many of us with pleasure, knowledge and a sense of community, whilst assisting talented disabled artists by providing opportunities which were far from evident in mainstream cultural organisations. I am sure that Colin Hambrook's sentiments on the loss of the London Disability Arts Forum (LDAF) echo those of many of us facing the demise of collective arts organisations: '[W]ithout LDAF it is also unlikely that I would have found myself amongst a community of disabled people with whom I felt I could share my own difference as someone who had spent a life in fear' (2008: unpaginated).

Disability arts often contribute to disability culture in ways which recognise and encompass the struggles and practical realities of the lives of disabled people, as a challenge to the hegemonic non-disabled 'norm', providing us with alternative forms of 'cultural capital' (Bourdieu and Passeron, 1973) to be shared, valued and used within disabled communities and beyond. Compelling arguments for the growth of disability culture can be found in the work of writers such as Darke (2003), Finkelstein (1987), Masefield (2006) and Sutherland (1997).

The second sense of the term 'disability culture' refers to the everyday realities and shared understandings we have of the collective (if often diverse) barriers we face. Vasey (2004) identified a number of everyday practices as an integral part of most disabled people's culture, such as the technologies, daily practices and rhythms which are crucial to our presence in the world (the time it takes and procedures involved in going to the toilet or getting washed, negotiating transport and non-disabled people's attitudes to us, for example). As many disabled people will know, these aspects of our lives are often fundamental to our being in the world, yet almost unknown and unacknowledged in wider culture.

However, some see the notion of disability culture as potentially problematic, in suggesting a unitary, fixed and essentialist disabled experience which does not and cannot represent the experience of all disabled people, and as such should be avoided. This is an important and serious consideration; and will be revisited after a brief look at these two different aspects of disability culture in relation to dominant culture.

Disability culture: Culture as lived experience

McDermott and Varenne (1995) recommend the value of understanding culture 'as the knowledge people need for living with each other' (p. 327). From this perspective, it becomes clear that there are a number of problems for disabled people in contemporary culture. How does the compulsion to go to bed three hours before you'd like to, because a social care professional has to operate a hoist, fit in with a wider cultural knowledge about how we should live with one another? And how does the mutability of an impairment such as MS or ME fit in with employers' and colleagues' expectations of you as a worker, your long-term employment trajectory, or the box-ticking required to meet the conditions for Employment Support Allowance? The knowledge that many aspects of our lives are outside the common everyday expectations of how people should live with one another is likely to have significant psycho-emotional and social implications. Most of us are painfully aware that the formal and implicit rules embedded in dominant culture work to position non-disabled people as 'normal', excluding the majority of disabled people as cultural outsiders (see Darke's work on normality theory, undated).

As studies of disabled people's everyday lives have demonstrated (e.g. Paterson and Hughes, 1999), our daily experiences of disablement render our knowledge as disabled people invalid [*sic*] in the majority of social circumstances (albeit in many different ways). The awareness that many aspects of our lives are outside the common everyday expectations of how people should live with one another is likely to have significant psycho-emotional and social implications for many of us, particularly in terms of how much we choose to hide or acknowledge any distinct ways of living and voice any unmet needs. At the same time, we have to grapple with dominant discourses of what is expected of us as disabled people. We are expected to accept other people's lives even though this respect is unreciprocated when we are stared at, or made the subject of other people's superstitions, fears or moral condemnations.

So how do highly personalised experiences of 'disability culture' fit within wider understandings of culture as the knowledge we need to live with one another? Geertz (1973: 5) suggests that our own views of wider culture are not neutral or objective but bound up with our own needs for actively and creatively making sense of our lives. I believe it is crucial to ask who has the power to create cultural knowledge and where, and how and why disability is implicated in these 'webs of significance' (1973: 5).

Disability arts and the forging of disability culture have come closest to answering these questions, providing ongoing and dynamic provocations to dominant culture. In a culture claiming the value of austerity (for some), it is an increasingly urgent matter that we understand the 'importance assigned to disability by dominant cultural discourses and whose interests these serve' (Peters, 2000: 588). These remain the most important questions to ask if we are to inform our understanding of, and strategies towards, disability culture as a form of cultural expression and resistance, especially in the face of growing media hostility (Briant et al., 2011).

Despite any limitations, it is undeniable that disability culture, particularly disability arts, has challenged much of the knowledge created about us as inaccurate, disabling and just plain wrong, and has done much to oppose a (non-disabled) normalised view of the world. I am arguing that, despite its paradoxes, innate limitations and the considerable obstacles to its survival, disability culture provides a valuable source of identification and remains crucial to disabled people's political identities and struggles.

The paradoxes of disability culture: A brief revisit

Despite the benefits disability arts and culture may have brought to disabled people and others, some scholars have questioned its value, often citing the problems of claiming a fixed, 'essentialist' or 'categorical identity', which could delimit other aspects of our identities and potentially serve as labels to oppress us further (Galvin, 2003).

The over-riding fear about disability culture is very understandable; it is crucial to the progress we make as disabled people that we should not fall into essentialist ideas of what disability culture is, and what disabled people are in our efforts to oppose and challenge old stereotypes. For example, in response to Peters's call for a syncretisation of three possible world views as a model for disability culture, Galvin asks:

> How can we claim unity without falling into the same exclusionary practices that have served to create our divisive identifications in the first place? Conversely, how can we relinquish practices of identification that are based on binary oppositions without losing the ability to claim identities at all? (2003: 675)

Galvin went on to argue against the creation of a more 'positive disabled identity', a reliance on the 'norm', and she called for the 'dissolution' of disabled identity, recommending that we work 'at the limits of ourselves' in an effort to work towards the removal of 'divisive identifications' (2003: 687). Certainly, the idea of 'positive disabled identities' and the imposition of disabling norms can be seen as detrimental to our well-being, both of these being fundamental to ideas which oppress us; cultural discourses on the imperative to 'get disabled people back to work' and 'off benefits' are a telling example of these dangers.

As ideals, of course, there can be little disagreement with these principles as key tenets of a non-disabling society (although we should expect considerable opposition from the 'disability industry'). However, our aspirations for 'the norm' are far from straightforward and our desire to occupy 'normal roles' in society often sit uneasily alongside our commitment to deconstruct the type of 'normality' which is at the root of our oppression. One example is the struggle many of us have faced to be treated as a 'normal' and deserving parent and to carry out our parenting roles free from external interference and judgements on our differences and perceived deficits whilst fighting for acceptance and support.

In these and other ways, Galvin's recommendations appear to be contradictory. She seems to misrecognise disability culture as a social grouping with a fixed set of ideas. It seems to me that one of the great strengths of disability culture is its capacity to address complexity and contradiction. The capacity of disability culture to maintain common goals and political identifications alongside diverse identities and conflicting interests remains strong, despite our inevitable divisions (seen, for example, in the growing internationalisation of disability arts).

Further, disability arts has often played a *leading role* in illuminating the cultural dilemmas we face in claiming a disabled identity that nourishes us without re-inscribing ourselves as 'Other'.

The story continues: The shape of disability culture in 2012

It is impossible to do justice to the expansive range of disability arts other than through a very brief sketch of the current landscape. Despite the demise of the disability arts forums four years ago and increasing erosion of disabled people's control in the arts (Darke, 2003) and elsewhere, disabled creativity seems to have flourished.

Digital culture has radically changed the shape of disability arts over the past ten years. Ten years ago, it was hard for people who live outside major cities to access many aspects of the arts or even to get news of such events. The Internet has provided far more opportunities to learn about, or participate in, disability arts for those of us who are able to access it. The growing internationalism of disability arts has fostered collaborations between many performers, potentially adding much to our cultural resources and understanding. Initiatives such as the International Guild of Disabled Artists and Performers (IGODAP) have grown from the collaborations of leading disabled artists and performers, and these international links are reflected in the number, quality and popularity of disability arts festivals. Dada is a good example of the strength of disability and Deaf arts, an organisation which emerged from Shape and the former North West Disability Arts Forum, particularly as it showcases disability arts whilst working to support and develop artists' work and provide training.

Much dialogue and knowledge sharing takes place on social networking sites (in dedicated groups and between individuals) and sites dedicated to disability arts and culture, including Disability Arts Online (www.disabilityartsonline.org.uk), Shape Arts (www.shapearts.org.uk), Disability Culture (www.disabilityculture.org/) and Disability Culture Watch (www.similinton.com/blog).

It is plain to see that there is a plurality of ideas in disability arts and that threads of disability culture are now discernible in wider culture. It can also be argued that our demands to be heard have had a considerable impact on mainstream culture, regardless of our continued marginalisation in dominant culture. Contrary to Galvin's claims, disability arts has been very successful at communicating hybridised identities without 'lionising' a fixed disabled identity (Galvin, 2003: 685), despite obvious political commitments. Examples abound. Many individual performers and organisations take mimetic approaches to disability in that they deliberately represent stereotypical views of disability in order to call them into question, a strategy which has often been adopted by the presenters of BBC's Ouch! podcast, where disabled people are often the (knowing) butt of jokes made by the (disabled) presenters.

Comedians such as Laurence Clark can also be seen to have strong affinities with the social model, yet, through the medium of comedy, he also conveys serious ideas about the barriers facing disabled people in everyday life. Like many other performers, he often turns the focus around to challenge common-sense attitudes towards disabled people, shedding light on the interests served by dominant stereotypes of disability. These strategies are epitomised in a series of clips (available on YouTube), which feature passers-by ignoring his pleas to deter them from putting money in his collection bucket for causes such as 'Kill the puppies'. At the same time, the avant-garde elements of disability art flourish, exemplified in the practices of Live Art as a 'space where the disenfranchised and disembodied can be visible and vocal' 'using their own bodies and site and material' (Keidan and Mitchell, 2012: 6–7).

Far from imposing a unified view of disability on us, disability arts has revealed a diversity of viewpoints and an appetite to learn from others, even where disagreements are rife. Alongside a multitude of accounts of impairment, disability and other dimensions of our lives, disability art also focuses on discourses of normality, revealing fundamental aspects of disabling culture.

Like Darke (2003), I remain concerned about particular aspects of contemporary disability arts and culture, not least in the dilution of more radical disability aesthetics, the impacts of an increasingly individualistic and potentially exclusionary framework on collectivist principles, and the neglect and potential absence of class- and ethnicity-based perspectives on disability. These latter concerns are of particular importance in the current climate of cuts to disabled people's income (Wood, 2012). For me, the issues of class and collective identity are of paramount importance to disability culture, in terms of social composition, cultural content and cultural capital.

Cuts in income and services for many disabled people have considerable implications for membership of a disability culture, exacerbating barriers to participation. Minimal collective opportunities for artistic expression and the erosion of disabled people's rights and incomes limit the opportunities for disabled people to enter their chosen field, or even become aware that it is possible for them to do so. The conditions of possibility for widespread participation in disability culture will remain scant or non-existent in the harsh and limiting circumstances which poverty, struggle and poor education force upon so many of us. Nonetheless, the resurgence of a radical disability culture is evident in the activities and associated networks of groups such as Disabled People Against the Cuts.

Conclusion

Disability culture and disability arts are important to us in many ways: as a distinct artistic aesthetic and a base for political and self-identifications, they enhance opportunities for disabled people's creativity and provide a sense of community, furthering our struggles for justice and human rights. They provide us with essential cultural knowledge that is needed for us all to live with and understand each other.

I do not think that disability arts and culture should be providing all the answers. Ideally, our efforts to answer the types of question Galvin raised should involve us all and be tempered with the knowledge that current political and material conditions exclude many disabled people further from these 'luxury' debates on culture and the collective struggle, in efforts to survive the changing culture of disablement.

Disability arts continues to raise the right kind of questions, however uncomfortable or unanswerable these might be – the ones that make us think. As my good friend Deborah Williams once said to me, explaining her own arts practice and position on disability culture: 'This is my position as a disabled person. First, always remember I'm disabled. Now, always forget I'm a disabled person.'

Acknowledgement

Massive thanks to Dr Steve Millett.

References

Barker, C. (2011) *Cultural Studies: Theory and Practice*. London: SAGE.

Bourdieu, P. and Passeron, J-C. (1973) 'Cultural reproduction and social reproduction', in R.K. Brown (ed.), *Knowledge, Education and Social Change*. London: Tavistock. pp. 71–112.

Briant, E., Philo, P. and Watson, N. (2011) *How the Newspapers are Reporting Disability*. Glasgow: Strathclyde Centre for Disability Research and Glasgow Media Unit, University of Glasgow.

Darke, P. (2003) 'Now I know why disability art is drowning in the river Lethe (with thanks to Pierre Bourdieu)', in N. Watson and S. Riddell (eds), *Disability, Culture and Identity*. Harlow: Pearson. pp. 131–42.

Darke, P. (undated) Introductory Essay on Normality Theory. Available at: www.outside-centre.com/darke/mycv/writings/normtheo/normtheo.html [accessed 8/07/12].

Finkelstein, V. (1987) 'Disabled people and our culture development', *Disability Arts in London*, 8 June.

Galvin, R. (2003) 'The paradox of disability culture: the need to combine versus the imperative to let go', *Disability & Society*, 18 (5): 675–90.

Geertz, C. (1973) *The Interpretation of Cultures*. New York: Basic Books.

Hambrook, C. (2008) Editorial: Arts Council Cuts. Available at: www.disabilityartsonline.org.uk/colins_blog?filter_by_month_added=2008-01&item=340&itemoffset=1 [accessed 1/07/12].

Keidan, L. and Mitchell, C.J. (eds) (2012) *Access all Areas: Live Art and Disability*. London: Live Art Development Agency.

Masefield, P. (2006) *Strength: Broadsides from Disability on the Arts*. Stoke-on-Trent: Trentham Books.

McDermott, R. and Varenne, H. (1995) 'Culture as disability', *Anthropology and Education Quarterly*, 26: 323–48.

Paterson, K. and Hughes, B. (1999) 'Disability studies and phenomenology: the carnal politics of everyday life', *Disability & Society*, 14 (5): 597–610.

Peters, S. (2000) 'Is there a disability culture? A syncretisation of three possible world views', *Disability & Society*, 15 (4): 583–602.

Storey, J. (2012) *Cultural Theory and Popular Culture: An Introduction*. London: Longman.

Sutherland, A. (1997) 'Disability arts, disability politics', in A. Pointon with C. Davies (eds), *Framed: Interrogating Disability in the Media*. London: British Film Institute. p. 159.

Vasey, V. (2004) 'Disability: the story so far', in J. Swain, S. French, C. Barnes and C. Thomas (eds), *Disabling Barriers – Enabling Environments* (2nd edn). London: SAGE. pp. 106–10.

Williams, R. (1983) *Keywords: A Vocabulary of Culture and Society*. New York: New York University Press.

Wood, C. (2012) 'For disabled people the worst is yet to come', *Destination Unknown: Summer 2012*. London: Demos. Available at: www.demos.co.uk/publications/destination unknown summer2012

17

'Race', Ethnicity and Disability

Yasmin Hussain

There continues to be severe disadvantages for disabled people from ethnic minorities. The disability movement has quite rightly focused on equality issues facing all disabled people. Debates within the disabled people's movement regarding inequalities based on 'race' emerged in the 1990s; however, these now need to be reconsidered in the light of more recent social and political developments. The 'War on Terror', for example, has highlighted the importance of state interventions in the everyday lives of ethnic minorities, and debates have moved on from a concern with race and ethnic identity to questions of religious identity. Discussions of ethnicity are increasingly concerned with religious differences.

These are the issues that now need to inform debates around racism, ethnicity and disability. South Asian groups have been the focus of much research, but Afro-Caribbean and other ethnic minority groups have been relatively neglected. Whilst highlighting religious discrimination for South Asians, we must not forget the continuing powerful forces of racialisation and racism affecting Afro-Caribbeans. The field of disability studies and ethnicity has also shown a tendency to focus on young people and children (Hussain, 2005; Islam, 2008) rather than adults who may have developed impairments later in life. How do older ethnic minority people, who have developed impairments and may be cared for by partners or younger family members, experience disability?

Furthermore, new diasporic communities have emerged due to new waves of migration since the 1990s. This has rendered the ethnic mosaic of the UK more complex so that some now speak of ethnic 'super-diversity' (Vertovec, 2007). New ethnic minority communities have emerged in recent years due to migration from Eastern Europe, sub-Saharan Africa and Latin America. These communities will doubtless have their own issues and concerns that will have implications for disabled people from these communities about which we know little or nothing.

This chapter is divided into three sections that sketch the development of research and thinking about racism, ethnicity and disability over the past 20 years, which are then followed by a section on new challenges. These new challenges reflect changes in public discourse about racism, ethnicity and religion, the emergence of new migrant groups and the ageing of established migrant populations. The key question here is how far the field of studies of racism, ethnicity and disability has responded to these challenges.

Disability, 'race' and racism

The focus of the first contributions to debates on ethnicity and disability was on the limits of the social model, the role of racism and studies of impairment seen as specific to particular racialised groups (e.g. Ahmad, 2000). This work was important in bringing a critical inter-sectionist perspective to disability studies. Many of the earliest contributions were of a theoretical agenda-setting kind. Very soon, empirical studies began challenging the stereotyped assumptions about ethnic minority communities 'looking after their own' as a reason for their lower levels of use of state services and benefits.

This early work criticised the social model as being Eurocentric (Ahmad, 2000). The challenge of diversity within the disabled people's movement was seen by some as risking fragmentation. Initial attempts to incorporate black people into the disabled people's movement were seen as either simply encompassing them under the challenge to the medical model and ignoring racism, or simply adding racism to produce a model of 'double oppression' (Stuart, 1993). In contrast, Stuart (1993) suggested that we needed to think in terms of simultaneous oppression where black disabled people were excluded from both white society and able-bodied black people. Disability thus had to be examined both in terms of relationships within ethnic minority communities, as well as in terms of ethnic minorities' relationships to wider society (Ahmad, 2000). This first wave of work criticised the tendency of some professionals to see impairments and long-term ill health amongst ethnic minorities as a product of their cultural practices, lifestyles and food. This was seen as a form of cultural racism that overlooked the socio-economic factors and racial exclusion affecting these groups (Stuart, 1993). Ethnic minority disabled people were seen as facing issues such as their citizenship status, language affecting access to services, professional stereotypes of 'caring ethnic minority families', etc. that were beyond the experiences of white disabled people (Ahmad, 2000).

Studies of the role of ethnicity and racism within the sphere of disability studies have since grown steadily. The academic debate initially centred on making visible the invisible ethnic minority experience within the disability sphere. This research created an awareness of the lack of knowledge of how minority ethnic disabled people and their families make sense of disability and caring. For instance, Chamba et al. (1999) raised the issue of inequalities within policy and practice, whereas the work of Katbamna et al. (2000) discussed service delivery and its failure to acknowledge the perspectives and needs of minority ethnic disabled people and their families. Atkin and Rollings (1996) also raised the question of how racist myths and stereotypes were dominating service support systems.

This work up to around 2000 both criticised the social model of disability for failing to take account of the distinctive positions and experiences of ethnic minorities
and criticised service providers for their failure to address the distinctive needs of
ethnic minority disabled people. From this point on, researchers began to expand on
and develop these concerns both theoretically and empirically.

Disability, ethnicity and cultural identity

Later contributions (e.g. Molloy et al., 2003; Hussain, 2005; Islam, 2008) were
influenced by the 'new ethnicities' paradigm which highlighted the contingent and
negotiated nature of ethnic identities (Hall, 1990), as well as by debates about
cultural hybridity (Modood et al., 1994). Rather than attempting to unify all ethnic
minority disabled people under the category of 'black' as was seen in the work of
Stuart (1993) and Banton and Singh (2004), these approaches increasingly recognised influential critiques of political blackness (Modood, 1994) and the lived
realities of different ethnicities and racisms. They thus brought insights from developments in ethnicity and racism studies to the examination of ethnic identities,
racism and disability.

Disability has a powerful influence on how ethnic minority disabled people
make sense of their lives, and it also mediates their sense of ethnic, religious and
cultural identity (Hussain et al., 2002). This suggests that a redefinition of the
social model is in order, and it was argued that impairment can only be made
sense of within the context of an individual's personal, cultural and social diversity. All disabled people, not just those from ethnic minorities, hold multiple identities, some more strongly than others, and many become particularly salient in
certain circumstances or places. In short, both disabled identities and ethnic identities are contingent, contextual and negotiated, their relevance and significance
being dependent upon the context and social relations involved (Islam, 2008). All
those with an impairment potentially have a number of identity claims – ethnic,
cultural, religious, age and disability among them. Disability has an important
influence on the way these people make sense of their lives, but this does not
occur within a vacuum. As many have argued more generally, identity can only be
made sense of as a complex and dynamic interplay between agency and structure
(see Archer, 2007).

The identification of disabled people from ethnic minorities also demonstrates
hybridity, a variety of historical, international, ideological and political factors
influencing their sense of self-hood and relationship with others. This is a distinctive product of their experience as members of a diasporic community of migrants
to the UK. Hybridity is not simply a question of choosing between, for example, a
'western' or 'Asian' identity – rather, it is a fusion of them (Modood et al., 1994).
Disabled people from ethnic minorities find a synthetic space to express a variety
of different and competing identity claims. These identifications, far from being dis-
connected from questions of power, structural inequalities and history, are closely

related to people assuming or rejecting identity claims. Both racism and disablism have important influences on the sense of identity of ethnic minority disabled people. Research into second-generation young disabled people from ethnic minority communities over the past decade or so has offered no support for notions of singular identities or of hierarchies of identification (Hussain et al., 2002). This work showed that the identity claims of disabled young people were negotiated and contingent, allowing freedoms within contexts in which ethnicity, religion, gender, social status, racism, generational relations and the meaning of being disabled were important considerations (Hussain, 2005; Islam, 2008).

Much of this research focused upon South Asian ethnic minority groups, so it is difficult to judge how far generalisations from them also apply to other ethnic minority groups such as Afro-Caribbeans or more recently formed diasporic communities. Furthermore, in reflecting the concerns of the time, there tended to be a focus on the experiences of younger second-generation disabled people from ethnic minorities, such as Islam's (2008) work which focused upon Bangladeshi and Pakistani young people, and Hussain et al.'s (2002) which focused upon South Asian families with disabled children. As a result, this has left us with a limited understanding of the positioning and experiences of the older first generation of migrants, who may only now as they get older be developing impairments, and may have very different experiences of the issues identified amongst the second generation.

Disability, ethnicity and religious practices

Like other aspects of racism and ethnicity studies since 2001, research has increasingly focused on religious difference, especially around Islam and Muslims (e.g. Ismail et al., 2005; Rhodes et al., 2008; Pestana, 2011). Much of this work has focused not so much on identity as on how ethnic minority people draw upon their religious beliefs to explain disability – especially amongst children. Religion seems to have become a new sign for ethnic minority as there seems to be less attention paid to the role of the religious beliefs of Christians in making sense of disability. It is almost as if only ethnic minorities had religious beliefs about disability. In particular, South Asian communities are thought of in this way, but what of Protestants from West Africa and Catholics from Eastern Europe or Latin America? There is a huge gap in our knowledge of how religion and ethnicity intersect in relation to disability in the present era of ethnic super-diversity.

Over time, it seems that the area has lost much of its critical edge, with the themes of racism giving way to concerns with identity and the religious practices of particular ethnic groups. This is despite increased concerns about Islamophobia (Abbas, 2005; Poole and Richardson, 2006; Hussain and Bagguley, 2012). Developments in this area have so far had a limited impact on the field of disability studies and ethnicity.

For example, Johnston and Lordon (2012) recently showed how discrimination against Muslims in England since 2001 has led to deterioration in their health in terms of stress, blood pressure, body mass index and cholesterol levels. These are all factors that have a propensity to produce impairments, especially later in life. This kind of work points to a key limitation of much current work on race, ethnicity and disability, which tends to take impairments for granted and explore the disabling, ethnic and religious constructions around them. What this work ignores is how disability, racism and Islamophobia may be intertwining processes over the life course.

New challenges

The first significant new challenge for researchers on disability and ethnicity arises from the ageing of established migrant populations from areas such as the Indian sub-continent and the West Indies. Many of the studies of ethnicity and disability have tended to focus on these communities, but less often on the relationship between ageing, emergent impairments and disability.

There is also a challenge in taking account of super-diversity (Vertovec, 2007) – more specifically, the development of new migrant groups from Eastern Europe, Latin America and various African countries – in relation to studies of ethnicity, racism and disability. As racialised groups, these are amongst the most excluded from the formal economy and state services. They are often small communities, not always settled in areas known for having ethnic minority populations, and have diverse socio-economic characteristics and legal statuses.

Disability studies is no different from most of UK social science by continuing to work on the assumption that ethnic minority means South Asian or West Indian in background and has been slow to catch up with this new super-diverse reality. Disabled people, like the rest of the UK population, are now characterised by a diversity of ethnic origins, community languages, religions and transnational connections. What is the situation in new migrant communities such as those from Eastern Europe and Latin America? In terms of official reports and routinely collected statistics, these are often 'invisible' ethnic minorities, so that even in terms of official data sources we have a very limited knowledge of the extent and patterns of disabilities among these groups.

Debates since 2001 in racism and ethnicity studies have reflected the impact of state responses to the riots of 2001 (Bagguley and Hussain, 2008) and terrorism (McGhee, 2008; Hussain and Bagguley, 2012). Themes of citizenship, Britishness, community cohesion and the failure of multiculturalism have become central issues. How far have studies of disability dealing with ethnic differences and racism taken on board the implications of these developments and debates? Multiculturalism in particular has been seen to be both a source of crisis and in crisis (McGhee, 2008).

Multiculturalism in the UK in relation to state agencies at least offered the hope of service delivery becoming more specific to the self-defined needs of disabled people from ethnic minorities, as was suggested by the findings of some early research with ethnic minority disabled people (Chamba et al., 1999; Katbamna et al., 2000). However, the reaction against multiculturalism, even amongst those such as the chair of the Equalities Commission who might be expected to be more supportive, might be seen as a threat to the creation of services more appropriate to the cultural and religious needs of ethnic minority disabled people. Some of the implications of the community cohesion agenda went against the idea of culturally and religiously sensitive or specific services, recommending that state funding should not be available for distinct ethnic minority communities (Community Cohesion Independent Review Team, 2001: 38). These kinds of developments, alongside attempts to link community project funding to gathering 'intelligence' on 'terrorists', have made many wary of state funding for voluntary organisations, especially in relation to Muslims and ethnic minority communities (Husband and Alam, 2011). How far disabled people and their carers might have been disadvantaged by these developments is unknown.

Conclusion

This chapter has provided an overview of developments in disability studies relating to ethnicity and racism. It has outlined the black critique in the 1990s of the disabled people's movement's unacknowledged assumptions of whiteness and its exclusionary effects. The social model of disability at that time was seen as Eurocentric, based on the white experience of disability overlooking the distinctive experiences and concerns of disabled ethnic minority people.

From this critique emerged a range of studies that sought to give voice to and analyse the experiences of ethnic minority disabled people. A key theme was the 'systemic failure' of state services to deal with the specific issues facing disabled people from ethnic minorities relating to cultural differences, religion and language. Reflecting wider intellectual developments, there was an increased concern with questions of identity, and studies increasingly recognised the complex and contingent character of identity for disabled ethnic minority people. More recently, research has focused more on how specific communities make sense of disability and how their cultural and religious accounts of disability may conflict with the medicalised accounts of the professionals they encounter.

However, there remain significant gaps in studies of ethnicity and disability, such as the experiences of the now older first-generation migrants who may have acquired impairments in later life. Many studies amongst established diasporic communities have tended to neglect Afro-Caribbeans who it is often assumed are more integrated into white society than some, despite continued racism. Finally, there is the challenge of understanding disability in an ethnically 'super-diverse' Britain with many new diasporic communities that have migrated here from many different parts of the globe.

References

Abbas, T. (2005) *Muslim Britain: Communities Under Pressure*. London: Zed Books.

Ahmad, W.I.U. (2000) *Ethnicity, Disability and Chronic Illness*. Buckingham: Open University Press.

Archer, M. (2007) *Making Our Way through the World: Human Reflexivity and Social Mobility*. Cambridge: Cambridge University Press.

Atkin, K. and Rollings, J. (1996) 'Looking after their own? Family care giving among Asian and Afro-Caribbean communities', in W.I.U. Ahmad and K. Atkin (eds), *'Race' and Community Care*. Buckingham: Open University Press. pp. 111–17.

Bagguley, P. and Hussain, Y. (2008) *Riotous Citizens: Ethnic Conflict in Multicultural Britain*. Aldershot: Ashgate.

Banton, M. and Singh, G. (2004) '"Race", disability and oppression', in J. Swain, S. French, C. Barnes and C. Thomas (eds), *Disabling Barriers – Enabling Environments* (2nd edn). London: SAGE. pp. 111–18.

Chamba, R., Hirst, M., Lawton, D., Ahmad, W. and Beresford, B. (1999) *Expert Voices: A National Survey of Minority Ethnic Parents Caring for a Severely Disabled Child*. Bristol: Policy Press.

Community Cohesion Independent Review Team (2001) *Community Cohesion: A Report of the Independent Review Team* (the Cantle Report). London: Home Office.

Hall, S. (1990) 'Cultural identity and diaspora', in J. Rutherford (ed.), *Identity: Community, Culture, Difference*. London: Lawrence and Wishart. pp. 222–37.

Husband, C. and Alam, Y. (2011) *Social Cohesion and Counter-Terrorism: A Policy Contradiction?* Bristol: Policy Press.

Hussain, Y. (2005) 'South Asian disabled women: negotiating identities', *The Sociological Review*, 53 (3): 522–38.

Hussain, Y. and Bagguley, P. (2012) 'Securitised citizens: Islamophobia, racism and the 7/7 London bombings', *The Sociological Review*, 60 (4): 715–34.

Hussain, Y., Atkin, K. and Ahmad, W. (2002) *South Asian Disabled Young People and Their Families*. Bristol: Policy Press.

Islam, Z. (2008) 'Negotiating identities: the lives of Pakistani and Bangladeshi young disabled people', *Disability & Society*, 23 (1): 41–52.

Ismail, H., Wright, J., Rhodes, P. and Smalll, N. (2005) 'Religious beliefs about causes and treatment of epilepsy', *British Journal of General Practice*, 55 (510): 26–31.

Johnston, D.W. and Lordon, G. (2012) 'Discrimination makes me sick! An examination of the discrimination–health relationship', *Journal of Health Economics*, 31: 99–11.

Katbamna, S., Bhakta, P. and Parker, G. (2000) 'Perceptions of disability and care giving relationships among South Asian Communities', in W.I.U. Ahmad (ed.), *Ethnicity, Disability and Chronic Illness*. Buckingham: Open University Press. pp. 12–27.

McGhee, D. (2008) *The End of Multiculturalism? Terrorism, Integration and Human Rights*. London: Open University Press.

Modood, T. (1994) 'Political blackness and British Asians', *Sociology*, 28 (4): 859–76.

Modood, T., Beishon, S. and Virdee, S. (1994) *Changing Ethnic Identities*. London: Policy Studies Institute.

Molloy, D., Knight, T. and Woodfield, K. (2003) *Diversity in Disability: Exploring the Interactions between Disability, Ethnicity, Age, Gender and Sexuality*. London: Department of Work and Pensions.

Pestana, C. (2011) 'A qualitative exploration of the life experiences of adults diagnosed with mild learning disabilities from minority ethnic communities', *Tizard Learning Disability Review*, 16 (5): 6–13.

Poole, E. and Richardson, J.E. (2006) *Muslims and the News Media*. London: IB Taurus.

Rhodes, P.J., Small, N., Ismail, H. and Wright, J.P. (2008) 'What really annoys me is people take it like it's a disability: epilepsy, disability and identity among people of Pakistani origin in the UK', *Ethnicity and Health*, 13 (1): 1–21.

Stuart, O. (1993) 'Double oppression: an appropriate starting-point?', in J. Swain, V. Finkelstein, S. French and M. Oliver (eds), *Disabling Barriers – Enabling Environments*. London: SAGE, in association with the Open University. pp. 93–100.

Vertovec, S. (2007) 'Super-diversity and its implications', *Ethnic and Racial Studies*, 30 (6): 1024–54.

18

Who is Disabled? Exploring the Scope of the Social Model of Disability

Dan Goodley

Introduction

Heightened debate is a sign of a political and intellectual movement's maturity. Major points of contention occur in disability studies, within and across the areas of academia and activism. A consistent area of debate relates to the explanatory powers of the social model of disability in accounting for the disabling experiences of *all* disabled people. In this chapter, I will argue that the social model of disability holds potential for the inclusion of *all* disabled people and disabled activists because it provides a 'sitpoint' from which to develop social, cultural and political responses to disablism. I will briefly examine key assumptions within British disability studies that have provided the impetus for the production of a social model of disability. In doing so, I will tease out – and challenge – some critiques, that are often made in relation to the social model, which have been used to point to the model's exclusionary nature. Then, I will consider the self-advocacy of people with learning difficulties and demonstrate how their activism and theorising contribute to social theories of disability – particularly interpretivist conceptions of 'impairment' as they are embedded in *storying the self* – thus opening up disability studies to be more inclusive.

Who is disabled in social model literature?

As with working-class, feminist, sexuality and critical 'race' movements, key moments can be identified in the origination of concepts and claims that gave rise to the formulation of the British disability movement's 'big idea' (Hasler, 1993): the social model of disability. By rendering disability as something outside of the impaired individual, this model has supported disabled activists and their allies in setting their sites on those disabling conditions of contemporary British life that need to be changed. Yet, questions still remain about the representative nature of this model. It is possible to identify a number of key criticisms that have been made by those whom Barnes (1998) and Roulstone et al. (2012) call 'second-wave' writers in disability studies.

Overly materialist

Corker and Shakespeare (2002) note that much of the associated key anti-theses of the social model of disability have adopted a Marxist or Gramscian stance, permitting disability studies scholars to theorise and change the material conditions of disablement (e.g. Abberley, 1987; Barnes, 1990, 1991, 1998; Finkelstein, 1981; Oliver, 1990, 1996). But what about those cultural artefacts that have more resonance for certain disabled people? For example, the very definition of 'learning difficulties' is crucially tied to cultural and professional forms of knowledge. For some observers, a materialist stance is theoretically unfit to deal with the more elusive discursive and culturally formulated meanings of cognitive impairments. In some cases, this has led critics to shun the social model of disability in favour of other social, cultural and minority models of disability (see Goodley, 2011 and Watson et al., 2012 for overviews of these approaches).

A Cartesian split of impairment/disability

A consequence of domineering materialist analyses has been the under-theorised biological body. While both Oliver (1990) and Abberley (1987) provide materialist accounts of capitalism's construction of 'mobility' and 'injured bodies' respectively, impairment-as-biological tends to remain theoretically untroubled. Hughes and Paterson (1997), Corker and French (1998), and Goodley (2001) argue that a materialist epistemology renders 'bodies' and 'minds' as static, unchanging phenomena: leaving impairment in medicalised realms of knowledge. A Cartesian distinction fails to accommodate some groups of disabled people precisely because their impairments need to be viewed socio-culturally and historically rather than in material and medical terms (Corker, 1999; Tremain, 2002). For others, the Cartesian split ignores the realities and predicaments of impairment (Shakespeare, 2006).

Impaired bodies only

A major political endeavour of the social model of disability is encapsulated in the rejection of categorising disabled people on the basis of 'impairment-specific' groupings (Oliver, 1996). The last 40 years of UK disability politics has concerned itself with

challenging impairment specificity and situating analysis in terms of common problems of disablement (Campbell and Oliver, 1996; Oliver, 1990). However, a call for
commonality may priviledge certain 'impairment-specific' concerns. Corker observes
in discussion with Thomas (Corker and Shakespeare, 2002: 29) that the dominance
of materialist and modernist thinking in disability studies is at risk of privileging the
body: 'My worry is that if the social theorization of impairment ... is conducted within
the modernist dichotomies of mind/body, individual/society and structure/culture ...
there will, given the current privileging of the physicality of the body in sociology and
related disciplines, be a sidelining of cognitive impairments accompanied by the erasure
of sensory impairments' (Corker and Shakespeare, 2002: 29).

Who is disabled in the social model? Following the critiques given above, one
would think only people with physical impairments (Ferguson, 1987). However, I
would suggest that a number of existing 'truths' should be kept in mind when interrogating the inclusive/exclusionary nature of the social model. First, it is important
to acknowledge that the social model is a product of its origins in British disability
politics. Whether or not this model is appropriate to other international contexts
is for others in these contexts to decide (Grech, 2009). Second, we are talking here
about a social model not a social theory (Oliver, 1996). While 'first-wave' writers
have promoted Marxist dialectical materialist accounts and Gramscian usages of
hegemony, these theoretical choices start from the *epistemological* stance of the
social model (Goodley, 2001). A model has no explanatory power but instead directs
us to theorise disability and concomitant phenomena such as 'impairment', 'exclusion' and 'activism'. Third, to borrow Thomas's (1999) phrase, 'social modellists'
have consistently made connections with a whole host of oppressions, including
race (Stuart, 1993), gender (Morris, 1991, 1996), class (Oliver, 1990), age (Zarb and
Oliver, 1993), childhood (Priestley et al., 1999) and sexuality (Shakespeare et al.,
1996). The social model has engaged with diversity. I find it helpful to keep four key
assumptions in mind:

- Disability studies continues to theoretically develop in ways that can and should
  encompass the experiences and ambitions of all disabled people.
- The social model is one philosophical and political stance from which a whole
  host of social theories and forms of activism can and should be developed.
- Disability studies is an arena in which social theories of disability and impairment
  can be developed to promote the inclusion of disabled people in mainstream life
  and the social model is one – *not the only one* – strong approach in this arena.
- Disability studies should seek to theorise and challenge disablism, which I think
  is usefully defined by Thomas (2007: 73) 'as a form of social oppression involving
  the social imposition of restrictions of activity on people with impairments and
  the socially engendered undermining of their psycho-emotional well being'.

In the remainder of this chapter, I will suggest that the social model of disability has
the potential to initiate the conception of an all-embracing arena for disabled people.
But, in order to demonstrate this inclusivity, it is necessary for social modellists to
widen their view of disability activism and disability theory to include the personal

and political actions of a whole host of disabled activists and to take seriously the experiences and views of disabled people whose voices may not be the loudest or strongest in the field.

People with learning difficulties are disabled: Storying impairment

British disability studies has become increasingly engaged with the lifeworlds of people with the label of learning difficulties (Stalker, 2012). More importantly, people so-labelled have much to offer social theories of disability and impairment. Indeed, within the wider arena of British disability politics, we can identify contributions by representative organisations of people with learning difficulties: particularly the self-advocacy movement. Members of this movement have had representation on the British Council of Disabled People (see Campbell and Oliver, 1996), contributed to discussions and formation of recent policy (e.g. the DoH 2001 White Paper *Valuing People*) and produced a whole host of literature which demands that service providers and professionals attend to the needs and ambitions of people with learning difficulties. Against this climate of activism, the movement boasts its own 'organic intellectuals' (Oliver, 1990). Members of self-advocacy groups are absorbed in debates that social modellists and disability studies can and should engage with. One example is the way in which self-advocacy groups have critically revisited notions of 'impairment' through their critiques of the label of 'learning difficulties'. In what I will term the project of *storying the self*, self-advocacy groups have contributed to an *interpretivist* model of disability and impairment (Atkinson and Williams, 1990; Bogdan and Taylor, 1976, 1982; Ferguson and Ferguson, 1995; Ferguson et al., 1992; Langness and Levine, 1986; Skrtic, 1995). Interestingly, North American formations of disability studies boast a long history of working alongside people with learning difficulties in promoting positive social change (see, for example, the University of Syracuse's Center on Human Policy). A key aim has been developing an interpretivist approach that conceives of disability as the product of voluntaristic individuals who are engaged in the creation of identities and the negotiation of roles. Such an epistemological stance recognises the disabling aspects of the world but approaches them through turning to the experiences, stories, interactions, scripts and social roles of non-disabled people. It is possible to view some of the activities of the British self-advocacy movement as contributing to this stance.

The self-advocacy movement has understandably been concerned with reappraising the very labels that have been foisted on them. Following Gillman et al. (1997), while physically impaired activists have celebrated 'bodily difference', self-advocacy groups have been engaged in a very different project: challenging the very label of 'learning difficulties' which constantly threatens to undermine notions of humanity. When self-advocacy groups name themselves 'People First' and promote slogans such as 'Label jars not people', they are suggesting that behind labels reside competence, humanity and voluntaristic personhood. Moreover, it is typical to see the use of oral history by members of self-advocacy groups in demonstrating their human worth. An example of this is offered by the following extract from the life story of the British self-advocate Joyce Kershaw:

> Two staff [in the Day Centre] would stand and say which row could go for dinner. But they used to eat their dinner in a little room. So I asked the boss if I could have a word with him. He said, 'Yes, what's the matter?' So I said, 'Aren't we good enough to eat with?' and he said, 'Yes, why?' I said, 'Well, it doesn't seem so – the staff eat in a little room of their own'. So he said he'd see what they'd say at the meeting. Then I asked him, 'Can we call the staff by the first name?' He said, 'Why don't you ask them?' So I did. Some said yes and some said no. Those who said no I said, 'Well, call me Mrs Kershaw'. (cited in Goodley, 2000: 93)

Kershaw's account articulates the very formations of difference between professional staff and centre 'user'. Note too how the story captures Kershaw voluntarily (but also as a reaction to the cultural context) challenging the practices around her that situate people with learning difficulties as different beings. In another extract from her story, Joyce reflects upon the label of learning difficulties: '"Learning disabilities" – I don't like that, disability makes you believe that we are in wheel chairs and we can't do anything for ourselves, when we can. We've got jobs now, we've got paid jobs' (cited in Goodley, 2000: 124).

This view suggests that impairment labels are open to interpretation and understood in relation to lived experiences. 'Who is disabled' in this sense depends on how identities, roles and labels are negotiated and constructed. For Joyce, certain labels and identities do not fit with her overarching aim to point out that learning difficulties do not amount to an 'insurmountable pathology'. The roles she identifies as crucial to her identity as an adult human being are not adequately captured by the label of learning disabilities. Some writers of disability studies have suggested that a turn to the personal, subjective, micro-level analysis – so characteristic of interpretivism – threatens to water down the potency of the social model:

> Writers like Jenny Morris have elevated the importance of personal psychological experience in understanding disability. Such work encouraged a shift away from thinking about the real world. Finding insight in the experiences of discrimination is just a return to the old case file approach to oppression, dressed up in social model jargon. (Finkelstein, 1996: 31)

Similarly, Barnes (1998) states that most of this writing represents either 'sentimental biography' or else a preoccupation with the medical and practical details of a particular condition (Hunt, 1966). Far from impairment being simply a personal experience (Oliver, 1996), stories about the construction of 'impairment' demonstrate how individuals are involved in the public creation of identities and the negotiation of roles that may exclude or empower: surely a key concern for the social model of disability and other approaches in disability studies.

Conclusion

Disability studies has the potential to be for *all* disabled people. Often, theoretical and political debate offers a view of disability studies as a fragmented arena. But the main aim of the social model of disability was always to understand and change disabling socio-political and cultural practices. I would suggest that the social model remains, at least for many in British disability studies, a 'sitpoint' (to borrow from Garland Thomson, 2005) from which to develop a social understanding of disability and disablism. However, like any vantage point we may scan the horizon in various ways, inspect different aspects and choose to traverse some roads over others. While the traditional social modellists push for a strict materialist analysis, we should not shy away from the possibilities offered by other social theories and forms of activism. While it is fruitful to remain committed to the socio-political tenets of the social model, we should not be precious about one particular theoretical orientation, if we are to hold on to the belief that disability studies matters to all disabled people and the world needs to be changed for the better. Perhaps then, disability studies – including the social modellists – will provide an arena from which to engage with a host of transformative and politicised theories and practices.

References

Abberley, P. (1987) 'The concept of oppression and the development of a social theory of disability', *Disability, Handicap and Society*, 2 (1): 5–21. [Reproduced in Barton, L. and Oliver, M. (1997) *Disability Studies: Past, Present and Future*. Leeds: The Disability Press.]

Atkinson, D. and Williams, F. (eds) (1990) *'Know Me as I Am': An Anthology of Prose, Poetry and Art by People with Learning Difficulties*. London: Hodder & Stoughton, in association with The Open University and Mencap.

Barnes, C. (1990) *The Cabbage Syndrome: The Social Construction of Dependence*. London: The Falmer Press.

Barnes, C. (1991) *Disabled People in Britain and Discrimination: A Case for Anti-Discrimination Legislation*. London: Hurst & Co. and University of Calgary Press, in association with the British Council of Organisations of Disabled People.

Barnes, C. (1998) 'The social model of disability: a sociological phenomenon ignored by sociologists?', in T. Shakespeare (ed.), *The Disability Reader: Social Science Perspectives*. London: Cassell. pp. 65–78.

Bogdan, R. and Taylor, S. (1976) 'The judged not the judges: an insider's view of mental retardation', *American Psychologist*, 31: 47–52.

Bogdan, R. and Taylor, S. (1982) *Inside Out: The Social Meaning of Mental Retardation*. Toronto: University of Toronto Press.

Campbell, J. and Oliver, M. (1996) *Disability Politics: Understanding Our Past, Changing Our Future*. London: Routledge.

Corker, M. (1999) 'Differences, conflations and foundations: the limits to "accurate" theoretical representation of disabled people's experiences', *Disability & Society*, 14 (5): 627–42.

Corker, M. and French, S. (1998) (eds) *Disability Discourse*. Buckingham: Open University Press.

Corker, M. and Shakespeare, T. (2002) (eds) *Disability/Postmodernity: Embodying Disability Theory*. London: Continuum.

Department of Health (DoH) (2001) *Valuing People: A New Strategy for Learning Disability in the 21st Century*. London: The Stationery Office.

Ferguson, P. (1987) 'The social construction of mental retardation', *Social Policy*, 18: 51–6.

Ferguson, P.M. and Ferguson, D.L. (1995) 'The interpretivist view of special education and disability: the value of telling stories', in T.M. Skrtic (ed.), *Disability and Democracy: Reconstructing (Special) Education for Postmodernity*. New York: Teachers College Press. pp. 104–21.

Ferguson, P.M., Ferguson, D.L. and Taylor, S.J. (eds) (1992) *Interpreting Disability: A Qualitative Reader*. New York: Teachers College Press.

Finkelstein, V. (1981) 'To deny or not to deny disabilities', in A. Brechin, P. Liddiard and J. Swain (eds) *Handicap in a Social World*. London: Hodder and Stoughton.

Finkelstein, V. (1996) 'Outside, "inside out"', *Coalition*, April, 30–6.

Garland Thomson, R. (2005) 'Feminist disability studies', *Signs: Journal of Women in Culture and Society*, 30 (2): 1557–87.

Gillman, M., Swain, J. and Heyman, B. (1997) 'Life history or "care history": the objectification of people with learning difficulties through the tyranny of professional discourses', *Disability & Society*, 12 (5): 675–94.

Goodley, D. (2000) *Self-advocacy in the Lives of People with Learning Difficulties: The Politics of Resilience*. Buckingham: Open University Press.

Goodley, D. (2001) '"Learning difficulties", the social model of disability and impairment: challenging epistemologies', *Disability & Society*, 16 (2): 207–31.

Goodley, D. (2011) *Disability Studies: An Interdisciplinary Introduction*. London: SAGE.

Grech, S. (2009) 'Disability, poverty and development: critical reflections on the majority world debate', *Disability & Society*, 24 (6): 771–84.

Hasler, F. (1993) 'Developments in the disabled people's movement', in J. Swain, V. Finkelstein, S. French and M. Oliver (eds), *Disabling Barriers – Enabling Environments*. London: SAGE, in association with the Open University. pp. 226–32.

Hughes, B. and Paterson, K. (1997) 'The social model of disability and the disappearing body: toward a sociology of impairment', *Disability & Society*, 12 (2): 325–40.

Hunt, P. (1966) *Stigma: The Experience of Disability*. London: Geoffrey Chapman.

Langness, L.L. and Levine, H.G. (eds) (1986) *Culture and Retardation*. Kluwer: D. Reidel.

Morris, J. (1991) *Pride Against Prejudice: Transforming Attitudes to Disability*. London: The Women's Press.

Morris, J. (ed.) (1996) *Encounters with Strangers*: *Feminism and Disability*. London: The Women's Press.

Oliver, M. (1990) *The Politics of Disablement*. Basingstoke: Macmillan.

Oliver, M. (1996) *Understanding Disability: From Theory to Practice*. London: Macmillan.

Priestley, M., Corker, M. and Watson, N. (1999) 'Unfinished business: disabled children and disability identity', *Disability Studies Quarterly*, 19 (2): 87–98.

Roulstone, A., Thomas, C. and Watson, N. (2012) 'The changing terrain of disability studies', in N. Watson, A. Roulstone and C. Thomas (eds), *Routledge Handbook of Disability Studies*. London: Routledge. pp. 3–11.

Shakespeare, T. (2006) *Disability Rights and Wrongs*. London: Routledge.

Shakespeare, T., Gillespie-Sells, K. and Davies, D. (1996) *The Sexual Politics of Disability*. London: Cassells.

Skrtic, (T.M.) (ed.) (1995) *Disability and Democracy: Reconstructing (Special) Education for Postmodernity*. New York: Teachers College Press. pp. 104–21.

Stalker, K. (2012) 'Theorising the position of people with learning difficulties within disability studies: progress and pitfalls', in N.Watson, A. Roulstone and C. Thomas (eds), *Routledge Handbook of Disability Studies*. London: Routledge. pp. 122–35.

Stuart, O. (1993) 'Double oppression: an appropriate starting point?', in J. Swain, V. Finkelstein, S. French and M. Oliver (eds), *Disabling Barriers – Enabling Environments*. London: SAGE, in association with the Open University. pp. 27–33.

Thomas, C. (1999) *Female Forms: Experiencing and Understanding Disability*. Buckingham: Open University Press.

Thomas, C. (2007) *Sociologies of Disability, 'Impairment', and Chronic Illness: Ideas in Disability Studies and Medical Sociology*. London: Palgrave.

Tremain, S. (2002) 'On the subject of impairment', in M. Corker and T. Shakespeare (eds), *Disability/Postmodernity: Embodying Disability Theory*. London: Continuum.

Watson, N., Roulstone, A. and Thomas, C. (eds) (2012) *Routledge Handbook of Disability Studies*. London: Routledge.

Zarb, G. and Oliver, M. (1993) *Ageing with a Disability: What Do They Expect After All These Years?* Greenwich: University of Greenwich.

19

Disabled People, Disability and Sexuality

Selina Bonnie

Over the past decade since this chapter was first written, a lot more disabled people have begun to enjoy the exploration and expression of their diverse sexualities; however, many continue to live in enforced celibacy. In 1992, disabled American activist and author Anne Finger said: 'Sexuality is often the source of our deepest oppression; it is also often the source of our deepest pain' (Finger, cited in Shakespeare et al., 1996: 5). Twenty years on, this statement is still relevant.

Historically, disabled people's sexuality and sexual expression have been oppressed in a variety of ways. Disabled children and teenagers have been dressed in androgynous or babyish clothes, denied relationships and sex education, and placed in segregated 'special' institutions and schools. Disabled adults have been infantilised, sterilised, prohibited from engaging in sexual activity and marriage, and excluded from mainstream social and leisure activities.

In this chapter, I have not set out to engage in an in-depth analysis of issues for disabled people and sexuality. I have written this chapter to provide an introduction to, and a synopsis of, the key issues facing disabled people's sexual expression.

Societal notions of disabled people's sexuality

According to the 2011 World Report on Disability, 'The prejudice that people with disabilities are asexual or else that they should have their sexuality and fertility controlled is widespread' (WHO, 2011: 78).

Society at best finds the thought of a disabled person being sexual repulsive and at worst presumes they are asexual. As a disabled person, this can be a very difficult reality to acknowledge; however, I would rather someone considered the thought of me being sexually active as distasteful rather than believing me to be asexual. At least with the former, they are thinking of me as a sexual being.

Traditionally, there has been a taboo around discussing sexuality, sexual expression and related matters in public. Sex was for marriage and procreation, and disabled people were not expected or encouraged to experience either. However, expressing one's sexuality is not just about sex. Sexuality is about relationships, confidence, self-image and choice making. It is about how we as human beings see and express our personalities and ourselves. Morris states: 'Many people assume we are asexual, often in order to hide embarrassment about the seemingly incongruous idea that such "abnormal" people can have "normal" feelings and relationships' (1989: 80).

Disabled people are rarely portrayed in the media, film, television and advertising industries. When they are, it is often as the recipients of charity, as evil characters in movies or as tragic victims of illness or accident. They are rarely, if ever, portrayed in relationships, as sexually active or as parents (see Chapter 16):

There is an unspoken taboo about relationships and disabled people. Disabled people's sexual and emotional needs are rarely included in any discussion or representation in everyday life, whether this is in the papers and magazines we read, or the movies we watch. This reinforces the public's attitudes and expectations towards disabled people as seeing them as 'sick and sexless' rather than participating in full sexual and family relationships. (Lamb and Layzell, cited in Shakespeare et al., 1996: 11)

Disabled people are guilty of this denial of disabled sexuality too. Historically, access to transport, housing, personal assistance, employment, education and getting rights enshrined in legislation have been the priority for the disabled people's movement. Social, leisure, relationships and sexual expression have been pushed way down the list of priorities, while disabled people have fought to achieve a better quality of life and independent living. However, as Liz Crow says, 'you can't get closer to the essence of self or more "people-living-alongside-people" than sexuality, can you?' (cited in Shakespeare, 2000: 165).

Sexual citizenship

Later in this chapter, I will highlight what I consider to be some key international debates. However, an issue, fundamental to sexuality and disability, which is currently being explored and advocated, is sexual citizenship.

With sexual citizenship comes not only the right to be free from harm and exploitation but also the right to satisfaction and pleasure. Enshrining these rights in international policy, such as the UN Convention on the Rights of Persons with Disabilities (Articles 23 and 25, 2006) and the UN Standard Rules for the Equalisation of Opportunities for Persons with Disabilities (Rule 9.2, 1994), strengthens disabled people's claim to sexual citizenship.

According to Plummer, sexual citizenship includes three main aspects: control, access and socially grounded choices (1995: 151). Given the historic widespread exclusion and oppression of disabled people, attaining sexual citizenship is fraught with barriers and complications. However, 'the right to full sexual citizenship has been taken up by disability activists who campaign for sexuality and sexual fulfilment as a human right' (Sanders, 2007: 450).

I believe that any discussion of disabled people and sexual citizenship would not be complete without addressing issues of identity: 'Citizenship is inseparable from identity, and sexuality is central to identity' (Bell and Binnie, 2000: 67). There are many events in life that influence how we identify with the world around us. A variety of elements fuse to form our identity, and our sexuality is an important part of that. People express their sexuality in many ways. How we dress, if we wear make-up, how confident we are in life and in the relationships we form are all influenced by, and in turn influence, the development and expression of our sexuality. Having the opportunity to express our sexuality in turn enables us to define our identity.

Sexual expression is just one part of the overall communication of our self. For many people, it is a very important part of their life and of how they express their identity. To travel throughout life constantly being denied this type of expression has had a detrimental effect on many disabled people's sense of self-worth. Disabled people are sexual beings and as such 'sexual wellness is important for overall health' (Browne and Russell, 2005: 375).

Access to expression

Disabled people encounter many barriers with regard to expressing their sexuality. I believe that the most significant of these are attitudinal, environmental and informational barriers.

Attitudinal barriers

Shakespeare et al. (1996) equated admitting that one is a disabled person with coming out as a gay, lesbian or bisexual person. I believe that even disabled people who are heterosexual go through a process of 'coming out' when they start to assert their sexuality.

'Parental overprotection is often cited as a hindrance to social experiences' (Baker and Donelly, 2001: 74). Parents tend to overprotect their disabled offspring, treating them as unable and childlike. We are not comfortable thinking of children as sexual beings and so parents find it difficult to see disabled offspring as such, and not as vulnerable, impressionable people at risk. Therefore, it is often a source of great concern for parents when their disabled offspring start to assert and express their sexuality.

It is particularly dangerous to deny that disabled children or young people are sexual beings. There have been numerous cases where young disabled people have been raped or sexually abused and did not know that what was happening was wrong, or what they should do, because sexuality had not been discussed with them, and they had not received any 'stay safe' education. People who are born with impairments or who become disabled in childhood become accustomed to numerous adults, such as parents or the medical profession, examining them. This can make it very difficult for young people to distinguish between appropriate and abusive behaviour from adults. By educating these young disabled people, I believe they would be more empowered to protect themselves.

Traditionally, disabled people have had to endure medical intervention to 'correct deformed bodies' or to 'cure' them and make them 'normal'. Furthermore, the combination of intrusive medical intervention, society's obsession with the perfect body and our denial as sexual beings has led to many disabled people having very low self-esteem, a lack of confidence and poor body image.

Historically, the arts have been a very influential vehicle used by groups to challenge oppression. In recent years, myths of disabled asexuality have been challenged through TV documentaries such as Laurence Clark's *We Won't Drop the Baby* (BBC, 2012), and through live shows such as *The Freak and the Showgirl* (a comic cabaret of striptease, freakshow and song) by Mat Fraser and Julie Atlas Muz.

Photography constitutes another form of media representation which has produced some powerful positive imaging of the sexuality of disabled people. *Intimate Encounters: Disability and Sexuality* is a touring exhibition featuring 30 photographic images, and essays by 40 people who collaborated with photographer Belinda Mason-Lovering, to express their desires, needs, love and affection, reflecting the diversity of their experiences of disability through the lens. *Bodies of Difference* is a collection of images which constitute part of an ongoing series of work by photographer Ashley Savage, documenting disability, sexuality and physical 'otherness'.

Environmental and informational barriers

Many never consider that disabled people also require access to services related to sexual expression, such as adult shops, family planning clinics and places where relationships are formed or services are provided. This widespread denial of sexual rights greatly impacts on disabled people's quality of life.

People with sensory impairments find it particularly difficult to interact and flirt in social places such as nightclubs, as the noise and lighting levels make it very difficult to be understood. Sencity (created by the Skyway Foundation in The Netherlands) is a unique multi-sensory touring event. Lyrics and music are translated through sign language, and a vibration floor responds to the frequency of the music. Aroma jockeys also convey the emotion of the music through scent.

Informational barriers can be as disempowering as environmental barriers. Access to information is absolutely vital, particularly in today's information-driven world, and the area of sexual expression should be no exception. In a truly inclusive society, adult literature would be available in accessible formats, adult websites would be built using the principles of universal design, and family planning services would have information both in accessible formats and appropriate to the needs of disabled people. Unfortunately, we do not live in a truly inclusive society and so disabled people's informational needs, and wants, are often unmet.

Examples of useful or inclusive publications which I have found include a chart on reproductive and contraceptive considerations for disabled women (Campion, 1990: 8–9); a Braille edition of *Playboy* (excludes pictorial representations); and *Tactile Minds*, a pornographic book complete with explicit text and raised pictures of naked men and women, created by Canadian artist Lisa Murphy.

The bigger picture: Current debates and issues

Thus far in this chapter, I have explored the issue of sexual citizenship and I have outlined key barriers facing disabled people's sexual expression. It is important to stress though that it is not all bad news. Over the past 20 years, many disabled academics have researched and written about issues of disabled people and sexuality (Morris, 1989; Shakespeare et al., 1996; Shakespeare, 2000; Tepper, 2000; Sanders, 2007, 2010). Disabled performers including Mat Fraser and Penny Pepper, who project quite strong sexualities, have broken into mainstream media. Organisations such as TLC Trust (www.tlc-trust.org.uk) and SHADA (Sexual Health and Disability Alliance) (www.shada.org.uk) in the UK and Touching Base in Australia have continued to develop. The 2005 'Time to talk sex survey' by UK magazine *Disability Now* was the first of its kind to collect data on the sexual experiences and needs of disabled people, and the growth of the worldwide independent living movement has led to a greater number of disabled people living their lives as they choose.

There are a number of debates taking place in varying degrees across the globe that are worth addressing. When considering these debates, it is important to remember that today, in the twenty-first century, these options for sexual expression are still only empowering a very small percentage of disabled people to explore their sexuality and realise their sexual desires.

Devotees are non-disabled men who are specifically aroused by women who have physical impairments. The devotee community is particularly big in the USA, with numerous websites and magazines devoted to the issue. This has also been referred to as 'disability fetishism' (Kafer, 2000) and has been the subject of much debate both in non-disabled society and the disabled people's movement. There are many facets to this debate. Two key strands have been that many people find devotees and their organisations distasteful and believe them to be exploitative of disabled women. However, many disabled women who are active in this community find the experience of being desired and considered more beautiful than non-disabled women extremely empowering. They believe that society should not judge the devotees as deviant just because they explicitly desire disabled women.

Surrogates are trained professionals who engage in sexual activity with people who experience difficulties with sexual expression/performance. The surrogate works at the direction of the therapist who prescribes this form of 'therapy' for the client. This system operates worldwide and is regulated by the Code of Ethics (2002) and Code of Practice from the World Association for Sexology (WAS) and the International Professional Surrogates Association (IPSA). These services are not specifically designed for disabled people, but do provide a supported opportunity to explore sexual expression. I would not advocate for disabled people to use this type of service because I believe it medicalises sexual needs. However, if a person is sexually oppressed and frustrated and has the opportunity to access such a service, I consider surrogacy a far healthier option than remaining frustrated!

Facilitated sexual expression in the independent living movement is based on the premise that if a disabled person (leader) who uses the services of a personal assistant (PA) has a significant impairment and needs their PA to assist them with tasks such as eating or washing, and so on, isn't it likely that they may also need assistance with sexual activity? (Shakespeare et al., 1996). Facilitation has many implications, particularly legal and ethical. For example, if a PA solicits a prostitute for their leader or assists with masturbation, they could find themselves in a very difficult legal situation. Equally, the leader, as an employer, could be breaching employment law and public policy by bringing facilitated sexual expression into the working relationship (Browne and Russell, 2005).

Apart from within the leader/PA realm, there are other examples of facilitation around the globe: many brothels in Australia have been made wheelchair-accessible; people with significant impairments are travelling to The Netherlands and Denmark to access sex services (established by the state specifically for disabled people); and a Swiss organisation is offering erotic massage to its members.

Disabled people experience many barriers in relation to becoming parents. Historically, there has been a worldwide practice of forcibly sterilising disabled people (particularly women) and administering contraceptives without consent (WHO, 2011). Although women with learning difficulties have been particularly targeted by these eugenic practices, people with physical, mental or sensory impairments have also endured such abuses.

Many parents with significant impairments have either had their children taken from them by social services or had the threat of this happening because they have been deemed unable to look after their children. For the majority of these parents, the provision of adequate personal assistance and support services would have enabled them to care for their children (Rush and Li, 2012) (see Chapter 16).

Conclusion

Disabled people are, and have a basic human right to be, sexual beings. A lot of disabled people lack the level of support they need to achieve the level of sexual expression to which they aspire. The barriers which disabled people face must be broken down and there are a number of key ways in which this should happen:

- Physical access and access to information in its broadest sense must be addressed. In today's modern age, there is no excuse for inaccessible design and service provision.
- Staff in day centres and rehabilitation settings should be trained to appropriately respond to disabled people's sexual expression.
- Peer support services for disabled people and support services for parents and guardians specifically in the area of sexuality and sexual expression should be adequately resourced.
- Appropriate relationships and sex education should be available to disabled people in schools and centres.
- Discourses of sexual citizenship that respect the sexual rights of all disabled people and not just male heterosexuals should be promoted.

Despite the difficulties, issues and implications explored in this chapter, it is important to remember that a lot of disabled people have fulfilling and fun sex lives, are enjoying long-term relationships, are becoming parents, and so on.

In 2000, Tepper stated:

Pleasure is an affirmation of life ... Pleasure adds meaning to our lives. Sexual pleasure is particularly powerful in making one feel alive. It is an antidote to pain, both physical and emotional ... Sexual pleasure can enhance an intimate relationship. It can add a sense of connectedness to the world or to each other. (2000: 288)

Sexual pleasure and freedom are truly powerful, and in the twenty-first century not one disabled person should have to endure enforced celibacy. Ultimately, my vision for the future is that society will accept us as sexual beings. This must start by disabled people taking ownership of the issue, debating it and engaging in personal and collective growth and development around their sexual expression and sexuality, and ultimately by claiming their rights as sexual citizens.

References

Baker, K. and Donelly, M. (2001) 'The social experiences of children with disability and the influence of environment: a framework for intervention', *Disability & Society*, 16 (1): 71–85.

Bell, D. and Binnie, J. (2000) *The Sexual Citizen: Queer Politics and Beyond*. Cambridge: Polity.

Browne, J. and Russell, S. (2005) 'My home: your workplace: people with physical disability negotiate their sexual health without crossing professional boundaries', *Disability & Society*, 20 (4): 375–88.

Campion, M.J. (1990) 'Reproductive and contraceptive considerations for women with physical disabilities', in *The Baby Challenge*. London: Routledge.

Kafer, A. (2000) 'Amputated desire, resistant desire: female amputees in the devotee community', *Disability World*. Available at: http://mailman2.u.washington.edu/pipermail/amp-l/2001-April/006350.html [accessed 01/05/12].

Morris, J. (1989) *Able Lives: Women's Experiences of Paralysis*. London: The Women's Press.

Plummer, K. (1995) *Telling Sexual Stories: Power, Change and Social Worlds*. London: Routledge.

Rush, C. and Li, A. (2012) Disabled Couple Thrilled They'll Be Able to Keep Their Baby. Available at: www.thestar.com/printarticle/1173602 [accessed 16/05/12].

Sanders, T. (2007) 'The politics of sexual citizenship: commercial sex and disability', *Disability & Society*, 22 (5): 439–55.

Sanders, T. (2010) 'Sexual citizenship, commercial sex and the right to pleasure', in R. Shuttleworth and T. Sanders (eds), *Sex and Disability Politics, Identity and Access*. Leeds: The Disability Press. pp. 139–53.

Shakespeare, T. (2000) 'Disabled sexuality: towards rights and recognition', *Disability & Society*, 18 (3): 159–66.

Shakespeare, T., Gillespie-Sells, K. and Davies, D. (1996) *The Sexual Politics of Disability*. London: Cassell.

Tepper, M. (2000) 'Sexuality and disability: the missing discourse of pleasure', *Sexuality and Disability*, 18 (4): 283–90.

United Nations (UN) (1994) Rule 9 of 'UN Standard Rules for the Equalisation of Opportunities for Persons with Disabilities'. Available at: www.un.org/esa/socdev/enable/dissre00.htm [accessed 23/04/12].

United Nations (UN) (2006) Convention on the Rights of Persons with Disabilities (CRPD). Available at: www.un.org/disabilities/convention/conventionfull.shtml [accessed 23/04/12].

World Association for Sexology (WAS) and The International Professional Surrogates Association (IPSA) (2002) Code of Ethics and Code of Practice. Available at: http://surrogatetherapy.org and www.worldsexology.org [accessed 23/04/12].

World Health Organization (WHO) (2011) 'General Healthcare: Box 3.6', in *World Report on Disability*. Geneva: WHO Press.

Part 3
Controlling Lifestyles

20

Challenging Barriers and Enabling Inclusion: The Role of Families

Dawn Benson and Sarah Keyes

Introduction

There are many ways in which families which include a person with impairment experience social, environmental, attitudinal and structural barriers that limit meaningful inclusion in society (Oliver, 1996). In this chapter, focusing on our experience of the UK, we share experiences, perspectives and strategies of such families and provide insights into some of the often disabling encounters that families can have with people, places and systems. We argue that whilst certain barriers disable individuals with an impairment, and indeed in the process often disable other family members too, there are empowering examples of families which include people with impairments who, during the ordinary course of life, act as agents for change in a disabling society. We have found that it is through attitude-changing interactions within and beyond such families, that changes in environments and policy for enablement of families begin to occur.

Our families and research

Our developing thinking around the often under-researched and under-theorised area of families, disability and inclusion draws on a combination of personal and research involvement with disabled people and their families, including some auto-ethnographic material from Dawn's ongoing doctoral work (Benson, forthcoming). Dawn is mother and stepmother to seven children, four of whom have impairments. Growing up as a disabled child herself, she spent three years in a children's hospital school. Since 2000, she has worked as a researcher and lecturer in Disability Studies

and Inclusive Education, thinking about, and conducting enquiries with, families
that include people with impairments. Her doctoral research, which provides powerful insights for this chapter, focused on the experiences of families where clinical
negligence at or around the time of birth had resulted in a child having an acquired
brain injury, and enabled her to come into contact with many families beyond her
own immediate networks. Sarah has worked with disabled people and their families
since 2007, using inclusive approaches to research (Keyes, 2010). Sarah has also
experienced impairment within her immediate family. Thus, note that our work is
grounded in experience.

Conceptualising family and disability

The concept of family is very much determined and influenced by society as it is
subject to variation through economic, demographic, political and cultural influences which impact directly upon the nature of families (Newman and Grauerholz,
2002). The word 'family' will have a different meaning for each reader. According
to Newman and Grauerholz (2002: xviii), 'everyone has grown up in one type of
family or another'. This may be so, as even those who have not grown up within
a biological family or traditional family structure will have lived in some way with
other people whom they have come to regard as family (Moore et al., 1996;
McLaughlin, 2012).

Sociological issues concerning family life have been well documented (for example, Newman and Grauerholz, 2002 and Chambers, 2012), particularly in relation
to marginalisation in terms of gender (Featherstone, 2004; Finch, 2007), economy
(Roosa et al., 2005), race (Fomby et al., 2010) and class (Gerstel, 2011). However, as
with other trends in sociological studies, disability and family has, and continues to
be in the main, neglected from debates, albeit with some limited representation from
social policy researchers such as Beresford (2008) and Burchardt and Zaidi (2008).
Nevertheless, since the emergence of disability studies as a specific branch of sociology (Thomas, 2007), an emerging discourse has evolved around differing aspects
of family life and disability, particularly recognising the achievements of families
which include disabled people in breaking down the barriers which threaten their
opportunity and desire to construct their own (usually ordinary) lifestyles (Ryan and
Runswick-Cole, 2008).

In contemporary Britain, flexible understandings are required of what a family is
and what ties people together. No longer does the notion of family relate necessarily
to kinship ties such as parents, offspring, siblings, grandparent lines, and so on. Many
families, such as Dawn's own, are newly constituted or re-constituted or even differently constituted on a day-to-day basis. A family including people with impairments
can be constituted from people with no biological link (Henretta et al., 2011). There
is evidence that families which include people who have an impairment are more
likely to experience family break-up and poverty than others (Beresford, 2008). But
there are also families with several disabled members who will not experience either

family break-up or poverty. One of the central messages of this chapter is that we must take great care not to stereotype and make assumptions about what families, which include disabled members, are like.

When exploring families and disability, researchers have tended to focus on specific topic areas, for example:

- Discrimination encountered by people with learning difficulties as they strive to engage in sexual relationships and to be parents (Booth et al., 2005).
- Discrimination experienced by parents of children with impairments as they try to maintain employment whilst meeting the inflexible appointment demands of statutory sector service providers (Magadi, 2010).
- Limited access to services, equipment and in particular suitable housing for families (Moore, 2004; Hemingway, 2011).
- Attitudinal barriers faced by families when they encounter others whose assumptions contrast with the way in which they value family members (Goodley and Runswick-Cole, 2010).
- Narratives from children and younger people (Robinson and Stalker, 2008) and older people (Bowers et al., 2011) describing the barriers that they encounter when professionals find it difficult to communicate with them.
- Lack of recognition of the support that family members provide for each other (Connors and Stalker, 2003: Mitchell, 2007; McLaughlin, 2012).

All of this work comprises useful reading for those interested in disability and family life. Yet we have found that when families that include disabled people tell their stories, they actually provide much more complex and tangled accounts of family life than research has typically conveyed.

Dismantling assumptions about families

When families with disabled members tell their stories, these are mostly linked, in our experience, to the ordinary events or activities that make up family life, such as support for going to school or work, relationships with health or social care systems, engagement with professionals, arranging and being included in ordinary leisure activities such as going on holiday or shopping – and any one of these topics crosses seamlessly into the next. We suggest that it is limiting to envisage the life of families which include people with impairments as neatly bounded into compartmentalised arenas of topic-related family life. The life of all families is complex and interwoven, and relationships within families and the role that individuals play can rarely be second-guessed. When considering these matters, we return to a realisation that it is attitudes towards families with disabled members that mostly shape our experience and which, in turn, shape the environments we live in and the policies we live by. It is also the attitudes of others that families including disabled people often influence deeply. Often, for example, families shape the attitudes of professionals through what Dawn describes as a 'gentle dance of enlightenment', whereby shifts in attitude alter environments and services, not only for the person doing the dance but also for those that follow them. In this regard, families which include a person who has an impairment can act as trailblazers.

Families pioneering enabling attitudes

When talking about and seeking to challenge disabling attitudes, some families consider their own attitude towards each other as acting like a mirror, reflecting to the outside world how they would like to be viewed. Dawn describes her world as a 'goldfish bowl, where lots of people think they have a right to stare in'. In this case then, she provides them with as many positive images of family life with disabled members as possible – i.e. 'look and learn'. At another level, negotiation around the values and ideas that professionals have about 'desired outcomes' for a family, for example, can be challenging and require families to be steadfast in their demonstration of alternative possibilities and viewpoints (Mason, 2008). There may be games to play, as one father highlights:

> you have to at least appear to consider what [service providers] are wanting otherwise you get labeled as difficult, so I always feel that I am playing a game where I give and take but eventually all I want is to be able to raise my daughter the way I want to – just like everyone who hasn't got a disabled kid. We get there in the end but I had to learn to be diplomatic. (cited in Benson, forthcoming)

Overcoming differing perspectives can be at the core of professional and family agendas and requires open communication to alter not only personal attitudes but also to shift professional agendas and goals (French and Swain, 2008). When talking about families 'having a coordinating role for the multi-disciplinary team that is involved with a disabled person', as is common in the UK at the time of writing, Dawn notes that different professional roles are subject to often conflicting agendas and even specific words are understood in different ways:

> We have to set an example to others about what we believe our disabled children are capable of. When professionals talk about 'independence' they are often talking about being able to go to the toilet or feed themselves. When I talk of 'independence' I am talking about the kids choosing who will wipe their bottom or cut their pizza up, when it should happen and how it should be done. It's about empowerment not some form of rehabilitation. (Benson, forthcoming)

Doing ordinary things as a family, like going to school, going on holiday, finding suitable housing, having a trip to the cinema, etc. often means negotiating attitudes within systems (Goodley and Runswick-Cole, 2010). This can include interaction with professionals who, though themselves may be constrained by the same systems, can also exacerbate inequality through opportunity-limiting attitudes that often require families to expect delays and barriers (Evans, 2008). Dawn draws attention to the need for families to be proactive about what service providers will need rather than the other way around:

> we needed to get the finance approved for the support for a summer activity and we would have paid for it, but because of the system it could only be funded through the Local Authority (they didn't take private clients). We were into week four of the holidays before it was approved – but fortunately we had expected that to happen so went away in the first part of the holidays.

Similarly, when discussing provision for their disabled son, a family member who was supporting an older uncle shared his strategy for getting what he knew his uncle needed: 'experience has taught me that if he needed 10 hours of support I need to ask for 20 then I stand a chance of getting 10 but if I ask for 10 I'll only get 5' (cited in Benson, forthcoming).

As Dawn knows from experience, getting support is a contentious process often feeling akin to 'running a gauntlet'. Understanding what professionals are actually offering to do presents a disabling conundrum:

> Eventually on one occasion when I was too tired to check myself I asked the social worker what I could do for her and she replied that rather it was she who was there to support me. I told her that, if that was the case, what I needed was some time to have a bath and sleep – I was utterly exhausted. She took her pen and pad out and began to make notes and explain how difficult it would be to get daily help to relieve me for long enough to have a bath. She suggested that it would be a number of weeks until the service could start, if at all, and she couldn't promise anything so not to build my hopes up. I handed her the baby and said 'well let's not waste time chatting. I'll make better use of your time and have a bath now while you're here.' I will never forget her expression. I didn't get my bath in the end because there was no hot water, but enjoyed making the point and did get to clean my teeth. (cited in Benson, forthcoming)

Ryan and Runswick-Cole (2008) advocate the benefits of parents (mostly they refer to mothers) of disabled children as 'activists', working in partnership with professionals in developing suitable services. However, the impact of involvement as an activist must not be underestimated:

> I was chatting to one of the other mums who said she had talked to mums with older kids and how you have to keep banging the drum but sometimes the energy dries up and that's what I don't want to happen, I don't want the energy to dry up. (Benson, forthcoming)

On the subject of activism, Dawn recalls several incidences in which her family have pioneered the way to changing services through direct action:

> I took all the children to County Hall 'cos no-one would phone me back. We took a packed tea, intending to sit there until somebody came to talk to me. They threatened to call the Police if I didn't move. I told them that I would call the press. In the end, I had an amicable conversation with a Senior SEN Officer, that resulted in my son going to the school that he wanted to: a positive result. (Benson, forthcoming)

It is not only in situations with statutory sector services that parents become activists but also with mainstream services and commercial organisations. Similarly:

> once, after months of talks with the railway about my son needing hand rails at our local station, I threatened to take a drill and fit the rails myself. I told them that I would then call the police to tell them that I had violated railway property – then I would call the press. It worked. (Benson, forthcoming)

Policy and legislation can often be useful tools for the support of families with disabled members (Roulstone and Prideaux, 2012), though families often discover that policy and legislation offer little recourse if not all stakeholders understand them. Families wishing to take disabled children on holiday, for example, may find they are more familiar with their rights and entitlements than service providers:

> We take seven kids and PAs and sometimes friends to [Holiday Park] every year – sometimes twice a year – and whilst it's by no means ideal it is relatively accessible once you're there. However just about every time I would have the same arguments with them around accessible lodges. They never have enough and so when they run out they try to sell you the more expensive one that's accessible. And every time I would quote them chapter and verse of the DDA and last year the Equality Act. Recently I went through the Equality Commission for help and even they didn't understand the legislation so I spent weeks involved with the Equality Commission and the legal team for [Holiday Park] to basically make sure that they changed their training so that the Equality Commission were giving out the right information and [Holiday Park] were training their sales team. (Benson, forthcoming)

It is situations such as this that can force people whose families include someone who has an impairment to become 'pseudo-professionals' (Clavering et al., 2006) or to turn themselves into professionals (Cole, 1990). Some go on to work in areas that challenge disabling barriers, including, like ourselves, becoming disability studies academics whose interest and passion are rooted in personal experience of disability within our families. It is through acts of resistance within families such as those we have shared in this chapter that barriers to inclusion are broken down, both individually and collectively. A parent of a disabled child articulates the experiences we have drawn upon in this chapter: 'What you want out of life is to be an ordinary family with an extra ordinary situation' (cited in Benson, forthcoming).

References

Benson, D. (forthcoming) For the Record: Parents' Experience of Pursuing a Claim for Clinical Negligence. Unpublished PhD thesis, University of Northumbria.

Beresford, B. with Rhodes, D. (2008) *Housing and Disabled Children – Round-up: Reviewing the Evidence*. York: Joseph Rowntree Foundation.

Booth, T., Booth, W. and McConnell, D. (2005) 'The prevalence and outcomes of care proceedings involving parents with learning difficulties in the family courts', *Journal of Applied Research in Intellectual Disabilities*, 18: 7–17.

Bowers, H., Mordey, M., Runnicles, D., Barker, S., Thomas, N., Wilkins, A. (National Development Team for Inclusion) and Lockwood, S. and Catley, A. (Community Catalysts) (2011) *Not a One Way Street: Research into Older People's Experiences of Support Based on Mutuality and Reciprocity*. York: Joseph Rowntree Foundation.

Burchardt, T. and Zaidi, A. (2008) 'Disabled children, poverty and extra cost', in J. Strelitz and R. Lister (eds), *Why Money Matters: Family Income Poverty and Children's Lives*. London: Save the Children. pp. 26–33.

Chambers, D. (2012) *A Sociology of Family Life*. Cambridge: Polity.

Clavering, E., Goodley, D. and McLaughlin, J. (2006) Parents, Professionals and Disabled Babies: Identifying Enabling Care. Available at: www.leeds.ac.uk/disability-studies/archiveuk (accessed 14/08/12).

Cole, B. (1990) *Mothers' Teachers: Insights into Inclusion*. London: David Fulton.

Connors, C. and Stalker, K. (2003) *The Views and Experiences of Disabled Children and Their Siblings*. London: Jessica Kingsley.

Evans, C. (2008) 'In practice from the viewpoint of disabled people', in J. Swain and S. French (eds), *Disability on Equal Terms*. London: SAGE. pp. 177–83.

Featherstone, B. (2004) *Family Life and Family Support: A Feminist Analysis*. Basingstoke: Palgrave Macmillan.

Finch, J. (2007) 'Displaying families', *Sociology*, 41 (1): 65–81.

Fomby, P., Mollborn, S. and Sennott, C.A. (2010) 'Race/ethnic differences in effects of family instability on adolescents' risk', *Journal of Marriage & Family*, 72 (2): 234–53.

French, S. and Swain, J. (2008) 'On equal terms', in J. Swain and S. French (eds), *Disability on Equal Terms*. London: SAGE. pp. 129–41.

Gerstel, N. (2011) 'Rethinking families and community: the colour, class, and centrality of external kin ties', *Sociological Forum*, 26 (1): 1–20.

Goodley, D.A. and Runswick-Cole, K.A. (2010) 'Parents, disabled children and their allies', in L. Dell and S. Leverett (eds), *Working with Children and Young People: Co-constructing Practice*. London: Palgrave Macmillan. pp. 69–79.

Hemingway, L. (2011) *Disabled People and Housing: Choices, Opportunities and Barriers*. Bristol: Policy Press.

Henretta, J.C., Soldo, B.J. and Van Voorhis, M.F. (2011) 'Why do families differ? Children's care for an unmarried mother', *Journal of Marriage and Family*, 73 (2): 383–95.

Keyes, S. (2010) Mutual Support: An Exploration of Peer Support for People with Learning Difficulties. Unpublished PhD thesis, University of Northumbria.

Magadi, M. (2010) 'Risk factors for severe child poverty in the UK', *Journal of Social Policy*, 39 (2): 297–316.

Mason, M. (2008) Dear Parents. Available at: www.inclusive-solutions.com

McLaughlin, J. (2012) 'Understanding disabled families: replacing tales of burden with ties of interdependency', in N. Watson, A. Roulstone and C. Thomas (eds), *Routledge Handbook of Disability Studies*. Abingdon: Routledge. pp. 402–13.

Mitchell, W. (2007) 'The role of grandparents in intergenerational support for families with disabled children: a review of the literature', *Child and Family Social Work*, 12 (1): 94–101.

Moore, M. (2004) 'The death story of David Hope', in D. Goodley, R. Lawthom, M. Moore and P. Clough (eds), *Researching Life Stories*. London: Routledge Falmer. pp. 26–39.

Moore, M., Sixsmith, J. and Knowles, K. (eds) (1996) *Children's Reflections on Family Life*. London: Falmer.

Newman, D.M. and Grauerholz, E. (2002) *Sociology of Families*. London: SAGE.

Oliver, M. (1996) *Understanding Disability: From Theory to Practice*. Basingstoke: Palgrave Macmillan.

Robinson, C. and Stalker, K. (1998) 'Introduction', in C. Robinson and K. Stalker (eds) *Growing up with Disability*, London: Jessica Kingsley. pp. 7–12

Roosa, M.W., Deng, S., Nair, R.L. and Lockhart Burrell, G. (2005) 'Measures for studying poverty in family and child research', *Journal of Marriage & Family*, 67 (4): 971–88.

Roulstone, R. and Prideaux, S. (2012) *Understanding Disability Policy*. Bristol: Policy Press.

Ryan, S. and Runswick-Cole, K. (2008) 'Repositioning mothers: mothers, disabled children and disability studies', *Disability & Society*, 23 (3): 199–210.

Thomas, C. (2007) *Sociologies of Disability and Illness: Contested Ideas in Disability Studies and Medical Sociology*. Basingstoke: Palgrave Macmillan.

21

Disability and Childhood: A Journey Towards Inclusion

John M. Davis

Introduction

During the 1990s, academics argued that we did not know what disabled children/ young people thought about public services and that this ignorance fostered stereotypes that depicted disabled children as passive victims who were incapable of making life choices and unlikely to progress to independent adulthood (Alderson, 1993; Shakespeare and Watson, 1998; Middleton, 1999). Since the 1990s, many authors have promoted participation and inclusion as solutions to disabled children's life issues. This chapter considers the extent to which disabled children experience inclusive services that recognise their ability to act in powerful ways and contribute to improving their own lives.

Education

In the main, studies in the 1990s that asked disabled children about their educational experiences painted a bleak picture of segregation, bullying and inequality (Corker and Davis, 2000, 2002). In the 1990s, it was argued that negative images of disabled children, league tables and personal prejudice fostered segregation, prevented professionals from recognising disabled children's abilities and restricted their opportunities (Armstrong and Galloway, 1994; Clark et al., 1997; Kenworthy and Whittaker, 2000; Davis and Watson, 2001). It was argued that processes of educational segregation had a strong bearing on disabled children's social and cultural experiences, such as the ability to develop friends at home, play in local spaces and mix with a variety of children in school:

> I wanted to go to my local school but when we went to see it ma mum realised it wasn't accessible, then we had to go to other schools until we found one. When I got there I didn't know any one at all. (Davis and Hogan, 2002: 12)

A distinction was drawn between integration (simply being integrated into the same buildings) and inclusion (having an equitable level of social and academic experience – Booth and Ainscow, 2000). Such ideas were incorporated into educational policy and acts in the devolved nations that make up the UK (Davis and Smith, 2012). At the heart of these policies was the presumption that disabled children would experience inclusion and that the process of inclusion would be supported by timely integrated assessment/planning that took account of pupils'/parents' views.

These new approaches in education were based on the realisation that inclusion was a process that required education professionals to experience training on inclusive practice, to share inclusive strategies through peer exchange, to review the structure/balance of the curriculum, to involve pupils and parents in genuine participation and to collaborate with other professionals (Munn, 2000; Evans and Lunt, 2002; Connors and Stalker, 2003; Allan, 2010; Davis, 2011).

The social model of disability has heavily influenced policies on inclusion and multi-professional working in the new millennium and service providers are now encouraged to recognise the positive nature of disabled people's diverse abilities, experiences and identities (Swain and French, 2000; Davis, 2011).

> Our school is better than my old school at my old school children who used wheel chairs wasn't allowed to do PE. Here is better, we play indoor cricket, and smack it and go and the teachers are very good at including every one. The teachers don't believe I'm disabled they always encourage me to do PE. (Davis and Hogan, 2002: 19)

An affirmative model of disability has emerged that seeks to encourage us to support disabled people's individual and collective aspirations, asserted value and validity to impairment; celebrate difference; and recognise disabled people's right to have control of what is done to their bodies (Swain and French, 2000). This idea (that we should question concepts of power and control) has been found to be particularly relevant in health settings where health professionals have traditionally ignored disabled children's diverse identities, sought to remove difference and produced generic solutions based on the assumption that all disabled children are the same (Connors and Stalker, 2003).

Health

In the 1990s, it was argued that parents and disabled children were initiated by medical professionals into a medical culture which did not allow space for them to challenge traditional orthodoxy and that failed to recognise conflicts of interest between children, parents and professionals (Shakespeare and Watson, 1998; Avery, 1999). Adults were deemed 'experts' and children were assumed to be unable to put forward their own solutions to their own life problems. This very often led adults to make decisions about children's lives without consulting them, or assume that they knew what was best for children. Children's problems were identified and resolved by parents and/or professionals, and ownership of their own choices was taken away from them (Davis and Watson, 2000). For example, in health settings too much emphasis was placed on adults'/parents' views at the expense of understanding the things that disabled children and teenagers wanted to change about the services that they encountered. In the most part, this occurred because a perception existed that disabled children lacked competency and agency and therefore were unable to put forward their own views (Shakespeare and Watson, 1998; Corker and Davis, 2000; Davis and Watson, 2000; Bricher, 2001). This perception came about because much of the health-based literature concentrated on illustrating the things disabled children could not do (such as how they failed to achieve developmental 'norms') rather than on understanding their skills and abilities (Woodhead and Faulkner, 2000; Bricher, 2001).

In contrast, it was argued that disabled children were very capable of making their views known about complex medical decisions when adults made the effort to learn the different ways that they communicated (Alderson, 1993; Bricher, 2001). Indeed, disabled children were able to differentiate between professionals who treated them with respect and those who did not:

> My consultant always talks to me and he is really funny like he makes jokes – the last time I was in he said, 'aren't you married yet?' and he just makes you feel that you are being treated like a grown up. (Davis, 2003: 8)

During the 1990s, a number of writers highlighted children's and teenager's abilities to make decisions about their lives (Alderson, 1993) and encouraged us to engage with children's views of the appropriateness of medical treatments (Middleton, 1999; Bricher, 2001). Subsequently, participatory approaches to children's health were contrasted with processes that sought to make profits for health companies (Singh, 2002; Davis, 2006; Lloyd et al., 2006). It was argued that medical professionals should be clearer about the benefits of their practice, critique their own diagnostic techniques and balance the utility of any medical treatment with the possibility that it could lead to the social isolation of disabled children (Davis, 2006, 2011). Policies in health responded to this critique by attempting to enshrine ideas of inclusion, participation and emancipation into practice (the National Service Framework, Health for All, etc.), however practice still lags behind policy and we have some way to go before professionals will feel confident about enabling and supporting inclusion (Noble and Davis, forthcoming).

Social services and transition

Research has suggested that there needs to be greater synergy between adult and children's services, particularly where adult service users are disabled parents (Morris and Wates, 2006). Writing on transition from services in the 1990s tended to concentrate on the transition from school to adult services (e.g. training, employment, unemployment) or from home/care to independence (e.g. couple-dom, adult sexuality, marriage, parenthood; or financial independence) (Morris, 1999). There was great concern that 30–40 per cent of disabled people had great difficulty in establishing independence. This was particularly the case for young disabled people from ethnic minority groups. A number of studies suggested that black and Asian disabled people had to contend with individual racism and insti-tutional racism, particularly in service provision in school and later in the working environment (Ali et al., 2001). Many young people felt that service providers did not take their aspirations seriously:

> 'I went to an interview for a computer post but the guy just asked me if I could tell the time I told him where he could stuff his job – he thought I was thick.'

> 'I went to the careers people and all they wanted to do was talk about what benefits I would get. I don't wanna talk about benefits a want to talk about a job.'

> 'The careers advisers think you don't have the brain. I wanted to work for youth service, which a now do. But they didn't help.' (cited in Davis and Hogan, 2002: 25–6)

Morris (1999) found that most local authorities did not collect information on disabled young people's health and support aspirations, that services were not user-led and that assessments often led to children receiving the support the local authority could afford rather than the services they had been assessed as requiring. Of particular concern were the high costs of moving away from home (which contrasted with the low incomes that were available to young disabled people) and a lack of accessible accommodation:

> 'I tried to do the independent living thing but it takes about a year to go through whole process and they are still deciding what I will get. In the end it all comes down to money.' (Davis and Hogan, 2002: 27)

> 'I got this new flat but I didn't get a PA so ma mum comes round everyday – that's not independent living.' (2002: 27)

Poor staff training and a lack of supported living projects have often restricted disabled young people in developing independence (Morris, 1999). The independent living movement promoted disabled people's rights to choose how they wanted to organise services to support their full participation in society (Morris, 1993). Yet in the 1990s, there was very little recognition of the ability of disabled children and young people to plan, develop and evaluate their own services (Davis and Smith, 2012).

   In recent times, research and policy has focused on a range of moments of transi-tion, including from early years to primary school, from primary to secondary and between services (e.g. hospitals and schools – see Noble and Davis, forthcoming). Policies have encouraged service providers to begin planning processes as early as possible and to include disabled children in these processes. Yet, recent research has suggested that transition literature produced by service providers is inadequate, that disabled children are rarely supported to take lead roles in transition processes and that approaches to transition could much more creatively utilise the abilities of disabled children (Noble and Davis, forthcoming). Such research has drawn from strength-based (as opposed to deficit model) approaches to service planning and delivery that have sought to enable service users to develop their own local/community-based solutions to their life problems, and promoted social justice perspectives that suggest service users require different things including recognition, respect, resources, legal support, swift responses and cooperative power sharing (Dolan, 2008; Davis, 2011; Davis and Smith, 2012). For example, disabled young people can be frustrated at the time it takes for changes to take place in local services and at the way adult power hierarchies (such as in-fighting between different budget holders) inhibit processes of change (Davis, 2011).

Conclusion: Disabled children in the new millennium

This chapter does not tell the whole story of disabled children's/young people's lives. There is a danger that by concentrating too much on the social problems that disabled children encounter, the chapter reproduces the passive, negative, victim stereotypes associated by authors with medical model images of disabled children/young people. The 2004 version of this chapter (in the second edition of this book) argued that what was lacking was an understanding that disabled children/young people did not always have negative experiences of services and that they were human beings first before they were service users. As we came out of the 1990s into the new millennium, more effort was put into understanding disabled children's views and into seeking out positive examples of change and sharing them.

In the 1990s, it was argued that not all disabled children were the same – some encountered supportive professionals and organisations, some were resilient and many wished to affirm their abilities (Alderson, 1993; Swain, 1993). In the first decade of the new millennium, a number of projects demonstrated that disabled children were very capable of confronting negative stereotypes, oppressive structures and entrenched attitudes (Davis and Watson, 2001; Connors and Stalker, 2003). It was concluded that disabled children could be adept at promoting their rights and the rights of others in educational, health and social service settings. It was also recognised that they could collaborate with adults and other children/young people to confront oppressive practices and promote individual, cultural and systemic change.

In the 1990s, there were some examples of change being supported by peer networks (Ahmad and Atkin, 1996; Morris, 1999). But it was also argued that local authorities should be better at gathering and responding to disabled young people's wishes. In the first decade of the new millennium, service providers began to develop more inclusive opportunities around the arts, TV, horticulture, etc. For example, in Liverpool the Children's Fund directed a significant part of its budget to fund new projects that enabled disabled young people and adults not only to organise art projects that promoted change but also to take up posts in the local authority to improve access audit, accessible play and inclusive leisure opportunities (Davis, 2011). Such changes were supported by studies that demonstrated disabled children/young people were fully capable of organising a multitude of leisure activities and accounting for different disabled children's/young people's tastes (Davis and Watson, 2000).

As we look forward, many innovative approaches are now under threat from a lack of local and national funding. It is incumbent on us all to ensure that hard-fought-for gains are not lost and that we continue to support disabled children and young people in having their voices and opinions heard (locally and nationally) by those in powerful positions. The development of children's health, education and social services is an intensely political process that requires sensitivity, reflexivity and creativity on the part of professionals, along with recognition of the diverse aspirations of disabled children (Davis and Smith, 2012). It can be a deeply inclusive process if professionals are willing to question their assumptions about disabled children and enable these children to design their own solutions.

References

Ahmad, W. and Atkin, K. (eds) (1996) *'Race' and Community Care*. Buckingham: Open University Press.

Alderson, P. (1993) *Children's Consent to Surgery*. Buckingham: Open University Press.

Ali, Z., Fazil, A., Bywaters, P., Wallace, L. and Singh, G. (2001) 'Disability, ethnicity and childhood: a critical review of research', *Disability & Society*, 16 (7): 949–67.

Allan, J. (2010) 'Questions of inclusion in Scotland and Europe', *European Journal of Special Needs Education*, 25 (2): 199–208.

Armstrong, D. and Galloway, D. (1994) 'Special educational needs and problem behaviour; making policy in the classroom', in S. Riddell and S. Brown (eds), *Special Educational Needs Policy in the 90's: Warnock in the Market Place*. London: Routledge. pp. 175–95.

Avery, D. (1999) 'Talking "tragedy": identity issues in the parental story of disability', in M. Corker and S. French (eds), *Disability Discourse*. Buckingham: Open University Press. pp. 116–26.

Booth, T. and Ainscow, M. (2000) *The Index for Inclusion: Developing Learning and Participation in Schools*. Bristol: CSIE.

Bricher, G. (2001) 'If You Want to Know About it Just Ask': Exploring Disabled Teenagers' Experiences of Health and Health Care. Unpublished PhD thesis, University of South Australia.

Clark, C., Dyson, A., Millward, A. and Skidmore, D. (1997) *New Directions in Special Needs Schooling: Innovations in Mainstream Schools*. London: Cassell.

Connors, C. and Stalker, K. (2003) *The Views and Experiences of Disabled Children and Their Siblings*. London: Jessica Kingsley.

Corker, M. and Davis, J.M. (2000) 'Disabled children: (still) invisible under the law', in J. Cooper (ed.), *Law, Rights and Disability*. London: Jessica Kingsley. pp. 217–38.

Corker, M. and Davis, J.M. (2002) 'Portrait of Callum: the disabling of a childhood?', in R. Edwards (ed.), *Children, Home and School: Autonomy, Connection or Regulation*. London: Falmer. pp. 75–91.

Davis, J.M. (2003) *Alderhay Consultation of Children and Teenagers Who Experience Complex Impairments and Their Parents*. Liverpool: Royal Liverpool Children's NHS Trust and the Liverpool Bureau for Children and Young People.

Davis, J.M. (2006) 'Disability, childhood studies and the construction of medical discourses: questioning attention deficit hyperactivity disorder – a theoretical perspective', in G. Lloyd, J. Stead and D. Cohen (eds), *Critical New Perspectives on ADHD*. London: Taylor & Francis. pp. 45–65.

Davis, J.M. (2011) *Integrated Children's Services*. London: SAGE.

Davis, J.M. and Hogan, J. (2002) *Diversity and Difference: Consultation and Involvement of Disabled Children and Young People in Policy Planning and Development in Liverpool*. Liverpool: Liverpool Social Services/Liverpool Children's Fund/Liverpool Bureau for Children and Young People.

Davis, J.M. and Smith, M. (2012) *Working in Multiprofessional Contexts: A Practical Guide for Professionals in Children's Services*. London: SAGE.

Davis, J.M. and Watson, N. (2000) 'Disabled children's rights in every day life: problematising notions of competency and promoting self-empowerment', *International Journal of Children's Rights*, 8: 211–28.

Davis, J.M. and Watson, N. (2001) 'Where are the children's experiences? Analysing social and cultural exclusion in "special" and "mainstream" schools', *Disability and Society*, 16 (5): 671–87.

Davis, J. M., Ravenscroft, J., McNair, L., and Noble, A. (2012) *FIESTA: A Framework For European Collaborative Working, Inclusive Education and Transition: Analysing Concepts, Structures and Relationships*. Report From the Facilitating Inclusive Education and Supporting the Transition Agenda Project Funded By The Education, Audiovisual and Culture Executive Agency (EACEA) Of The European Commission Project Number 517748-LLP-1-2011-IE-COMENIUS-CNW.

Dolan, P. (2008) 'Social support, social justice and social capital: a tentative theoretical triad for community development', *Community Development*, 39 (1): 112–19.

Evans, J. and Lunt, I. (2002) 'Inclusive education: are there limits?', *European Journal of Special Needs Education*, 17 (1): 1–14.

Kenworthy, J. and Whittaker, J. (2000) 'Anything to declare? The struggle for inclusive education and children's rights', *Disability & Society*, 15 (2): 219–32.

Lloyd, G., Stead, J. and Cohen, D. (2006) *Critical New Perspectives on ADHD*. Abingdon: Routledge.

Middleton, L. (1999) *Disabled Children: Challenging Social Exclusion*. Oxford: Blackwell Science.

Morris, J. (1993) *Independent Lives*. London: Macmillan.

Morris, J. (1999) *Hurtling into a Void: Transition to Adulthood for Young Disabled People*. York: Joseph Rowntree Foundation.

Morris, J. and Wates, M. (2006) *Supporting Disabled Parents and Parents with Additional Support Needs: Adult Services Knowledge Review 11*. London: Social Care Institute for Excellence.

Munn, P. (2000) 'Can schools make Scotland a more inclusive society?', *Scottish Affairs*, 33: 116–31.

Shakespeare, T. and Watson, N. (1998) 'Theoretical perspectives on disabled childhood', in K. Stalker and L. Ward (eds), *Growing Up With Disability*. London: Jessica Kingsley. pp. 13–28.

Singh, I. (2002) 'Bad boys, good mothers and the "miracle" of Ritalin', *Science in Context*, 15 (4): 577–603.

Swain, J. (1993) 'Taught helplessness? Or a say for disabled students in schools', in J. Swain, V. Finkelstein, S. French and M. Oliver (eds), *Disabling Barriers – Enabling Environments*. London: SAGE, in association with the Open University. pp. 155–62.

Swain, J. and French, S. (2000) 'Towards an affirmation model of disability', *Disability & Society*, 15 (4): 569–82.

Woodhead, M. and Faulkner, D. (2000) 'Subjects, objects or participants? Dilemmas of psychological research with children', in P. Christensen and A. James (eds), *Research with Children*. London: Falmer. pp. 9–36.

22

Housing and Independent Living

Laura Hemingway

Housing plays a vital role in people's lives. It can be a place of independence, control and security, or (if inaccessible or unsuitable) it can restrict an individual and their family, leading to dependency and negatively affecting lifestyle choices. Although housing circumstances are significant elements of life for everybody, for disabled people they can be especially crucial in the achievement of independent living. In the early 1980s, disabled people identified appropriate housing as the third most important essential need for independent living (which, in logical order, lists information, peer counselling, housing, technical aids, personal assistance, transport and access) (Davis, 1990). Identifying the ways in which disabled people's housing options and pathways can be constrained, conditioned or assisted, is therefore fundamental to ensuring that housing needs are met and independent living is achieved.

This chapter draws on insights from the current author's research, which examined opportunities and barriers within housing for disabled people (Hemingway, 2011). The study focused especially on disabled people from the UK, but the findings are also applicable elsewhere. Investigating aspects of the lives of disabled people in a direct way was seen as fundamental to the study, and so experiences and opinions were gathered in disabled people's own words. Some of these are included below (names have been changed to ensure anonymity). These were complemented by accounts from disabled people's organisations, as well as mortgage and housing industry representatives to explore how barriers might work. The research uncovered the difficulties that disabled people encounter in relation to inaccessible environments, income and labour market position, and attitudes, assumptions and institutional practices, which negatively impact upon opportunities to access housing. These factors were found to affect not just housing choices and pathways, but also experiences, or meanings, of home.

Experiences of 'home'

The meaning attributed to 'home', or a person's ability to achieve a sense of 'home' within a dwelling, is central to considering housing needs. Whilst the home means different things to different people, it often symbolises more than a shelter or physical space. Various factors can impact on a person's ability to feel at home in a dwelling, and whilst literature on this subject is extensive, there is a tendency to focus on the role of relationships, tenure, work, responsibilities, time, place and culture. Although these can be applicable for both disabled and non-disabled people, certain variables may specifically apply for disabled people, including issues of accessibility, safety, professional intervention and inclusion in the community. The time spent in a dwelling can also be significant, for as Hamer (2005: 5) points out, 'low incomes, low rate of employment and lack of mobility mean [disabled people] are likely to spend more time at home than non-disabled people'. This is likely to also be the case for older people.

Inadequately designed housing which fails to reflect diversity in the human body and experience, can affect common associations with home such as security, safety and comfort (Heywood, 2005; French and Swain, 2006), or may reinforce feelings of 'otherness' (Burns, 2004). Several informants in the current author's research reported the importance of an accessible environment which facilitates independence in achieving a sense of home. As 'Ellen' explained:

> a property where I can be one hundred per cent independent is just about everything ... I suppose that's what having the home that I've got now means to me, in that it allows me to be the person that I want to be because I'm not having to rely on other people, I'm not having to ask people to do things for me, I can do everything that I need to do, whereas for the first twenty years of my life, my life was the absolute opposite to that. Everything had to be done by other people because things were inaccessible, always having to ask, always having to be grateful, always having to seek permission. But in a property where I have everything at the right level, I can, in a sense, have choice and control.

It should be noted that accessibility is about more than the dwelling itself, and can include accessibility of the local environment, public services and amenities, and the proximity of good transport links (Hemingway, 2011). Furthermore, the more accessible (and affordable) accommodation is typically provided by the social rented sector, and has commonly focused on targeting specific or individual access needs, often under the label of 'special needs' housing. This tends to be located in areas which are segregated from mainstream housing, separating disabled people from family, friends and the community. Thus, whilst independence may (in some cases) be exercised within the dwelling, with inaccessible environments everywhere else, disabled people can become socially isolated or restricted to their dwelling. In such circumstances, the dwelling might not necessarily constitute 'home' for the inhabitant, but rather a place of confinement (Imrie, 2006).

There are various other factors which can affect meanings of home for disabled people, outside of physical issues (Hemingway, 2011). In terms of 'care' and support, for instance, interactions with professionals and providers of support within the dwelling may be important to achieving a greater sense of home, but can also negatively impact on control, privacy, safety and notions of 'retreat', which may be central to feelings of home. The relationship an individual has with home may also be affected by notions of 'recovery' or rehabilitation, with 'home' providing emotional or psychological security for some. Furthermore, a sense of inclusion within the neighbourhood and community may be important in achieving a sense of home, but can be negatively affected by 'nimbyism' (not in my back yard) or harassment and social exclusion. Issues of tenure have been widely discussed in literature on meanings of home and can be especially important for disabled people, particularly as disabled people are likely to be found 'under-represented' in the owner-occupied sector and 'over-represented' as social renters, without a large share of private tenancies. Finally, it is worth noting that life experiences vary considerably by time and place and from person to person, and so personal attributes such as age, ethnicity, sexuality or socio-economic position may be significant in these experiences.

Accessing housing: Barriers and constraints

As we have seen, the way in which housing is experienced by an individual is extremely important, but also significant is a person's acquisition of, or access to, accommodation. Using a social model approach to disability, the current author examined the various opportunities and barriers that disabled people encounter within a range of housing options (Hemingway, 2011). Constraints identified included aspects of housing design and construction (especially the general inaccessibility of the physical environment), the limited availability and inadequate presentation of information on housing options, economic disadvantage (affecting general affordability and the ability to secure housing finance), and the role of 'actors' involved in the process of building, selling and allocating housing. These factors can be categorised as physical, communication, financial and attitudinal barriers.

The various physical (or access) barriers that can affect housing opportunities for disabled people – and not just people with mobility impairments – represent aspects of the environment which do not cater for a variety of bodily forms. Accessible properties, for instance, which cater for a diversity of bodies, tend to be lacking within the general stock of housing across all tenures. This may cause difficulties when visiting family and friends, or, more importantly, when trying to find a property to either rent or buy. 'Katie', for example, found few accessible properties in private renting, and so felt forced into purchasing a property before she had planned to do so. Finding a property to buy (or at least one that could be adapted), however, proved just as difficult. Thus, one of the most significant issues for her was: 'the loops you have to go through to just find accessible housing ... just finding somewhere to buy that you can make accessible'.

Furthermore, when a suitable flat had been located, the inaccessible communal step and the refusal of the management committee to agree to the erection of a ramp (despite her offer to pay for it), meant that she once again had to continue her search. There have been some developments relating to inaccessible housing, such as Part M of the building regulations in 1999 (and the equivalent regulations in Northern Ireland and Scotland) and 'Lifetime Homes' standards, but these strategies have been insufficient in many ways (Imrie, 2003; Milner, 2005). Adaptations and assistive technology may provide a short-term solution to inaccessible environments for some, but lack of information on available support and exclusions, and the complex adaptations process, can cause difficulties here. Additionally, as mentioned earlier, an accessible home environment is about more than the dwelling itself, and includes the accessibility of the outside space (including the garden and communal areas), as well as the surrounding neighbourhood.

The communication (or information) barriers that disabled people encounter within housing have long been recognised, and disabled people have been active in addressing the problems in different ways. These have included setting up Centres for 'Independent', 'Inclusive' or 'Integrated' Living (CILs), and the Disablement Information and Advice Line (DIAL) (Barnes and Mercer, 2006). Nonetheless, gaps remain in the availability of accessible information from housing and allied service providers. There are four key issues here. First, there is limited available general information on housing options, entitlement and support for disabled people. Second, the language used tends not to be straightforward or in plain English. Third, information is not always available in different formats, making it inaccessible for different audiences. Whilst there has been progress here since the 1995 Disability Discrimination Act (DDA) made it a legal requirement to produce materials in a range of different formats, responses to the requirements have varied amongst housing providers. Private landlords, for instance, have been less likely to have made adjustments than social landlords, and there is evidence that other housing and mortgage providers have fallen short of meeting these requirements. 'Carol' discussed her experiences of dealing with a mortgage lender:

> I was very clear from my very first interview that I had a visual impairment so any information would be needed in .14 font. And he said that shouldn't be a problem because he'd be printing quotes off the computer. Of course, he'd forgotten about the brochures. But actually, when he tried to print things off the computer, it wouldn't do it. So I didn't get anything accessible. Even when I was dealing with head office, I kept reminding them and saying could you please write to me in an accessible way, and they'd say oh yes. But I never got a single thing from them that actually followed my requests.

Finally, service providers can fail to make equipment or support available to ensure information is communicated effectively for different audiences. This has been shown especially for people with hearing impairments, disabled people from black and minority and ethnic groups, and – in the current author's research – for people with speech impairments.

Financial factors are extremely significant in the housing and disability relationship, and include employment security and history; income (including receipt of benefits); additional costs relating to impairment, disabling environments and life insurance; and issues associated with risk assessment in the mortgage application process. Whereas some of these factors (such as income and employment) affect access to all housing tenures, others (such as life insurance and risk assessment for housing finance) are more specific to owner-occupation. In terms of the income and employment situations of many disabled people, it is well known that disabled people experience disadvantage in the labour market, which results in limited resources for participating in the private sector and weaker positions in the housing market. The additional costs of impairment and disability-related expenses can further reduce available resources. The receipt of state benefits as income can also be viewed negatively by some housing providers, such as private landlords and mortgage lenders, affecting access, in particular, to private sector housing. 'Paul', for example, who was applying for a mortgage with his partner, approached a large high street lender. Despite earned income, as well as several different benefits between them, and an established relationship with the lender, they were declined a mortgage on the basis that the benefits would not be accepted. What was interesting about this case was that this particular lender had previously been described by the financial services informants as being one of the most likely lenders to accept benefits. Clearly, actual practice suggests otherwise.

Examination of risk assessment processes by the current author also indicated that some institutions may (informally) consider impairment within mortgage applications, particularly in relation to perceptions about the applicant's capacity to understand the contract or commitment, and the assumed effect on employment circumstances (or ability to earn). As one informant explained:

Learning difficulties for us, as a financial services organisation, is probably the most difficult barrier to overcome, because how can you possibly understand how much an individual understands about the process, of whether they are mentally capable of entering into a contract?

It was evident that certain impairments may be both perceived and treated differently by some institutions, which could have a negative effect on some disabled people's applications for a mortgage. People labelled with 'learning difficulties', mental health service users and people with progressive impairments, for instance, were discussed as either being difficult to assess or as being potentially perceived as higher risk. It also appeared that applications could be rejected, or considered higher risk, if mortgages on adapted properties were requested. The mortgage industry might therefore play a role in creating and reinforcing the barriers encountered by disabled people through risk assessment practices for mortgage application. The recent and ongoing economic crises are likely to exacerbate many of these financial difficulties for disabled people.

The attitudes, assumptions and practices of various housing providers, organisations and 'gatekeepers' can be just as 'disabling' as the physical and financial environment. The assumptions and knowledge of professionals, such as planning regulators, property developers and house builders, for instance, are extremely important in the availability of accessible housing (and especially private sector housing). Research has shown that understanding of barrier-free housing can be limited and disabled people's housing needs are rarely considered (Imrie, 2003), and where they are, assumptions have been based on a limited conception relating to mobility impairments (Burns, 2004), or individual understandings of disability. There is also some suggestion that disabled people can be subject to negative attitudes and practices in the private rented sector, with a tendency for private landlords to lack knowledge of disabled people's housing needs or their obligations under the DDA, or to employ practices which may exclude some disabled people. In terms of owner-occupation, we saw earlier how processes of risk assessment and perceptions of impairments can affect the ability to secure a mortgage for owner-occupation (Hemingway, 2010, 2011). Previous research has also shown that those in the industry often fail to regard disabled people as customers of the sector (Thomas, 2004).

Assumptions and practices within the social rented sector also play important roles in disabled people's housing opportunities. Disabled people may actually be prioritised in some housing allocation systems, but with many procedures being influenced by medical assessments, this does not always mean that needs are met. Some housing associations use matching systems to allocate suitable dwellings to people with particular impairments, but – among other problems (Hemingway, 2011) – these can limit choice for disabled people. Choice-Based Letting (CBL) may eradicate some of these issues, but not all local authorities solely use CBL, constraints arise in relation to supply and demand, and assessments of priority need (as determined by the landlord) remain in place. The latter can rest on medical assessments, which contrast with the goal of supporting or enforcing independent living. Thus, judgement of the severity of a person's impairment may be considered more important in applications for housing than experiences of inaccessible dwellings, poor support or neighbourhood harassment (Crowther, 2000). Assessments of risk might also affect provision, with evaluations of housing need focusing on 'risk of harm' to the individual, or exclusion from eligibility for housing on the grounds of risk to housing providers or the community (especially for mental health service users). Assumptions about capacity (particularly for people labelled with learning difficulties) and differential treatment relating to ethnicity can also have an impact on housing allocation.

As we have seen, the social model of disability provides an important tool in the identification of barriers, discrimination and oppressive practices. It can also be taken further to show how barriers work, by looking at differences in relation to perceptions of impairment and risk. This is about understanding disabling practices and perceptions, rather than disadvantage related to individual difference. If we apply or extend social model thinking to risk, we can say that risk is likely to be crucial for disabled people through institutional responses to disability, which inform the perspectives and practices of institutions, and have implications for particular groups of people. As mentioned earlier, people with different impairments can be perceived as more vulnerable or 'risky' by both the rented sectors and the owner-occupation industry, or classified and measured according to risk. These institutional practices may have a negative impact on disabled people's opportunities to access particular housing options.

Conclusion

It is hoped that this chapter has made evident the ongoing difficulties faced by disabled people within housing, not just in terms of housing choices, opportunities and pathways, but also in their experiences of housing or meanings of 'home'. The social model approach to disability has been central in identifying these barriers, demonstrating the ways in which systematic processes and perspectives impact on disabled people's housing opportunities, but also highlighting the importance of using disabled people's own voices to present their opinions and experiences. Housing practitioners and policy makers would benefit from assessing institutionalised practices from this perspective to inform developments in policy, practice and processes. With disabled people constituting such a large percentage of the population, and with an ever-increasing ageing population, ensuring that housing needs are met is crucial. Without radical change, the situation is unlikely to improve, and so the urgency of developing more appropriate housing strategies, and accessible housing for all, must be recognised.

References

Barnes, C. and Mercer, G. (2006) *Independent Futures: Creating User-Led Disability Services in a Disabling Society*. Bristol: Policy Press.

Burns, N. (2004) 'Negotiating difference: disabled people's experiences of housebuilders', *Housing Studies*, 19 (5): 765–80.

Crowther, N. (2000) *Overcoming Disability Discrimination: A Guide for Registered Social Landlords*. London: RNIB and the Housing Corporation.

Davis, K. (1990) A Social Barriers Model of Disability: Theory into Practice – The Emergence of the 'Seven Needs'. Paper prepared for the Derbyshire Coalition of Disabled People, The Disability Archive UK. Available at: www.leeds.ac.uk/disability-studies/archiveuk/archframe.htm

French, S. and Swain, J. (2006) Housing: The Users' Perspective. The Disability Archive UK. Available at: www.leeds.ac.uk/disability-studies/archiveuk/archframe.htm

Hamer, R. (2005) *House Hunting for All: Opening up Property Search Systems to Disabled People*. Edinburgh: Ownership Options in Scotland.

Hemingway, L. (2010) 'Taking a risk? The mortgage industry and perceptions of disabled people', *Disability & Society*, 25 (1): 75–87.

Hemingway, L. (2011) *Disabled People and Housing: Choices, Opportunities and Barriers*. Bristol: Policy Press.

Heywood, F. (2005) 'Adaptation: altering the house to restore the home', *Housing Studies*, 20 (4): 531–47.

Imrie, R. (2003) 'Housing quality and the provision of accessible homes', *Housing Studies*, 18 (3): 387–408.

Imrie, R. (2006) *Accessible Housing: Quality, Disability and Design*. London and New York: Routledge.

Milner, J. (2005) 'Disability and inclusive housing design: towards a life-course perspective', in P. Somerville and N. Sprigings (eds), *Housing and Social Policy: Contemporary Themes and Critical Perspectives*. London and New York: Routledge. pp. 172–96.

Thomas, P. (2004) 'The experience of disabled people as customers in the owner occupation market', *Housing Studies*, 19 (5): 781–94.

23
Changing Technology

Alison Sheldon

Technology is constantly changing and the pace of change seems to accelerate by the year. That which seems ordinary today would have been the stuff of science fiction as little as 50 years ago. In 50 years' time, we will doubtless be excited, perturbed and baffled by yet more new developments. The technology now available to disabled people is extraordinary and its ability to compensate for our perceived deficits seems to hold a particular fascination. Figures such as Stephen Hawking and Oscar Pistorious are perhaps as well known for the technology they use as for their achievements. The focus here though is not on technology developed *for* disabled people (although such technology is crucial for many disabled people). Here, the discussion will centre on the taken-for-granted information and communication technology (ICT) that has found its way into our working environments, our domestic spaces and, increasingly, our coat pockets. Such technology is arguably changing the society in which we live, and, with it, the social category of people we consider 'disabled'. It thus has the potential to impact on disabled people's lives whether or not they are willing and able to use it themselves.

Many extravagant claims have been made about such technology's potential role in the lives of disabled people. However, the area is still lamentably under-researched. This is a curious omission, since, as one commentator has cogently argued: 'studying the use (and non-use) of technologies can provide valuable insights into the meaning of disability' (Blume, 2012: 349). It seems clear though that many disabled people are finding ways to use ICT to their advantage – to access information and services, to affiliate with others and to find new means of self-expression and dissent (see Chapter 36). At the same time, recent developments are disempowering others yet further. Current trends are likely to present particular problems for certain segments of the disabled population, such as those with learning difficulties, those outside the world of paid employment, the growing number of older disabled people and others who simply 'don't get on with computers' – a group including many who are not currently deemed disabled. Hence, we may see increasing polarisation between the technological 'haves' and 'have-nots' in the disabled population and shifts in the 'disabled' category itself (Sheldon, 2001).

Disabled people's complicated relationship with technology will be briefly considered, before the crucial issue of access to technology is examined. The liberatory potential of ICTs will then be briefly evaluated in relation to two key areas – accessing information and services, and communication and self-organisation.

Changing technology and disabled people: Emancipation or oppression?

Technology is not neutral. It is created by the same oppressive society that turns those with impairments into disabled people. Whilst 'stamped with the desires and needs of the ruling class' it is, at the same time, 'produced amidst conflicting social relations, and thus holds the possibility of being a tool for liberation as well as for social control' (Davis et al., 1997: 6). It is no surprise, then, that disabled people have a complicated relationship with technology. We are often excluded from mainstream technology, a factor said to have contributed to our current labour force exclusion and, indeed, to the creation of the modern 'disability' category (Finkelstein, 1980; Oliver, 1990). At the same time, we have become the recipients of an ever-growing business involved in developing and marketing technologies specifically for our ascribed needs. Many of us have been impaired as a direct result of modern technology. Others would not be alive today without it. *All* of us are now dependent upon it to satisfy even our most basic needs (Illich, 1973).

Every new technological breakthrough is invariably hailed as a saviour for disabled people, as a way of minimising our 'deficits' and thus making us less dependent on other people. This despite the fact that dependency on others is a part of life for *everyone*, and may well be preferable to dependency on unreliable technology. ICT is capable of delivering a myriad of services directly into disabled people's homes, thus reducing the need to travel or rely on others for assistance. It is here that its main benefits are often assumed to lie. Like their non-disabled peers though, disabled people want *choice* in how they make contact with the world. Access to the latest technology, though regarded as increasingly necessary, is not considered the highest priority for many. The removal of more traditional disabling barriers is generally thought to have greater urgency. This creates concerns that technology might be provided as a cost-cutting exercise, reducing the need to make more meaningful social changes and effectively segregating disabled people in their own homes (Sheldon, 2001). There is a very real danger that such 'technical fixes' could create further disadvantage, since with the increasing power of technological tools one has a 'barring of alternatives' (Illich, 1973: 23). Many may thus find themselves more isolated than before and less capable of satisfying their needs in other ways. As one commentator suggests, this uncritical faith in technology, underpinned by an individual model of disability, 'is often reflected in laws, policies, institutional arrangements and social attitudes which privilege technological solutions to the problems faced by disabled people' (Gleeson, 1999: 99). It is clear, then, that technology should not be pushed onto people as a sticking-plaster solution to deeper social problems. It is also clear that this could easily happen in the current political climate.

It is proposed that a less over-optimistic analysis of technology's implications for disabled people would come from the disabled people's movement, which may be 'central to ensuring that technology is used to liberate rather than further oppress disabled people' (Oliver, 1990: 126). Whether the movement can rise to this difficult challenge remains to be seen, however. Many disabled activists have been equally enthusiastic about our future prospects, claiming, for example, that with the appropriate technology we can become part of the 'main-stream of life' and 'contribute fully in society' (UPIAS, 1981: 1). Some though emphasise technology's 'double-edged nature' (Oliver, 1990) and stress that it can be 'both oppressive and emancipatory, depending on the social uses to which it is put' (Gleeson, 1999: 104). Taking such an approach, we can identify a number of potential pitfalls and promises for disabled people that are associated with the increasing reliance on technology in today's world. The first, most significant and perhaps most easily forgotten pitfall relates to inequitable access to technology.

Access all areas?

Disabled people have long been denied access to the technology that others take for granted, and there is little evidence that this exclusion is dissipating. Figures from 2012, for example, suggested that over 4 million disabled people in the UK had never used the Internet – just under half of the country's adult 'non-users' (ONS, 2012). Similarly, there is evidence to suggest that mobile phone ownership is less likely amongst disabled adults (Goggin and Newell, 2006; Ofcom, 2006). Despite this, the issue of access to technology is often obscured because of the undue emphasis placed on its *potential* for improving disabled people's lot (Roulstone, 1993).

A number of barriers stand in the way of disabled people's beneficial use of computers, the Internet and mobile communications. Of these, finance looms largest. Whilst ICTs are now more affordable, disabled people and their families are 'grossly over-represented amongst poor people' (Beresford, 1996: 53) and their poverty is set to increase yet further as austerity measures take their toll (Edwards, 2012). It is difficult then to stay abreast of technological developments. The adoption of smartphones and tablets – the stuff of fantasy even a decade ago – has reportedly 'surpassed that of any consumer technology in history' (Meredith, 2012: unpaginated), with one model rapidly replaced by the next. Since the profits of major corporations depend on persuading consumers to upgrade or replace their old devices, they stand accused of deliberately using strategies of 'built in obsolescence' in order to maximise sales (Hern, 2012). Thus, the pace of change itself presents a huge barrier to those with limited means, with newer, 'better' models of perfectly serviceable devices constantly renovating poverty (Illich, 1973).

Disabled people share many characteristics of the non-disabled poor population (Thomas, 2005) but further barriers to access are created through discriminatory design. Despite organisational rhetoric to the contrary, disabled people are not 'designed in' to products from the outset, often making expensive add-ons necessary. Whilst it is true that certain gains have been made, it is unlikely that the free market will ever guarantee access for a relatively small social grouping with little disposable income. Effective regulation is urgently required to ensure that corporations attend to the accessibility of the equipment they develop (Sheldon, 2001). We must not be distracted, however, into denying the socio-structural origins of the problem. Access to technology is *not* simply a technical issue with technical solutions. The inaccessibility of technology is just one more symptom of disabled people's continuing oppression. In the UK, the disabled people's movement has organised around the premise that no one aspect of the disablement of people with impairments should be treated in isolation (UPIAS, 1976). This approach suggests that as well as considering access to technology as a purely *technological* problem, other aspects of disabled people's exclusion must also be considered – access to the wider world of employment, education, housing, transport, the built environment, and so on. Equal access to the beneficial use of technology can only be secured alongside the removal of these more traditional disabling barriers (Roulstone, 1998).

Whilst a consideration of access is vital, it is not sufficient. We cannot assume that all disabled people want to use technology or, indeed, see any utility in doing so. The potential value of ICTs for disabled people will now be considered in relation to just two crucial areas – information and services, and communication and self-organisation. Here too, however, the issue of access still looms large.

Informed consumers?

Open access to information, considered vital for *all* in today's society, is a particular concern for disabled people, who are isolated by a variety of other barriers. ICT provides new ways for them to obtain the information they need, in formats which are accessible to them. It also enables them to take control of information, through, for example, blogging (Kuusisto, 2007). Without substantial changes though, 'easy access to the information that can really empower and liberate people still looks likely to be the preserve of an affluent minority' (Haywood, 1998: 26). Furthermore, the increased use of ICT for disseminating information may have an adverse effect on other means of information provision. This may mean that accessing information in traditional ways becomes even more problematic. Thus, the Internet is not the panacea that many suggest. There is still a need for appropriate and accessible information to be disseminated to disabled people in other ways, or the disabled community may become yet more polarised. Similar issues arise in relation to online shopping.

Approximately 30 per cent of people in OECD (Organisation of Economic Cooperation and Development) countries are said to use the Internet to buy goods and services. This figure leaps to 60 per cent in the UK which has the most enthusiastic online shoppers in the OECD (OECD, 2011). The 'phenomenal growth of online retailing' and the 'rise of mobile retailing' have been blamed (at least in part) for the collapse of many long-established retail chains and the demise of the British high street (Portas, 2011: 2). The high street offers far more than the opportunity to purchase products, providing various other resources 'for people who are at risk of marginalisation' (Yuill, 2009: unpaginated). For isolated disabled people then, shopping excursions can give a sense of belonging to a larger community, whether or not purchases are made. Whilst online shopping is undoubtedly welcomed by many disabled people who are effectively segregated in their homes by a multitude of disabling barriers, there is a risk that the increased reliance on this kind of purchasing will make other means of consumption less possible and reduce the pressure to make the environment more accessible for disabled people. Again then, many people – both disabled and non-disabled – may find themselves more isolated than before, and less capable of satisfying their needs in other ways (Sheldon, 2001).

Networking for change?

The potential for otherwise isolated 'housebound people' to maintain and initiate friendships from their homes is one of the main advantages said to be gained from the use of ICT (Haywood, 1998). It is further suggested that disabled people, excluded from their geographic communities, might find themselves included in online communities – communities untainted by 'the contaminating effects of physicality, prejudgement, or prejudice' (Avery, 1998: 2). Many disabled people have little contact with others and live very isolated lives. In the absence of more meaningful social transformation, the Internet can provide another means of communicating and connecting with others, a means that circumvents many of the barriers to disabled people's mobility. For others though, mediated communication provides a poor second-best to actually *being* with people and may actually increase feelings of isolation (Sheldon, 2001: 225).

ICT enables more than just interpersonal interaction however, offering the opportunity for disabled people to gain a political 'voice' and to organise collectively to improve their world. One of the Internet's potentials has long been said to lie in its ability to advance 'the interests of politically and socially disadvantaged groups' (Fitzpatrick, 2000: 386), and it is here that technology might offer the most to disabled people globally. The disability blog has been celebrated as 'a powerful and dynamic contemporary force in the disability community' (Kuusisto, 2007: unpaginated), and it has been highlighted that ICTs 'have become essential to reformers, revolutionaries and contemporary democracy movements. They serve as venues for the shared expression of dissent, dissemination of information, and collective action' (Youmans and York, 2012: 315).

It is vital for activists within the disabled people's movement to use any means at their disposal to make a better world, and it seems that technology is becoming an important part of the disability activist's toolkit. ICT is enabling new forms of dissent by disabled people, as well as facilitating the organisation of other more traditional forms of direct action. High-profile protests have been staged in response to government spending cuts, such as the Twitter campaign to raise awareness of the 'responsible reform' (aka 'Spartacus') report (Campbell et al., 2012). New and vibrant disabled people's organisations, such as Disabled People Against Cuts (DPAC), are also making use of social networking technologies, using Facebook and Twitter to 'engage disabled people' and setting up an 'online protest page for people unable to attend rallies' (Lisney in Peck, 2010). It must be remembered though that the activists who are setting the political agenda are those with access to the requisite technology. This elite group must find ways to include those without such access in order to mitigate the disabling impact of the digital divide within the disabled population.

Conclusion

Being part of the mainstream of society currently entails keeping up with that society's changing technology, something that is not possible for many disabled people, or indeed for many of their non-disabled peers. The disabled community risks becoming more polarised as the technological 'haves' leave their less fortunate contemporaries behind. The boundaries of the 'disabled' category may even be redrawn in the future. Whilst this might be liberating for some currently disabled people, those disabled by the society of the future will not be so enthusiastic. We cannot then assume that the 'problem' of disability will be solved with each new technological innovation. Instead, we need to transform society – the society that created the Internet, the society that oppresses. Nonetheless, the latest ICT also offers great potential for disabled people's self-emancipation, enabling access to essential information and providing new means to affiliate and express dissatisfaction with the world. It remains to be seen whether the increasing use of such technology by a disabled elite will facilitate the emergence of effective new strategies for improving that world for everyone. The success of ICT as a political tool cannot be measured by the number of Facebook friends or Twitter followers. Instead, we must look to the effects produced outside cyberspace.

References

Avery, D. (1998) 'Electronic parenting or, it takes a (listserv) village to raise families with disabilities', *CMC Magazine*, January, 1–11. Available at: www.december.com/cmc/mag/1998/jan/avery.html [accessed 04/09/00].

Beresford, P. (1996) 'Poverty and disabled people: challenging dominant debates and policies', *Disability and Society*, 11 (4): 553–66.

Blume, S. (2012) 'What can the study of science and technology tell us about disability?', in N. Watson, A. Roulstone and C. Thomas (eds), *Routledge Handbook of Disability Studies*. London: Routledge. pp. 348–60.

Campbell, S.J., Marsh, S., Franklin, K., Gaffney, D., Dixon, M., James, L., et al. (2012) Responsible Reform: A Report on the Proposed Changes to Disability Living Allowance (Diary of a Benefit Scrounger). London: Spartacus. Available at: http://wearespartacus.org.uk/spartacus-report/ [accessed 19/09/12].

Davis, J., Hirschl, T.A. and Stack, M. (1997) 'Introduction: integrated circuits, circuits of capital, and revolutionary change', in J. Davis, T.A. Hirschl and M. Stack (eds), *Cutting Edge: Technology, Information, Capitalism and Social Revolution*. London: Verso. pp. 1–10.

Edwards, C. (2012) The Austerity War and the Impoverishment of Disabled People. Norwich: NCODP. Available at: http://documents.ncodp.org.uk/news/3%20September%20 2012%20The%20Austerity%20War%20and%20the%20impoverishment%20of%20 disabled%20people.pdf [accessed 19/09/12].

Finkelstein, V. (1980) *Attitudes and Disabled People*. New York: World Rehabilitation Fund.

Fitzpatrick, T. (2000) 'Critical cyberpolicy: network technologies, massless citizens, virtual rights', *Critical Social Policy*, 20 (3): 375–407.

Gleeson, B. (1999) 'Can technology overcome the disabling city?', in R. Butler and H. Parr (eds), *Mind and Body Spaces: Geographies of Illness, Impairment and Disability*. London: Routledge. pp. 98–118.

Goggin, G. and Newell, C. (2006) 'Disabling cell phones', in A.P. Kavoori and N. Arceneaux (eds), *The Cell Phone Reader: Essays in Social Transformation*. Oxford: Peter Lang. pp. 155–88.

Haywood, T. (1998) 'Global networks and the myth of equality: trickle down or trickle away?', in B.D. Loader (ed.), *Cyberspace Divide: Equality, Agency and Policy in the Information Society*. London: Routledge. pp. 19–34.

Hern, A. (2012) 'Does Apple build in obsolescence?', *New Statesman*, 15 June. Available at: www.newstatesman.com/blogs/technology/2012/06/does-apple-build-obsolescence [accessed 21/11/12].

Illich, I.D. (1973) *Tools for Conviviality*. London: Calder and Boyars.

Kuusisto, S. (2007) 'Introduction: a roundtable on disability blogging', *Disability Studies Quarterly*, 27(1): unpaginated.

Meredith, L. (2012) 'Smartphones and tablets poised to take over the world', *TechNewsDaily*, 27 August. Available at: www.technewsdaily.com/4762-smartphones-and-tablets-poised-to-take-over-the-world.html [accessed 21/11/12].

Ofcom (2006) *Media Literacy Audit: Report on Media Literacy of Disabled People*. London: Office of Communications.

Oliver, M. (1990) *The Politics of Disablement*. London: Macmillan.

ONS (2012) *Internet Access Quarterly Update, 2012 Q1*. Office for National Statistics Statistical Bulletin.

Organisation for Economic Co-operation and Development (OECD) (2011) The Future of the Internet Economy: A Statistical Profile, June 2011 update. Paris: OECD. Available at: www.oecd.org/internet/interneteconomy/48255770.pdf

Peck, S. (2010) '"Cuts kill" drives protest agenda', *Disability Now*. Available at: www.disabilitynow.org.uk/article/cuts-kill-drives-protest-agenda [accessed 21/11/12].

Portas, M. (2011) The Portas Review: An Independent Review into the Future of our High Streets. London: Department for Business, Innovation and Skills. Available at: www.gov.uk/government/uploads/system/uploads/attachment_data/file/31797/11-1434-portas-review-future-of-high-streets.pdf [accessed 21/11/12].

Roulstone, A. (1993) 'Access to new technology in the employment of disabled people', in J. Swain, V. Finkelstein, S. French and M. Oliver (eds), *Disabling Barriers – Enabling Environments*. London: SAGE, in association with the Open University. pp. 241–48.

Roulstone, A. (1998) *Enabling Technology: Disabled People, Work and New Technology*. Buckingham: Open University Press.

Sheldon, A. (2001) Disabled People and Communication Systems in the Twenty-first Century. Unpublished PhD thesis, University of Leeds.

Thomas, P. (2005) Disability, Poverty and the Millennium Development Goals: Relevance, Challenges and Opportunities for DFID. Available at: http://digitalcommons.ilr.cornell.edu/cgi/viewcontent.cgi?article=1257&context=gladnetcollect [accessed 07/02/11].

UPIAS (1976) *Fundamental Principles of Disability*. London: UPIAS.

UPIAS (1981) *Policy Statement*. London: UPIAS.

Youmans, W.L. and York, J.C. (2012) 'Social media and the activist toolkit: user agreements, corporate interests, and the information infrastructure of modern social movements', *Journal of Communication*, 62: 315–29.

Yuill, C. (2009) 'The credit crunch and the high street: "coming like a ghost town"', *Sociological Research Online*, 14 (2): unpaginated.

24

Communication Barriers: Building Access and Inclusive Relationships

Alan Hewitt and Carole Pound

'Through aphasia erm, we are so isolated ... we as a group are exiled. You know, that's erm, we are other, not the same.' (Binda)

'Aphasia, as foreign in ones language, as a minority group, colonized by some kind of brain invading insult and often prejudized/discriminated in society. An invisible group has little power, few resources and often isolated. So we need strong allies.' (Ireland, in Ireland and Pound, 2003: 160)

This chapter draws on the experience of individuals living with aphasia, a communication disability affecting the ability to use and comprehend spoken or written words. Our illustrations draw on the views and experiences of people with aphasia who contribute to peer-led services at Connect and act as co-researchers in a participatory action research project exploring the friendship experiences of younger people with aphasia. (See www.ukconnect.org and http://friendshipandaphasia.weebly.com)

Aphasia is a common consequence of stroke, itself the major cause of long-term disability in the UK. Few people know what it is or how to respond to the challenges it presents. Communication difficulty belongs equally to those with the impairment and those who struggle to communicate with them. Aphasia places the spotlight on language and communication both as the source of disablement and improved access. To have a voice within social and political discourse, to enjoy access to equality, citizenship and social belonging, reminds us of the central importance of language. With hidden impairments affecting communication, cognition, mental health and energy, the experience of living with language difficulty challenges the social model of disability to grapple with discussions of access, inclusion, identity and impairment.

The trouble with communication: Getting your head around it

> The trouble with communication – real communication – is that it's all around you … I only realised about five years into aphasia that I was on shaky ground. With the realisation that I'd got this language disability that was with me for life – all I wanted to do was to shout 'I've got aphasia – do you know what that means?' Of course I couldn't shout, couldn't make sense of the things around me, I was adrift in a sea of language. I couldn't see the way out. (Alan)

Discussing the impact of communication disability on their ability to engage with the world and locate themselves within it, people with aphasia consistently describe the 'other-worldliness' of aphasia. They use metaphors of fog, mist, swimming underwater or dreamlike fantasy worlds to describe their struggles to get a fixed hold on identity and everyday life: 'a different world … weird, weird … me and silent movie … Marcel Marceau! … like a veil … I'm here but not here' (Jeff).

People with aphasia also talk about the complexity of describing or explaining their aphasia to others:

> with aphasia I get a sense of an idea and it remains opaque, like seeing through a frosted glass, without precise definition. Or a concept wrapped in cellophane seen from afar. There is so much effort involved in finding the word that often I will forget why I was looking for it in the first place. (Khosa, 2008: 118–19)

The dual dilemma of personal disorientation, alongside the loss of words to describe or explain the experience, does little to bridge understandings between those who struggle to live with aphasia and those who struggle to imagine or comprehend its impact: 'Erm, well, I don't think really other people really know. Because erm, you can't ex-, you can't explain aphasia and, and how how, how you explain it, doesn't sound like, does it!' (Trisha)

For many individuals, the consequence is a pervasive experience of social exclusion operating at personal, interpersonal and infrastructural levels (Parr, 2007). The source of exclusion is often in the hands of individuals and organisations at a loss for how to respond to altered abilities to convey and receive verbal messages. But the difficulty in identifying and problem-solving communication barriers may be equally obscure to those who live with communication difficulty (Hammel et al., 2006).

Barriers and communication disability

Seminal interview and ethnographic studies by Parr and colleagues (Parr et al., 1997; Parr, 2007) outlined four overarching types of communication access barriers faced by individuals living with language impairment:

- environmental
- structural

- attitudinal
- informational.

Environmental barriers

People with aphasia talked of being sidelined by the noisy blare of social environments – for example, the impossibility of going to shops, restaurants or pubs without the assault of background music: 'People talking all at once … the noise … I can't cope with that' (Parr et al., 1997: 128).

A key environmental barrier for people with aphasia is the presence or absence of skilled communication supporters in the everyday environment, enabling access, for example, to health services, transport, work, relationships (Howe et al., 2008).

Structural barriers

> I always say, you know, I had a stroke. Duhduhduh duh … Don't, what's in my head, what's the question, slowly, slowly. In the hobsitals I say 'hang on', because … 'slowly' because I can't understand the question. (Shana)

Access to resources, services and opportunities so often depends on understanding and navigating letters, forms, telephone calls, websites and electronic communications that are the gateway to those services. People with language impairment frequently have difficulty with numbers, with writing and with memory for instructions. The use of automated telephone systems, call centres and online forms may be part of changing communications but they disadvantage people with language impairment. The need for more time and face-to-face explanation does not tally with the growing lack of access to 'real live people'.

The experience of welfare assessments for many is one of double disadvantage. People with language impairments find themselves at the mercy of unclear and incomprehensible assessment procedures and a failure to recognise that it is the poor communication skills and practices of others which operate as the primary source of disablement.

> If the assessment goes the wrong way – which I assume is the case because it's geared at people **with** language, **by** people with language – I'll have to up sticks from London and go to a part of the country which I don't want to be because of the way that I'd have to be financially, for no other reason … all my friends here I'll have to say goodbye to all of it … horrendous. I'll have to start all over again … I get tired thinking about it. (Alan)

Many people with aphasia want to be employed but they encounter huge infrastructural challenges arising from the mesh of communication barriers implicit in working. These begin with verbally dependent job application processes, and continue, for example, with the requirements of creative line management support, the challenge of

filtering overwhelming volumes of electronic communications and the subtle understandings and adaptations required of the entire workforce around communicatively
inclusionary practices.

Attitudinal barriers

The equation of communication disability with 'having nothing to say' and a perception of incompetence are well documented: 'Some of them actually thought I
think you are an imbecile' (Parr et al., 1997: 128).

Participants with hidden cognitive and communication impairments in Hammel
et al.'s (2006) study noted the negative reactions of others when they claimed disability benefits, used accessible transport seats or requested help using the Internet
in libraries.

Many disabled people are subject to the disabling assumptions and attitudes of other
people. But somehow the greater visibility of certain disabilities will give clues or suggestions as to possible reactions. People with aphasia may not have the luxury of using
speech to direct more common-sense reactions from their communication partners.

Informational barriers

'Why, what, how'; 'You cannot always ask.' (Parr et al., 1997: 129)

Recent years have seen a welcome acknowledgement of the importance of accessible
information as the entry point to services. Production of easy-read and large-font
summaries, alternative formats such as DVD and audio description, and the use of
icons and images supporting written text and web-based material have revolution-
ised the production of more diverse and accessible information. Improvements in
signage have helped navigation around unfamiliar and confusing geographies. However, consultations about service shortcomings and improvements consistently highlight lack of information as a major hurdle.

Documents (including texts, leaflets, letters, reports, websites) may have features of
clarity relating to fonts and format but attention to tone, structure and honing down
of information requires a second wave of 'translation'. Consultations with people
with cognitive and communication impairment invariably prioritise welcoming and
warmth from a person with time and information navigation skills over 'death by
leaflets' or the tsunami of Internet information which they are unable to read.

Temporal barriers and communication disability

'It's very very difficult. How can you ask the world to slow down the pace?'
(Alan)

The rapid rhythm and tempo of everyday life make few allowances for a calmer, slower, more deliberate form of interpersonal communication. Contemporary living is characterised by speed, busyness and time-poor lifestyles where people juggle jobs, families, relationships, long distances and multiple ways of communicating. For people with communication disabilities, a slower tempo is not a choice but is the only accessible pace.

As Ireland explains, the consequence of non-adjusted conversational tempo is frustration, pain and missing out on meaning:

> Yes, sometimes I foreign in my own language. People don't have time for deep listening. You grab conversations with people. On the hop conversations. I hate them. They hurt me. Stressed out my brain, too much in. Your head goes everywhere ... On the hop, there is so much moulted stuff ... multi ... multi-layered stuff. Not enough time to check what they really mean by it. (Ireland, in Black and Ireland, 2003: 25)

Experience of involving people with aphasia in recruitment, research, consultation meetings and as co-workers at Connect[1] highlight a range of temporal barriers to equal participation. Additional time may be needed to:

- find words
- formulate and express ideas
- process ideas and respond to questions
- revisit and recall previous discussions
- negotiate choices and decisions.

For the person without aphasia, additional time is required to:

- listen and tolerate silence
- develop a relationship of communicative trust and ease
- research and prepare useful communication props or ramps ahead of time, e.g. agendas and meeting documents written in a clear and accessible style with key concepts highlighted and lengthy documents summarised
- develop their own skills as conversation partners and communication supporters
- negotiate and inform themselves about individuals' communication preferences
- problem-solve the communication breakdowns, e.g. when words or ideas suddenly go missing
- record discussion and decisions in a communicatively accessible way, e.g. 'aphasia-friendly' minutes emphasising key points and supported with relevant images.

As Alan remarks, 'it's a fine line between being over the top and leaving people completely floundering'. Aphasia manifests so differently from one person to the next, requiring communication supporters to manage a skilful interplay of time, learnt skills and relaxed, one-on-one relationships.

'It's all about individual relationship' – time and relationships

In a study reviewing the friendship experiences of younger people with stroke and aphasia (see http://friendshipandaphasia.weebly.com), time and the ability to manage time and effort creatively emerged as prominent factors in whether friends maintained friendships when one of them acquired aphasia. In addition to an inability at a conversational level to adapt their communication tempo, friends' busy lives, lack of 'sincere patience' and an inability to 'drift with the silence' were all perceived as major barriers to maintaining relationships: 'Time yeah! But the, the thing with some people is that they're, they don't have the time to (...). Yeah. Yeah. Don't make the effort. Yeah. The effort' (Anthea).

Conversely, many people in our projects who accessed peer support groups or virtual communities suggested it was not just the shared experience of stroke and aphasia which cemented new friendships. In the company of peers, individuals could 'hang out' with the stories of exiled others, often just watching and listening, quietly exploring different ways of 'being' and belonging (Pound, 2011). Peer support offered unpressurised time to communicate and to evolve new understandings:

> We understand each other. We care for each other. We communicate with our photos, our music and art as well as words. So we become confident with other. Gradually we are more confident with everyone. (Hussey, 2010: 9)

A decade of change? Time and technology

Radical advances in technology have introduced exciting possibilities for manoeuvring around language barriers. In our research group, people with aphasia spoke about the benefits of smartphone technology for communicating and expressing identity, for example using keyboards to spell out hard-to-pronounce words, photos on phones to tell jokes, Facebook thumbs up/down to highlight likes and dislikes, IPads and smartphones for backing up fragmentary speech with photos, images and explanatory Google maps. Others use Skype to partially address the challenge of the telephone through face-to-face interaction or text-to-speech software to circumvent some aspects of reading.

However, technology can impose still more barriers. Successful implementation requires time, additional support, communication and cognitive skills: 'its yes and no ... its double whammy ... the talking and the computer ... its learning ... its time ... its slow ... example I thought "oh twitter"... its short ... but twitter its more time to learn it' (Jeff).

The rapid communication exchange of social networking can be a tool for connecting and reconnecting socially but it can equally reinforce perceptions of 'falling behind' or being left to observe from the sidelines: 'Facebook and Twitter ...

lots and lots of stuff ... there is a kind of fear that you've been left out ... a little bit excluded ... again' (Priya).

So despite technological solutions, changes in awareness levels and improved disability legislation, 20 years into his lifetime as a person with aphasia and 10 years on from the first version of this chapter, Alan contends:

> For me on a day to day basis in my life the change has been miniscule ... almost imperceptible for me. Maybe apart from a little bit more awareness of communication access by health and social care providers. My life when I go out, use transport, go to the bank ... it's the same – people don't know what communication disability is or what to do in the case of communication 'breakdown'.

Conclusion: A vision for communication access

Alan states: 'if you can't get into a building physically you can't participate in the discussions and activities that happen there. If you can't get into a conversation or understand the papers for a meeting you can't participate in the important decisions. You're lost' (Hewitt, in Parr et al., 2008). Communication access offers a 'way in' to discussion, information and influence for people with communication disability.

Communication access is about everyone developing communication which is clear, comfortable and easy to understand and interact with. It will cover communication in spoken and written form, communication that is face to face or remote, conversations about everyday happenings or complex debate about strategic and theoretical issues. It will attend to an interweaving tapestry of written documents (including all forms of electronic communications), environments and personalised interactions (Parr et al., 2008).

How might this look in practice? Communication access training focusing on written documents will support everyone in an organisation from receptionist to finance officer to volunteer to therapist to reword complex, abstract documents and information into clear, jargon-free language. Communication partners will attend not just to format, layout and design but to the amount and tone of language.

Accessible interactions will build on communication skills training and induction programmes for those without communication disability – for example, developing a personal kitbag of supported conversation techniques (Kagan, 1998), such as slowing down, supplementing spoken conversation with key word writing or bringing relevant communication props to the interaction. Training should be prioritised and statutory in the way that basic health and safety requires knowledge of 'lifting and handling'. These basic communication skills would enable everyone to share responsibility for respecting and involving people with communication disability.

Accessible buildings will be those where thought has been given to signage and information design as well as physical layout. Consideration of communication and temporal barriers in meetings and group discussions will ensure that those who take more time to have a voice in the debate have their access accommodations met (Parr et al., 2008).

Progress over the next decade must embrace these sharper understandings of communication access and the skills, relationships and technologies which underpin it. As Simmons-Mackie and Damico (2007) caution:

Promoting communicative inclusion and access can require significant consumption of time and energy for all parties. Participants must have internalised the values to support communicative access and be willing to dedicate the effort required to support participation. (2007: 93)

Note

1 Connect – the communication disability network promotes innovative support services for people living with stroke, brain injury and aphasia. By working with people with aphasia to explore creative approaches to communication access, Connect aims to influence other service providers to improve the lives of people with aphasia and communication disability and support re-connecting with life.

References

Black, M. and Ireland, C. (2003) 'Talking to ourselves: dialogues in and out of language', in S. Parr, J. Duchan and C. Pound (eds), *Aphasia Inside Out*. Maidenhead: Open University Press. pp. 21–31.

Hammel, J., Jones, R., Gossett, A. and Morgan, E. (2006) 'Examining barriers and supports to community living and participation after a stroke from a Participatory Action Research approach', *Topics in Stroke Rehabilitation*, 13 (3): 43–58.

Howe, T., Worral, L. and Hickson, L. (2008) 'Interviews with people with aphasia: environmental factors that influence their community participation', *Aphasiology*, 22 (6): 618–43.

Hussey, M. (2010) 'I'm no longer Silent', *Topics in Stroke Rehabilitation*, 17 (1): 6–9.

Ireland, C. and Pound, C. (2003) 'Cebrelating aphasia poetry power', in S. Parr, J. Duchan and C. Pound (eds) *Aphasia Inside Out: Reflections on Communication Disability*. Maidenhead: Open University Press. pp.144–62.

Kagan, A. (1998) 'Supported conversation for adults with aphasia', *Aphasiology*, 12: 816–30.

Khosa, J. (2008) 'Personal testimony', in J. Swain and S. French (eds), *Disability on Equal Terms: Understanding and Valuing Difference in Health and Social Care*. London: SAGE. pp. 115–19.

Parr, S. (2007) 'Living with severe aphasia: tracking social exclusion', *Aphasiology*, 21 (1): 98–123.

Parr, S., Byng, S. and Gilpin, S. with Ireland, C. (1997) *Talking about Aphasia*. Buckingham: Open University Press.

Parr, S., Wimborne, N., Hewitt, A. and Pound, C. (2008) *The Communication Access Toolkit*. London: Connect Press.

Pound, C. (2011) 'Reciprocity, resources and relationships: new discourses in healthcare, personal and social relationships', *International Journal of Speech Language Pathology*, 13 (3): 197–206.

Simmons-Mackie, N. and Damico, J. (2007) 'Access and social inclusion in aphasia: interactional principles and applications', *Aphasiology*, 21(1): 81–97.

25

Controlling Exclusion in Education

Michele Moore

Introduction

In this chapter, I will discuss the critical importance of controlling exclusion in the education of disabled children and young people. In the UK, imperative to talk on *exclusion* are newly embedding UK policies and practices which make plain there is little commitment to discussion of inclusion and that it is its oppositional force, exclusion, that dominates discourses of education across recent and current decades (Barton, 2003, 2012; Wertheimer, 1997).

Interpretations of inclusive education are, and always have been, problematic (Allan, 2003, 2008; Barton and Armstrong, 2007; Moore and Slee, 2012; Slee, 2011). In this chapter, I will work with the assumption frequently made by Barton (e.g. 2003, 2004, 2012) that inclusive education is always 'hard work'. Inclusive education is not simply about children with impairments attending neighbourhood schools alongside their contemporaries (Hemingway and Armstrong, 2012). The minutiae of inclusion is deeply complicated and must be attended to in every last detail if exclusion is not to surface in so-called inclusive education settings. In my experience of researching inclusive education in schools around the world, it is true that the willingness of teachers to attend to the minutiae of exclusion often means it can be in segregated settings that some of the most inclusive education can actually be observed. This, however, comprises an invidious circumstance since segregated settings arise out of discrimination – they recycle injustice and their very existence denies disabled children equality and their human rights. A helpful proposition to use to make sense of diverse cross-cultural meanings attached to inclusive education around the world, and to the beleaguered landscape of inclusive education arising from a history of special and inclusive education that Armstrong has described as a 'wild profusion of entangled events' (Armstrong, 2002), can be drawn from the idea that a school can never be satisfactory if it cannot welcome, value and respect every individual child (CSIE, 2012).

Voice

In the second edition of this book, French and Swain (2004) pointed to difficulties created for the agenda of inclusive education when commentators are non-disabled people claiming to talk on behalf of disabled children and young people, prescribing experiences of teaching and learning without reference to the inside perspectives of disabled children and young people who will themselves encounter those experiences. Here, I have to start by acknowledging a contested position as another of those non-disabled commentators.

In previous writing (Moore, 2010), I have claimed some lines of credibility for my reflections on the imperative to control exclusion in education for children with impairments. Being the mother of children with impairments, for example, means the consequences of my engagement in schools impact on my own children's destinies. In my work, I can never afford the detachment of an outsider's gaze because my own children live with the consequences of barriers which impede a global vision of inclusive education. The key requirement for those who have any power to control inclusion and exclusion in education, whether at the level of creating policy or of day-to-day organisation of the resources in children's school bags or on their desks, is that we are always reflective about the limitations of our own positions and open to the seldom heard voices of children with impairments, especially those for whom communication is neither an easy or comfortable process. Ways must always be found of foregrounding the voices of disabled adults, children and young people so that their aspirations for their education and learning are not overlooked. And so, with the parameters of my own position made clear, I claim that in critical ways I share experiences and hold commitments which perhaps lessen the remoteness of my reflections on the importance of controlling exclusion in the education of disabled children.

There is no doubt that there is much to learn from taking seriously the voices of disabled children and young people when thinking about whether to include or exclude (Billington and Pomerantz, 2004). To start with, as many disabled teenagers know:

It is not impairments – which are what we have – that make us disabled children. For me, my impairment will always be with me and is a part of me and I can live with that. It is society which makes me disabled by not letting me join in (Claire, aged 14 years). (ODPM, 2003: 11)

This idea, that exclusion creates disablement, not impairment is not difficult to grasp. Both of my children have impairments: my son is partially ambulant and a sometimes wheelchair user; my daughter has an auditory processing hearing impairment, but 'disability' is part of their experience only if they encounter diminishing or oppressive attitudes, inaccessible environments or resource limitations which create exclusion (Moore, 2011). In school, if my son is asked to sit out of tennis lessons then he is an excluded and disabled child. If a creative teacher can find a mode of participation that will include him as a wheelchair user then he is an enabled child. This is not rocket science. I often think back to clarity offered on this point in the observations of the head of a segregated school for children with hearing impairments in Trinidad who explained to me: 'Kentry can hear but he's come to this school because he has speech and language difficulties and people can't understand what he says.' It is clear that for Kentry, impairment, even lack of it, has nothing to do with the reasons for his placement in a segregated school. In Kentry's case, other people's listening difficulties and disabling attitudes turn into justifications for exclusion. I was recently struck by the simplicity with which a young practitioner in Oman, in the very earliest days of her practice as one of a new cadre of Inclusive Education Practitioners, made plain a deep practical and theoretical understanding of the link between disabling environments and disablement when she explained, 'I said to the teacher "I cannot stay in that room with him all alone everyday – otherwise I will get autism too". So I found another boy and I took them to the zoo.' The link between exclusion in education and disablement is not difficult to fathom. It is essential to realise, however, that the link has very little, if anything at all, to do with impairment.

'Children who can't be included'

I wish to argue on the basis of personal experience, professional observation and the writing of other parents (e.g. Bartley, 2010; Mason, 2008; Runswick-Cole, 2007) that there is nothing essentially sensible, meaningful or appropriate about the separation of any child with impairments from their peers. A day spent in another school, again in the Caribbean, helps to make this crystal clear. The head teacher explained that her segregated school is for 'children who can't be included'. She said the school was formerly a school for deaf children but rubella vaccines and improved interventions for meningitis led the incidence of deafness to decrease. With falling rolls, the school looked set to close until the principal found herself inadvertently operating as one of the world's unsung pioneering advocates of inclusive education. Another teacher recounted:

> It all started when the Principal agreed to take in the child of a friend of hers who wasn't doing very well in the regular secondary school and the Principal said 'well, some of our deaf children are going a little slower so let her come here'.

Changes in intake followed as first one, then another, then another child came to the school NOT for the purposes of special education for children with hearing impairment, but because the school for 'children who can't be included' was self-evidently delivering inclusive education. One morning, I watched the children go about their school day. I saw John, a wheelchair user with little spoken language, being helped up the stairs by three ambulant boys, all of whom had learning difficulties. John was skillfully directing his more ambulant peers, laughing at their confusion when his limbs were hard to control and making them laugh. The boys made it to the top corridor in the manner of any four friends enjoying a challenge.

It seemed to me that if this group of children with many and complex impairments between them could be inclusive of each other then we must ask ourselves 'how hard can the project of inclusive education be?' What could children without impairments do to include John and what could being with John and his friends do to promote the learning and development of other children?

Breaking down barriers

So, what *are* the barriers to inclusive education?

Expertise?

It is often suggested that 'lack of professional expertise' is a barrier: perhaps teachers without specialist training will not be able to include children with impairments in teaching and learning. It may be that to effectively include a child with hearing impairment in teaching and learning, for example, it is necessary to have an in-depth knowledge of pediatric audiology or of sign language. Or is it, more realistically, that the drivers of inclusion will be found within any teacher who will work tirelessly to understand and remove the day-to-day disabling barriers that might create exclusion in the classroom? Again in Oman, I saw these possibilities brought to life recently when a young practitioner overcame immense fear and trepidation in coming to teach a group of profoundly deaf sign-language users for the first time, deciding to get on with the job of understanding and dismantling disabling barriers:

> Immediately I needed to access some kind of sign language or any kind of strategy for enabling communication. I had no chance for training so I used drawing and acting and finger spelling and joking and everything I could think of because I had to learn a way to become familiar with all the children in the school ... And I did!

This is not to denigrate the role of specialists in inclusive education. The role of speech and language therapists, physiotherapists, occupational therapists, and so on can be instrumental in dismantling barriers when practice is steeped in commitment to inclusive education. But, given the reality of funding for schools around the world, and the lightning speed at which children's lives flash by, it is very often essential to make inclusive education happen wherever we are and with whatever resources we happen to have to hand. Whilst there are no 'quick-fixes', *The Index for Inclusion* (Booth, 2011) and *Community-Based Rehabilitation: CBR Guidelines on Making International Development Inclusive for Disabled People* (WHO, 2011) both offer practical guidance on this.

Resources?

It is often suggested that resources required for inclusive education are prohibitive, yet in East Caribbean schools, where I have seen some excellent inclusive practice, only the salaries of teachers are provided for by the Ministry; infrastructure, resources and all other expenses relating to the school have to be raised through charitable efforts or by parents. Teachers tell me, as if this were a fact of all teachers' lives, that they 'sponsor the children who are too poor to travel here; some pay for a child's travel for years to keep a child coming' … 'if I have a little extra something at home I bring it in to share'. All over the world in the most under-resourced schools, there are teachers and teaching assistants getting on with the everyday job of minimising the barriers that create exclusion (Miles, 2009; Moore, 2008). Teachers are to be found working consistently and diligently to overcome structural, economic, organisational, political and any other barriers to inclusion which disabled children face, even though they frequently operate in a context visibly bereft of resources.

Risk?

It is often thought that inclusive education is 'too risky' for children with impairments – they might be bullied, knocked down or ridiculed, for example. 'All of these things', said Emma, contemplating how to manage her visual impairment and severe arthritis in a busy secondary school, 'could happen in any school'; 'I'd rather take the risk of being included and getting some more broken bones', says my son, 'than be Billy-no-mates.' Disabled scholar Paul Doyle looks back on his days in a segregated residential school: 'I hated this school. Nothing was happening academically for me. The evenings and weekends were worse. I did not really have any friends.' French et al. (2006) present many disturbing recollections of visually impaired adults thinking back to their years in segregated schools. Doyle's doctoral research sheds light on parallels between retrospective narratives of disabled adults who survived segregated settings, and feelings of marginalisation, oppression and despair being expressed by young disabled people about to leave segregated schools today (Doyle, forthcoming). In Doyle's study, disabled people leaving segregated schools articulate fear of an isolated future and lament the continued absence of relationships with non-disabled peers which has characterised their childhoods and which they know will consequently shade their life beyond school. Desire for inclusion is one of the most uppermost priorities in the lives of disabled children across the world and their parents and teachers and allies know it.

Of course, concerns about safe and respectful inclusion of children with impairments must always be embedded in any school culture and ethos. Again, in the words of a young Omani practitioner: 'I taught the non-disabled children to be inclusive. I just took them aside and talked to them. One girl said "I didn't know disabled children were the same as us but now I will play with them and I will tell everyone I know."' Risk is an integral part of ordinary development and campaign groups stress that disabled children would rather encounter risk than exclusion (Dunn and Moore, 2005).

Conclusion

There is no doubt that making education inclusive is inordinately hard work. Inclusion can mean different things to disabled children and young people, and their sense of what it means can change at any time.

In the Middle East, where for centuries gender, religion and poverty have functioned as determinants of exclusion layered on top of impairment, it is deeply encouraging to observe the first cohort of professionals being trained to work with disabled children and their families developing an infectious belief in both the value and possibility of inclusion for disabled children:

> I have learned not to stop when I find myself in front of the barriers that create exclusion. I must break them down ... I taught the teacher; I said 'don't expect that the disabled children won't achieve, just try'. I said 'don't expect the children will be afraid ... it might be we who are afraid.' (University of Nizwa, 2012)

They are passionate advocates of the unheard voices of disabled children and young people:

> Disabled children HAVE power and strength and they want to be in the community. The children hidden away in Class 3 say 'we are like you and we want to share with everything you do. We are human like you. We have the right to study and work and help build our country with you.' I want to take their message forward. (University of Nizwa, 2012)

Raising children's voices is never straightforward; they may be embarrassed to say what they want, they may say what they think adults want to hear, they may be differently articulate and those listening may have limited skills for accessing their views (Clough and Barton, 1998; Moore, 2000; Pomerantz et al., 2007). The more difficult it is to raise insider perspectives, the more we must endeavour to do so in order that disabled children can create their own recipes for inclusive education. In Jordan, a student teacher told me:

> people said Fajar would never talk and she would never speak but I wanted to try and I talked to her every day. And after six weeks I noticed that when she was with the other children she was excited and she would sort of sing. And her teacher said to me 'this is the first time in all of the year I have heard her voice'.

Herein lie the power and significance of resisting exclusion in education.

References

Allan, J. (2003) *Inclusion, Participation and Democracy: What is the Purpose?* Dordrecht: Kluwer.

Allan, J. (2008) *Rethinking Inclusion: The Philosophers of Difference in Practice.* Dordrecht: Springer.

Armstrong, F. (2002) 'The historical development of special education: humanitarian rationality or "wild profusion of entangled events"', *History of Education: Journal of the History of Education Society*, 31 (5): 437–56.

Bartley, J. (2010) That isn't Choice. Centre for Studies on Inclusive Education. Available at: www.csie.org.uk/news/index.shtml#120510 [accessed 30/07/10].

Barton, L. (2003) *Inclusive Education and Teacher Education: A Basis of Hope or a Discourse of Delusion.* Stevenage: Pear Tree Press.

Barton, L. (2004) 'Foreword', in F. Armstrong and M. Moore (eds), *Action Research for Inclusive Education: Changing Places, Changing Practices, Changing Minds.* London: RoutledgeFalmer. pp. x–xi.

Barton, L. (2012) Inclusive Education: What's in a Name? The Necessity of a Politics of Hope. Paper presented at the Centre for Disability Studies conference, 'Future Bright or Future in Crisis?', University of Leeds, 2 April.

Barton, L. and Armstrong, F. (2007) *Policy, Experience and Change: Cross-cultural Reflections on Inclusive Education.* Dordrecht: Springer.

Billington, T. and Pomerantz, M. (eds) (2004) *Children at the Margins.* Stoke-on-Trent: Trentham Books.

Booth, T. (2011) *The Index for Inclusion: Developing Learning and Participation in Schools* (3rd edn). Bristol: CSIE.

Clough, P. and Barton, L. (1998) *Articulating with Difficulty: Research Voices in Inclusive Education.* London: Paul Chapman.

CSIE (2012) *Centre for Studies on Inclusive Education: supporting inclusion, challenging exclusion.* Information Leaflet. Bristol: Centre for Studies on Inclusive Education.

Doyle, P. (forthcoming) Beyond Segregated School: Voices of Disabled School Leavers. PhD thesis to be submitted, University of Sheffield.

Dunn, K. and Moore, M. (2005) 'Developing accessible playspace in the UK: what they want and what works', *Children, Youth and Environments*, 15 (1): 331–53.

French, S. and Swain, J. (2004) 'Controlling inclusion in education: young disabled people's perspectives', in J. Swain, S. French, C. Barnes and C. Thomas (eds), *Disabling Barriers – Enabling Environments* (2nd edn). London: SAGE, pp. 169–75.

French, S., Swain, J., Atkinson, D. and Moore, M. (eds) (2006) *An Oral History of the Education of Visually Impaired Children: Telling Stories for Inclusive Futures.* Lampeter: Edwin Mellen Press.

Hemingway, J. and Armstrong, F. (2012) 'Space, place and inclusive learning', *International Journal of Inclusive Education*, 16 (5–6): 479–83.

Mason, M. (2008) *Dear Parents.* London: Inclusive Solutions.

Miles, S. (2009) 'Engaging with teachers' knowledge: promoting inclusion in Zambian schools', *Disability & Society*, 24 (5): 611–24.

Moore, M. (ed.) (2000) *Insider Perspectives on Inclusion: Raising Voices, Raising Issues.* Sheffield: Philip Armstrong.

Moore, M. (2008) 'Inclusive relationships: insights from teaching assistants on how schools can reach parents', in G. Richards and F. Armstrong (eds), *Key Issues for Teaching Assistants: Working in Diverse and Inclusive Classrooms.* London: Routledge. pp. 84–95.

Moore, M. (2010) 'Inclusion, narrative and voices of disabled children in Trinidad and St Lucia', in J. Lavia and M. Moore (eds), *Cross-cultural Perspectives on Policy and Practice*. London: Routledge. pp. 101–15.

Moore, M. (2011) 'Including parents with disabled children', in G. Richards and F. Armstrong (eds), *Teaching and Learning in Diverse and Inclusive Classrooms*. London: Routledge. pp. 133–44.

Moore, M. and Slee, R. (2012) 'Disability studies, inclusive education and exclusion', in C. Thomas, N. Watson and A. Roulstone (eds), *Routledge Handbook of Disability Studies*. London: Routledge. pp. 225–39.

Office of the Deputy Prime Minister (ODPM) (2003) *Developing Accessible Play Space: A Good Practice Guide*. London: ODPM/Twoten.

Pomerantz, K.A., Hughes, M. and Thompson, D. (eds) (2007) *How to Reach 'Hard to Reach' Children: Improving Access, Participation and Outcomes*. Chichester: Wiley.

Runswick-Cole, K. (2007) 'The experience of families who go to the Special Educational Needs and Disability Tribunal (SENDisT)', *Disability & Society*, 22 (3): 315–28.

Slee, R. (2011) *Irregular Schooling*. London: Routledge.

University of Nizwa (2012) *Quotations from Student Presentations, Diploma in Inclusive and Special Education*, University of Nizwa, Oman in association with Institute of Education, University of London.

Wertheimer, A. (1997) *Inclusive Education: A Framework for Change – National and International Perspectives*. Bristol: CSIE.

World Health Organization (WHO) (2011) *Community-Based Rehabilitation: CBR Guidelines on Making International Development Inclusive for Disabled People*. Geneva: WHO.

26

User Involvement in Services for Disabled People

Sally French

Robson et al. define user involvement as 'the participation of users of services in decisions that affect their lives' (2003: 2), and Croft and Beresford believe that 'speaking and acting for yourself and being part of mainstream society, lies at the heart of … service user involvement' (2002: 389). The concept of 'user involvement' is now well established within professional and managerial practice, in both health and social care, and enshrined within legislation and policy such as the Mental Health Act 2005 and the NHS Constitution (DoH, 2009). Although this can be viewed as progress, Martin (2012) reminds us that partnership is not necessarily linked to either influence or equality. Indeed, the enmeshment of user groups within mainstream policy can be regarded as a process of deradicalisation as user groups are compelled to work within professional, managerial and academic frameworks. As Martin states, 'influence comes at the cost of ceding control of agendas to the state rather than holding on to autonomy' (2012: 51).

Despite the legislation which pertains to user involvement in health and social care, it would be a mistake to imagine that government is entirely committed to it. In a report by the Labour Party's Public Administration Select Committee, for instance, it is stated:

> Involving service users is not always appropriate. In some circumstances it could create inequalities in services, as well as being risky and expensive. In other situations people may simply be unwilling or unable to engage in this way. A key challenge for the government and public service providers will therefore be to establish where user involvement is desirable and in what form. Service providers also need to ensure that user involvement complements – rather than conflicts with – the contribution made by public service workers. (2008: 8)

It is not surprising, therefore, that many service users are sceptical of government commitment to user involvement. There is much reported dissatisfaction with the process of user involvement among disabled people. For instance, Duffy (2008) reported the results of a questionnaire on user involvement in health and social care where 127 respondents out of 143 (89 per cent) reported dissatisfaction. A service user interviewed by Branfield states: 'The government is driving for user involvement, but a lot of it is not real ... They want passive user involvement' (2007: 11). Barnes and Gell (2012) believe that user involvement is frequently based on terms dictated by the organisation, and Cotterell and Morris (2012) believe that user involvement may be embarked on for reasons of professional legitimation rather than as a mechanism for change.

Methods of user involvement

Methods of involving users in health and social care can take many forms. Brown (2000) lists the following methods:

- residents' committees
- user panels
- customer surveys
- suggestion boxes
- involvement in management committees
- involvement in forums and working parties
- focus groups
- public meetings.

Goss and Miller (1995) depict user involvement as a ladder, with the top rung giving total control to users and the bottom rung giving no control at all (see Figure 1.2).

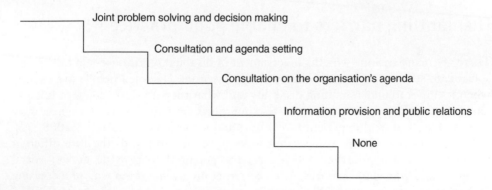

Figure 1.2 The Ladder of User Involvement

Bewley and Glendinning (1994) warn against relying heavily on any one method or model as none are perfect and a variety is needed to reach all disabled people. They note a heavy reliance on formal meetings in user involvement which, according to Duffy (2008), can reinforce power inequalities. Evans and Carmichael are particularly critical of the widespread use of public meetings in user involvement initiatives. They state:

> To engage in public meetings … demands, on the whole, familiarity and confidence with the normal style, format and language of these meetings. In addition very practical issues of physical access, transport, interpreters, signers, personal assistance and so on must be addressed by social and health services if disabled people are to be enabled to take part in consultation meetings. (2002: 20)

Swain et al. (2005) undertook a study on user involvement for a large charity which provides residential care for disabled people. Although it had in place various formal mechanisms for user involvement, such as committees and a disabled people's forum with paid disabled staff, formal involvement was viewed by many residents as ineffective within existing power relations and management structures. Although formal methods and structures may be necessary, Finlay et al. warn against the tendency to regard user involvement only in these terms rather than in regard to everyday interaction. They state:

> Empowerment is not just about choosing to take this kind of support rather than that or providing input into the evaluation and process of a service in structured situations, but is about what happens between people moment by moment, the mundane details of everyday interaction. Power permeates everyday life – it is exercised in the way people talk to each other, in what utterances are taken up and what are ignored, in how and what options are offered, in how information is presented, how spaces are opened up for people to express preferences and in how spaces are shut down. (2008: 350)

Dismantling barriers to enable good practice

There are many reasons why the involvement of disabled service users in health and social care services is not only necessary but essential. Disabled people are experts when it comes to understanding disability and what they need to achieve a full and happy life. As Dow, a service user states, 'our views are valuable, they are necessary and are based on real experience, real hurt and sometimes real anger' (2008: 52). Lester and Glasby (2006) believe that users of services bring to the fore different perspectives and approaches which have the potential to provide greater social inclusion and 'joined up' services. At its best, user involvement is a way of increasing the rights and dignity of disabled people.

However, many practical, organisational and cultural barriers need to be addressed if the involvement of disabled people in the management, planning and delivery of health and social care services is to become a reality. A central issue is the unequal power relationship between service users and professionals and managers. Dow states:

Power issues underlie the majority of identified difficulties with effective service led change. The message is that any service user participation initiative requires continual awareness of the context of power relations in which it is being conducted. (2008: 14)

People who are powerless and marginalised within society may not be able readily to express themselves, to make complaints or to effect change. Disabled people have frequently been disempowered by previous experiences, for example time spent in institutions, and need time, support and resources to build up sufficient confidence to participate fully. As O'Sullivan says:

A principle of sound decision-making practice is for clients to have the highest feasible level of involvement, but they may not always feel sufficiently empowered to make decisions ... Stakeholders need to consult with each other to share information but the presence of clients at these meetings is not sufficient in itself to ensure their involvement. Active steps may be required to prevent them being excluded from meaningful participation. (2000: 86)

Rice and Robson (2006) believe that membership by service users within governing bodies in health and social care is key to successful user involvement, although there is sometimes a level of seniority above which service users are not permitted to go (Straniszewska et al., 2012). Robson et al. (2003) note that a controlling style of management can be a strong and destructive barrier to user involvement and, conversely, a facilitatory style can be beneficial. Influential allies within the power structure can enhance the potential of service users to influence decisions, as can external groups such as disabled people's organisations.

'Knowledge is power' but all too often accessible information is lacking. Information needs to be accessible to all disabled people, regardless of impairment, if user involvement is to succeed. This may include information in Braille, in pictorial form or on audio CD. Disabled people, like all people, also need background information in order to participate meaningfully. Disabled people, however, face numerous barriers to accessing information, and are consequently marginalised unless this issue is resolved. Being unable to access information is, for instance, a problem faced in all areas of life by visually impaired people. Stereotypical responses to what people need, for instance assuming that all blind people read Braille, are also common.

A frequent complaint that disabled people make when they take part in user involvement initiatives is the lack of feedback they receive from researchers or managers about the impact of consultation (Duffy, 2008). Carr states that: 'lack of feedback can result in frustration and cynicism about the practice of service user participation as well as potential disengagement from the process altogether' (2004: 9). Duffy (2008) believes that user involvement must be related to tangible outcomes, and McSloy, a service user, says: 'Any involvement that does not value the use of people's time and wastes that time by not using the outcome to influence change should be questioned' (2008: 44). However, Straniszewska et al. (2012) believe that, at the present time, organisations, rather than users, predominantly define the outcomes of user involvement. These issues have led disabled people to become more selective in deciding when, how and to whom they will give their time, effort and views (Carmichael, 2004).

Services to people with learning difficulties have a history of being very poor. It is important that the views of people with learning difficulties and their allies are heard and that they are part of the user involvement movement in health and social care. This may take time and imagination but without it services are unlikely to improve. As Mencap states:

> the NHS has a poor track record in dealing effectively with people with a learning disability. As a result people with a learning disability have poorer health, greater health needs and shorter lives. There is a real concern that negative discriminatory attitudes and poor communication skills among healthcare staff contribute to this unfortunate state of affairs. (2004: 31)

One of the problems that is frequently mentioned in relation to the poor health status of people with learning difficulties is 'diagnostic overshadowing', where any problems or symptoms the person may have are viewed in terms of their learning difficulty (Mencap, 2004; DRC, 2006). This makes it difficult for people with learning difficulties, and those trying to assist them, to be taken seriously by health and social care professionals. An example of this is given by the mother of James, a man with learning difficulties:

> James kept telling me that he could see a 'funny black thing'. I took him along to see the optometrist, but he didn't seem to take us seriously. I knew that there was something wrong, so I kept taking him back. On our fourth visit James said: 'Black blob bigger'. This finally prompted the optometrist to have a look at the back of James' eyes. He found two detached retinas, which it has so far not been possible to repair. James has now been registered blind. (Mencap, 2004: 16)

Examples such as this illustrate the importance of including people with learning difficulties in the process of user involvement.

Disabled people are constantly accused of being unrepresentative when they express their views or when they attempt to speak on behalf of other disabled people (Lester and Glasby, 2006; Barnes and Cotterell, 2012; Beresford and Branfield, 2012). As Evans and Carmichael say: 'Representatives from organisations of disabled people, including self-advocacy groups, were sometimes dismissed by social and health service officers as being unrepresentative of users because they appeared to be too articulate to be "real" users' (2002: 22).

Similarly, Brown notes that 'users who represent the movement may not be representative in the sense of being "typical" ... this may be used to challenge the legitimacy of their position in speaking for others' (2000: 105). Lindow (1999) contends, however, that users are more likely to be representative than professionals and asks whether professionals would choose to send their least confident and articulate members to speak for them.

Furthermore, disabled people are often used in a tokenistic way, such as having just one disabled person on a committee, where they may feel isolated and have little or no power, although the service may be seen to be 'doing what it has to do' (Evans and Carmichael, 2002; Cotterell and Morris, 2012). Carers are also asked to represent disabled people, especially people with learning difficulties or those who cannot speak English even though their views may differ. Duffy (2008) found, for instance, that disabled children sometimes express differing views from their parents. Beresford and Campbell believe that managers and professionals, who follow such practices, are in no position to criticise the representativeness of disabled people. They state:

> Questions about the mandate of disabled people and service users ignore or deny the validity of the large and growing number of democratically constituted and controlled local, regional, national and international disabled people's, service users and self-advocacy groups and organisations to which they belong and which they are elected or chosen to represent. (1994: 316–17)

Conclusion

Disabled people are becoming empowered within society and are no longer prepared to have decisions made on their behalf. It is the challenge of professionals and managers in health and social care to ensure, not only that the involvement of disabled people is possible, but that it is extensive, meaningful and translated into practice with positive outcomes for disabled people's lives. Robson et al. make the point that 'When user involvement is second nature to enough people in an organisation it becomes "the way we do things round here" and, in a sense, ceases to exist as a separate or optional activity' (2003: 23). However, user involvement must aim to bring about change on disabled people's terms rather than being an 'add-on' which merely tinkers with decisions already made by those in power.

References

Barnes, M. and Cotterell, P. (2012) 'Introduction: user movements', in M. Barnes and P. Cotterell (eds), *Critical Perspectives on User Involvement*. Bristol: Policy Press. pp. 1–6.

Barnes, M. and Gell, C. (2012) 'The Nottingham advocacy group: a short history', in M. Barnes and P. Cotterell (eds), *Critical Perspectives on User Involvement*. Bristol: Policy Press. pp. 19–32.

Beresford, P. and Branfield, F. (2012) 'Building solidarity, ensuring diversity: lessons from service users' and disabled people's movements', in M. Barnes and P. Cotterell (eds), *Critical Perspectives on User Involvement*. Bristol: Policy Press. pp. 33–46.

Beresford, P. and Campbell, J. (1994) 'Disabled people, service users, user involvement and representation', *Disability & Society*, 9 (3): 315–25.

Bewley, C. and Glendinning, C. (1994) *Involving Disabled People in Community Care Planning*. York: Joseph Rowntree Foundation.

Branfield, F. (2007) *User Involvement in Social Work Education*. London: Shaping Our Lives National User Network.

Brown, H. (2000) 'Challenges from service users', in A. Brechin, H. Brown and M.A. Ely (eds), *Critical Practice in Health and Social Care*. London: SAGE. pp. 96–116.

Carmichael, A. (2004) 'The social model, the emancipatory paradigm and user involvement', in C. Barnes and G. Mercer (eds), *Implementing the Social Model of Disability: Theory and Research*. Leeds: The Disability Press. pp. 191–207.

Carr, S. (2004) *Has Service User Involvement Made a Difference to Social Care Services?* London: Social Institute for Excellence.

Cotterell, P. and Morris, C. (2012) 'The capacity, impact and challenge of service users' experiential knowledge', in M. Barnes and P. Cotterell (eds), *Critical Perspectives on User Involvement*. Bristol: Policy Press. pp. 57–69.

Croft, S. and Beresford, P. (2002) 'Service users' perspectives', in M. Davies (ed.), *Companion to Social Work* (2nd edn). Oxford: Blackwell. pp. 393–401.

Department of Health (DoH) (2009) *The NHS Constitution: The NHS Belongs to Us All*. London: Department of Health.

Disability Rights Commission (DRC) (2006) *Equal Treatment: Closing the Gap*. London: Disability Rights Commission.

Dow, J. (2008) 'Our journey: perspectives from people who use services', in M. McPhail (ed.), *Service User and Carer Involvement*. Edinburgh: Dunedin Academic Press. pp. 49–59.

Duffy, J. (2008) *Looking Out from the Middle: User Involvement in Health and Social Care in Northern Ireland*. London: Social Care Institute for Excellence.

Evans, C. and Carmichael, A. with members of the Direct Payment Best Value Project Group of Wiltshire and Swindon Users' Network (2002) *Users' Best Value: A Guide to User Involvement Good Practice in Best Value Reviews*. York: Joseph Rowntree Foundation.

Finlay, W.M.L., Walton, C. and Antaki, C. (2008) 'Promoting choice and control in residential services for people with learning disabilities', *Disability & Society*, 23 (4): 349–60.

Goss, S. and Miller, C. (1995) *From Margin to Mainstream: Developing User- and Carer-centred Community Care*. York: Joseph Rowntree Foundation.

Lester, H. and Glasby, J. (2006) *Mental Health Policy and Practice*. Basingstoke: Palgrave Macmillan.

Lindow, V. (1999) 'Power, lies and injustice: the exclusion of service user voices', in *Ethics and Community in the Health Care Professions*. London: Routledge.

Martin, G.P. (2012) 'Service users and the third sector: opportunities, challenges and potentials in influencing the governance of public services', in M. Barnes and P. Cotterell (eds), *Critical Perspectives on User Involvement*. Bristol: Policy Press. pp. 47–56.

McSloy, N. (2008) 'Expert knowledge: a carer's perspective', in M. McPhail (ed.), *Service User and Carer Involvement*. Edinburgh: Dunedin Academic Press. pp. 40–8.

Mencap (2004) *Treat Me Right: Better Healthcare for People with a Learning Disability*. London: Mencap.

O'Sullivan, T. (2000) 'Decision making in social work', in M. Davies (ed.), *The Blackwell Encyclopaedia of Social Work*. Oxford: Blackwell. pp. 85–7.

Public Administration Select Committee (2008) *User Involvement in Public Services: Sixth Report of Session 2007–08*. London: House of Commons.

Rice, B. and Robson, P. (2006) *Tipping Point: User Involvement Project*. Executive Summary. London: University of East London/RADAR.

Robson, P., Begun, N. and Locke, M. (2003) *Developing User Involvement: Working Towards User Centred Practice in Voluntary Organisations*. Bristol: Policy Press.

Straniszewska, S., Mockford, C., Gibson, A., Heron Marx, S. and Putz, R. (2012) 'Moving forward: understanding the negative experiences of patient and public involvement in health service planning, development and evaluation', in M. Barnes and P. Cotterell (eds), *Critical Perspectives on User Involvement*. Bristol: Policy Press. pp. 129–41.

Swain, J., Thirlaway, C. and French, S. (2005) *Independent Evaluation: Developing User Involvement in Leonard Cheshire*. London: Leonard Cheshire.

27

User-Led Organisations: Facilitating Independent Living?

Hannah Morgan

Introduction

That there has been a proliferation of organisations controlled and run by disabled people across the UK since the early 1980s is 'an indicator that the disability movement has come of age' (Harris and Roulstone, 2011: 119). These include centres for independent/inclusive living (CILs), local coalitions of disabled people, service user organisations and, more latterly, social enterprises and community interest companies. What unites these diverse organisations is a commitment to the social model of disability and to having a constitutional structure that ensures control rests with disabled people. The movement has been bolstered by successive governments' commitments to greater choice and control for disabled people and to promoting the development of user-led organisations encapsulated in the (still unmet) 2005 commitment that 'by 2010, each locality (defined as that area covered by a Council with social services responsibilities) should have a user-led organisation modelled on existing CILs' (Cabinet Office, 2005: 91).

The language used to describe disabled people's organisations has, and continues, to evolve. The terminology used varies and some terms are used interchangeably. Different documents refer to DPOs (Disabled People's Organisations), ULOs (User Led Organisations) and increasingly to DPULOs (Disabled People's User Led Organisations). The following definitions capture the essence of the way in which the first two terms are used:

- A disabled people's organisation is 'an organisation whose constitution requires it to have a membership and management board with a majority of disabled people and whose objectives are the rights and equality of disabled people' (Disability Listen Include Build, 2008: 11).

- A user-led organisation is 'one where the people the organisation represents (or provides a service to) have a majority on the Management Committee or Board, and where there is clear accountability to members and/or service users' (Morris, 2006: 3).

Some organisations will be both a DPO and a ULO, while others, such as *Shaping Our Lives* which is a national network of service users and disabled people, draws in non-disabled people who use services, such as children and young people in the care system. The term DPULO is used throughout this chapter to refer to organisations that are controlled and run by disabled people.

This chapter begins by outlining what independent living has come to mean in the UK before moving on to consider why it has been viewed as essential by the disabled people's movement that the practical application of this approach should be controlled and implemented by disabled people. There is then an overview of the nature, scope and purpose of DPULOs, focusing especially on what distinguishes them from other ostensibly similar organisations. The discussion focuses on the distinctive contribution DPULOs make to the lives of disabled people and to challenging disablism on a wider scale. The chapter ends by considering the current position of the ULO community and in particular the challenges they face at a time when many in the wider disability field are appropriating the language and style of the disabled people's movement.

Independent living

Life is more than just a house and getting up and going to bed. Independent Living is about the whole of life and it encompasses everything. We want equal opportunities. We want citizenship. These are the issues that drive the independent living movement. It is philosophical, it is political, it is about integration and disabled people becoming a part of this world and not separate, segregated and second class. That is what we are actually after and that is why independent living is so important. (Evans, 1993: 63)

As this quote from John Evans, one of the leaders of the independent living movement, suggests, independent living is a way of combatting the oppression and discrimination disabled people endure. Independent living can be viewed as both a philosophy and a practice. As a philosophy, it shares many of the central tenets of the social model of disability and questions the way in which an individualistic understanding of 'independence', meaning people have to be able to do everything themselves, has come to dominate policy and practice in western industrial societies.

Understandings of disability which assume that disabled people are inherently and inevitably dependent and requiring 'care' to meet their needs have been so dominant that the resulting *hegemony of care* has pervaded policy and practice cultures. This has meant that the ways in which services and other forms of support are organised have created and perpetuated the physical, financial and psychological dependency of large numbers of disabled people in a way that would be unacceptable to non-disabled people. This has usually occurred through the provision of 'special' and usually segregated services that take disabled people's dependency for granted and view it unproblematically. The result is that disabled people are excluded from exercising many of the rights and responsibilities that most non-disabled people take for granted, such as having a job or raising a family.

The alternative understanding of disability provided by a social model analysis enables disabled people and their allies to turn traditional and taken-for-granted assumptions about disability on their heads. As a result, independent living groups have pioneered innovative and effective ways of working to enable disabled people to exercise choice and control in their lives and to allow them to participate within society on equal terms with non-disabled people.

In contrast to the independent living movement in the USA where the focus was more on the individual and on self-help, in the UK independent living 'entailed collective responsibilities for each other and a collective organisation. Independent living wasn't about individual empowerment; it was about individuals helping one another' (Campbell and Oliver, 1996: 204). Thus, DPULOs have tended to focus on collective forms of action such as campaigning and placed a particular emphasis on peer support. Peer (or peer-to-peer) support is where one disabled person draws on their own experience, knowledge and skills to support another disabled person. Peer support recognises the value of sharing the lived experience of disability and the contribution disabled people can make to one another. A review of peer support undertaken for the Department of Health found that it is frequently 'an effective method of achieving a range of goals', especially in relation to making choices about support needs where 'Such support would appear to be an essential element in giving people opportunities to control their own lives' (NCIL, 2008: 32). Peer support has been at the heart of all DPULOs.

Defining characteristics of disabled people's user-led organisations

The most essential characteristic of a DPULO is that it is an organisation *of* rather than *for* disabled people. There has been a sustained and successful critique of the dominance of organisations for disabled people, often large well-funded charities such as Scope and Mencap, who seek to both represent disabled people in policy discussions and to provide services to meet their needs. Until relatively recently, these organisations adopted what Oliver (2004) termed a *humanitarian approach* to the welfare of disabled people. This approach privileged the knowledge and expertise of professionals who provided services to disabled people on the basis of individualised and medical understandings of disability. Disabled people became dependent on services over which they had no control, that frequently did not meet their needs and which were contingent on the assessment of professionals. Inherent in this approach was a paternalistic 'we know best' assumption about the needs and aspirations of disabled people, an assumption that has been refuted by disabled people since the early work of Paul Hunt (1966).

There is consensus that DPULOs should be social model organisations, that is they should have a formal commitment to the principles of the social model and be controlled by disabled people (Barnes and Mercer, 2006: 83). Participants in an evaluation of DPULOs identified five criteria that they should aspire to:

- adopt a social model approach to the development and operation of services
- provide disabled people with meaningful choice and control
- be flexible and responsive to the needs and wishes of local disabled people
- be inclusive and offer services based on the common experience of disability
- meet a range of core services, while it was agreed that CILs should also respond to local needs. (Barnes et al., 2000: 8)

The way in which this is implemented on the ground varies considerably, with DPULOs providing a diverse array of services and campaigning on a wide range of topics at a local and national level.

Derbyshire CIL produced a list of *seven needs* that need to be met if disabled people are to achieve independent living:

- information
- counselling/peer support
- housing
- technical aids and equipment
- personal assistance
- transport
- access to the built environment (Davis, 1990).

Hampshire and Southampton CILs added a further five areas, which they termed *basic rights*:

- inclusive education and training
- adequate income
- equal opportunities for employment
- advocacy
- appropriate healthcare provision (Woodin, 2006).

These combined lists have been adopted by many DPULOs as the framework for their activities. Writing in 2007 as the result of a project that mapped the capacity of ULOs in England, Maynard-Campbell et al. identified a range of expertise contained within the ULO community that includes:

- peer support, mentoring and empowerment
- direct payments advice and support

- knowing what accessible features, environments and facilities are required for participation to be physically inclusive to all
- support for consultation and involvement
- provision of interpreting and transcription services
- employment and education support
- access auditing
- Disability Equality and diversity training
- knowledge of the Disability Discrimination Act and other disability-specific legislation
- accessible housing and transport
- delivery of research, consultancy and training (2007: 8).

The manifold services and facilities provided by DPULOs span the whole gamut of disabled people's lives, from promoting inclusive education and providing support to disabled people and their families seeking to navigate the complex health and welfare terrain, to assisting mainstream providers of services in meeting their obligations to disabled customers and being a proactive voice of disabled people in policy discussions. DPULOs now occupy, formally at least, a central and influential position in shaping and leading disability policy and the provision of services seeking to meet the needs and aspirations of disabled people.

Threats and challenges facing DPULOs

However, while DPULOs enjoy significant levels of support, particularly at a national and policy level, their position often remains precarious (Barnes and Mercer, 2006; Maynard-Campbell et al., 2007). As with the social model of disability, the concept of independent living has been adopted as a goal by many disability organisations. A wide range of service providers in the public, voluntary and private sectors claim that independent living for disabled people is now their guiding principle. However, there is often a gap between the aspirations of disabled people to be in control and the ways in which some 'independent living' services have been implemented. Jenny Morris (2011), amongst others, warns of the dangers of the language and ideas of the disabled people's movement being appropriated by policy makers and service providers.

   This creates a tension at the heart of the DPULO movement. As more local authorities and traditional service providers and charities adopt the formal trappings of a DPULO (such as commitment to the social model and a majority of disabled people on the management committee), it is becoming increasingly difficult to tell them apart. The result is frequently to the detriment of genuinely user-led organisations which rarely attract the levels of funding and high-level policy access enjoyed by the large disability charities (Barnes and Mercer, 2006). The result is that 'these organizational wolves in sheep's clothing are then able to compete with DPOs for scarce resources, threating the very existence of some DPOs' (Disability Listen Include Build,

2008: 13). While, as Morris argues, 'adjusting one's language to suit the prevailing discourse' may be a pragmatic and often effective strategy to adopt, it does leave the ULO community and wider disability movement vulnerable to colonisation.

Gibbs, formerly an influential member of staff at DCIL, asserts that social model services provided by statutory and traditional providers are an oxymoron, that is, a contradiction in terms. He contends that such providers are locked into an approach that is at odds with the philosophy and principles of independent living. He goes on to argue that:

> the social model is non-reducible, it cannot be implemented by any programme of services that is separate from other functions. Even within the disabled people's movement, it is commonly believed that 'service provider' and 'lobbying' functions are incompatible in a single organisation. To the contrary, the social model cannot be applied by either on its own. (2004: 158)

This is illustrated by the way in which one of the original Centres for Independent Living in Derbyshire has evolved (DCIL, undated). Derbyshire Coalition of Disabled People was established in 1981 as a democratic representative organisation of disabled people. It received funding from the county council and focused on campaigning and peer support. The Coalition worked in collaboration with the local authority to set up a Centre for Integrated Living (CIL) in 1986, with a commitment to the social model and the seven needs of disabled people underpinning the venture. The CIL provided a range of services, including the training and provision of peer counsellors, direct payment support and an employment service, as well as providing employment and volunteering opportunities for local disabled people.

The functions of the two organisations were separate although the membership overlapped; the Coalition was a campaigning organisation while the CIL developed 'practical applications' of a social model perspective. This arrangement was felt to give the Coalition freedom to pursue campaigns that targeted the local authority while also allowing the CIL to develop the more formal structures required of a service provider. A review was undertaken in 1996 when it became clear the funding and political landscape was making it difficult to 'safeguard the original wide-ranging objectives and community emphasis' of the organisations (DCIL, undated). The result was the formation of Derbyshire Coalition for Inclusive Living, a title that was felt to be a more accurate description of the county-wide work of the organisation, while the shift from integrated to inclusive was seen to resonate more closely with a social model emphasis on challenging disablism rather than integrating disabled people into society (Barnes and Mercer, 2006: 78). DCIL describes itself as a DPULO and is run by a board of directors elected by members.

While the value and contribution of DPULOs have been acknowledged in key policy documents and in independent evaluations of DPULOs (such as Barnes and Mercer, 2006), providing formal evidence of the added value provided by DPU-LOs has been less easy. Methods such as calculating the 'social return on investment' explored by Lewis and Roulstone (2010) have the potential to capture the less tangible benefits created by DPULOs in a format funders and commissioners understand. Becoming increasingly 'savvy' in terms of their engagement with policy makers and commissioners may run the risk of incorporation or naturalisation, however, without it, DPULOs are in danger of appearing marginal, amateurish or overtly political.

Conclusion: The future of DPULOs in an age of austerity

While an emphasis on the 'big society' and the priority afforded to DPULOs by government appear to offer great potential to DPULOs, disabled people have been amongst the hardest hit by the swingeing cuts to public sector services and implementation of 'welfare reform' by the Coalition government (Wood, 2012). There is a contradiction between policy rhetoric that says DPULOs have a vital role to play and the still relatively minor funding they secure compared to traditional disability charities. Moreover, austerity creates very real threats for disabled people and their organisations, most obviously in relation to crises in funding opportunities. However, it also has the potential to open up new opportunities. Resistance to the cuts offered by disabled people has reinvigorated the campaigning element of DPULOs and their allies (see Disabled People Against the Cuts at www.dpac.uk.net, for example). Local and national government are having to think much more creatively about how to 'do more with less', and this provides the scope for DPULOs who have an established track record in providing innovative and effective solutions.

References

Barnes, C. and Mercer, G. (2006) *Independent Futures: Creating User-Led Disability Services in a Disabling Society*. Bristol: Policy Press.

Barnes, C., Mercer, G. and Morgan, H. (2000) *Creating Independent Futures: An Evaluation of Services Led by Disabled People – Stage One Report*. Leeds: The Disability Press. Available at: www.leeds.ac.uk/disability-studies/archiveuk/Barnes/Report.pdf.

Cabinet Office (2005) Improving the Life Chances of Disabled People. Available at: www. dh.gov.uk/en/Publicationsandstatistics/Publications/PublicationsPolicyAndGuidance/ DH_4101751

Campbell, J. and Oliver, M. (1996) *Disability Politics: Understanding Our Past, Changing Our Future*. London: Routledge.

Davis, K. (1990) A Social Barriers Model of Disability: Theory into Practice – The Emergence of the 'Seven Needs'. Available at: www.leeds.ac.uk/disability-studies/archiveuk/DavisK/ davis-social%20barriers.pdf

Derbyshire Coalition of Inclusive Living (DCIL) (undated) History. Available at: www.dcil. org.uk/about-us/history-of-ddcil/history [accessed 16/07/12].

Disability Listen Include Build (2008) *Thriving or Surviving: Challenges and Opportunities for Disabled People's Organisations in the 21st Century*. London: Scope. Available at www.disabilitylib.org.uk/images/stories/DisabilityLIB_report.pdf

Evans, J. (1993) 'The role of centres of independent/integrated living', in C. Barnes (ed.), *Making Our Own Choices: Independent Living, Personal Assistance and Disabled People*. Clay Cross: BCODP. Available at http://disability-studies.leeds.ac.uk/files/library/Barnes-making-our-own-choices.pdf.

Gibbs, D (2004) 'Social model services: an oxymoron?', in C. Barnes and G. Mercer (eds), *Disability Policy and Practice: Applying the Social Model*. Leeds: The Disability Press.

Harris, J. and Roulstone, A. (2011) *Disability, Policy and Professional Practice*. London: Sage.

Hunt, P. (ed.) (1966) *Stigma: The Experience of Disability*. London: Geoffrey Chapman. Also available at: www.leeds.ac.uk/disability-studies/archiveuk/Hunt/Foreword.pdf

Lewis, R. and Roulstone, A. (2010) The Social Return on Investment of User Led Organisations: Final Report. Commissioned by Vision Sense, on behalf of the North East User-Led Organisation Network.

Maynard-Campbell, S., Maynard, A. and Winchcombe, M. (2007) *Mapping the Capacity and Potential for User-Led Organisations in England: A Summary of the Main Findings from a National Research Study Commissioned by the Department of Health*. London: Department of Health.

Morris, J. (2006) Centres for Independent Living/Local User-Led Organisations. A discussion paper. London: Department of Health. Available at: www.dh.gov.uk/en/publicationsandstatistics/publications/publicationspolicyandguidance/DH_078838

Morris, J. (2011) *Rethinking Disability Policy*. York: Joseph Rowntree Foundation. Available at: www.jrf.org.uk/publications/rethinking-disability-policy

National Centre for Independent Living (NCIL) (2008) *Review of Peer Support Activity in the Context of Self-Directed Support and the Personalisation of Adult Social Care*. London: NCIL. Available at: www.ncil.org.uk/imageuploads/Peer%20support%20Final%201.doc

Oliver, M. (2004) 'The social model in action: if I had a hammer', in C. Barnes and G. Mercer (eds), *Implementing the Social Model of Disability: Theory and Research*. Leeds: The Disability Press. pp. 18–32.

Wood, C. (2012) 'For disabled people the worst is yet to come', in *Destination Unknown: Summer 2012*. London: Demos. Available at: www.demos.co.uk/publications/destinationunknown summer2012

Woodin, S. (2006) Mapping User-Led Organisations: User-Led Services and Centres for Independent/Integrated/Inclusive Living. A literature review prepared for the Department of Health. Available at: www.leeds.ac.uk/disability-studies/archiveuk/woodin/v2%20 user%20led%20-%20CIL%20Literature%20Review%203.pdf

28

Accessing Social and Leisure Activities: Barriers to Inclusion Experienced by Visually Impaired People

Donna Marie Brown, Pauline Gertig and Maureen Gillman, with Joyce Anderson, Cathy Clarke and Simon Powell

The Social In-Sight project is a disabled people's user led research project based at Newcastle Society for Blind People. It seeks to understand, identify and dismantle disabling barriers faced by Visually Impaired people when attempting to access mainstream social and leisure activities. Members of the project include the named authors of this chapter as well as Martin Horsley, Lee Cawkwell, Lisa Charlton, Julie Irvine, and Pam Satterthwaite.

Introduction

This chapter will discuss the themes that have emerged from the first stage of a piece of user-led research into the barriers experienced by visually impaired people when accessing social and leisure activities. The Access to Social and Leisure Activities Group is a collaborative project supported by Newcastle Society for Blind People (NSBP) in partnership with Northumbria University and the local Sensory Support Team of Newcastle City Council. The project began in March 2011 and is ongoing.

The aim of the first stage of the project is to explore visually impaired people's experiences of accessing mainstream social and leisure activities. The initiative for this project came from visually impaired people themselves who wanted to investigate these issues. The project is driven by visually impaired people who have designed and conducted the research.

The project is user-led and is informed by, and adheres to, the social model of disability. Many visually impaired people experience barriers to inclusion when attempting to access mainstream social and leisure activities in their local communities. These include, but are not limited to:

- inaccessible information
- inaccessible environments
- disabling attitudes, for example, stereotypical attitudes, such as perceptions of visually impaired people as a health and safety risk, as objects of pity or patronage, or as people who are dependent on others.

The case studies emerging from the research begin to explore what these barriers mean in real terms for visually impaired people. As social and leisure activities are now acknowledged as being essential to a person's health and well-being, it is important to identify and dismantle these barriers so that visually impaired people can enjoy the same mainstream facilities as non-disabled people.

The remainder of this chapter will discuss the unique nature of the research activity with specific reference to the emancipatory approach taken (see Chapter 6). It will then go on to discuss narrative accounts that have been generated by visually impaired people in relation to the barriers that they have faced in accessing mainstream social and leisure activities.

Research methodology: The emancipatory approach

As opposed to producing research *on* or *for* visually impaired people, the project aims to be fully participatory, working *with* volunteers and providing training and support, to enable them to design, conduct, analyse and disseminate social research themselves. This project is qualitative in nature due to the everyday life experiences that it aims to capture. Oliver, one of the key proponents of the emancipatory approach, suggests that it 'is about the facilitating of a politics of the possible by confronting social oppression at whatever levels it occurs' (1992: 110). This approach is essentially about the empowerment of disabled people through changing both the research process and production, and addresses the key characteristics of accountability, the role of the social model of disability, and the choice of methods and outcomes (Barnes, 2003).

The key steps that have been taken to ensure that this research is emancipatory are:

- The research topic, aims and questions were all designed by visually impaired people. They therefore seek to be meaningful to the participants and demonstrate a key area that they feel deserves further attention.
- The research methods used were chosen by the volunteer researchers to ensure that they were accessible. The volunteer researchers will be at the centre of the data generation phase as traditional boundaries between the 'researcher' and the 'researched' are collapsed (Duckett and Pratt, 2011).
- The narrative accounts that were produced at stage one are reflective of the personal stories of the research volunteers. They serve as a medium through which people's everyday experiences can be told.
- The volunteer researchers will go on to play a central role in the next stages of the research project, including completing data generation, analysis and dissemination.

The role of the University team is to support volunteer researchers in becoming the main drivers in the construction of knowledge. As Oliver argues:

> The issue then for the emancipatory research paradigm is not how to empower people but, once people have decided to empower themselves, precisely what research can then do to facilitate this process. This does then mean that the social relations of research production do have to be fundamentally changed; researchers have to learn how to put their knowledge and skills at the disposal of their research participants, for them to use in whatever ways they choose. (1992: 111)

The key way that this issue has been addressed is by responding to the requests of the visually impaired research volunteers and ensuring that the skills of the Northumbria University team are used to train them to conduct the primary investigation themselves as opposed to being the subjects of the research. Training and support, in this project, are therefore pivotal to the emancipatory approach. The project aims to develop the research capacity of the volunteer researchers so that their skills can continue to be used once this particular project has been completed.

In phase one of the study, visually impaired volunteer researchers produced narrative accounts of their own experience of accessing social and leisure activities. The next section of this chapter will discuss the accounts in relation to the barriers encountered.

Narrative accounts: The key themes emerging from everyday experience

Non-disabled people are probably not aware of the degree of preparation and planning required by visually impaired people before accessing a social or leisure experience. Whilst non-disabled people are often able to be spontaneous about going out to the cinema or for a meal at a restaurant, they may be surprised at the degree of organisation required for a visually impaired person to access the same activity. Joyce describes her attempts at organising a trip to a cinema that offered audio description:

I first telephoned the cinema and spoke to a young lady who told me that they had a Loop System and Sub Titled films and when I again pointed out that I was visually impaired not deaf she went off to seek assistance. She kept me hanging on for several minutes then returned to inform me that the technical manager was not available. I left my email address and asked him to contact me which he did the next day. However, he said that because of technical problems they were unable to offer audio-described films. Finally using a premium rate telephone number (10p per minute) I rang another cinema and after pressing many numbers and choosing numerous options I actually managed to speak to a human. After much to-ing and fro-ing and being put on hold for what seemed like an hour she informed me that there was no audio described films at their cinema in Newcastle but they were available in their cinema 10 miles away. So persistence does work but after all that telephoning and emailing I do not have any energy left for a cinema visit.

Although there are sometimes concessions available in certain venues, rules and procedures for accessing concessions are not consistent. As Maureen described:

I wanted to see an Irish folk singer at a local venue. I phoned to ask about concessions and was told that I would have to produce a letter from my GP confirming I was blind. When I said that I could show them the letter from the local authority confirming my registration 14 years ago, I was told that this was out of date and that I might have been cured since then!

Preparation for accessing leisure activities includes negotiating with service providers and organisers about the 'reasonable adjustments' required in order to access the facility. This is in direct contrast to non-disabled people who are able to turn up at the venue with the expectation that all will be well. A common experience for the people involved in this study was that despite such negotiations, the staff seemed curiously unprepared for a visually impaired person to join the activity. As Simon discussed:

I stood in the gym for about 5 minutes and guess what, no greeting, no challenge by staff, nothing at all. I would have imagined that, if someone was standing in the doorway, looking lost, dazed and somewhat apprehensive, a question or two might have been in order. This was despite the fact that I had telephoned the gym prior to going and I had explained that I was blind.

Even prior knowledge of the barriers that a visually impaired person might face in a particular activity does not always help. As Maureen noted:

I had been in a choir before so could anticipate some of the barriers I would meet when trying to join another choir. I contacted the choir leader and told her that I would like to join and that I was visually impaired. I explained that I was unable to read print on paper so would need the lyrics of the material each week sent electronically so that I could learn the words. It is impossible to learn a part in the choir if you do not have access to the words. The choir leader promised to let me have the lyrics in good time to learn the words. The choir is on a Monday evening and by Saturday I had not received any lyrics. I emailed her and eventually got the lyrics on Sunday evening – so 24 hours to learn 3 pieces of music and I was out most of Monday!

For many visually impaired people, the first barrier they face when attempting to access a leisure facility is actually getting there. Transport is a major headache for many and encompasses a variety of disabling barriers. Structural inequalities in the lives of many disabled people include the inadequacy of benefits to allow them to use taxis, which, for many, are essential and not a luxury. Simon commented that:

Getting to the gym has become relatively easy these days. I am the proud owner of a Taxi card. This gives me up to £125 a year off taxis. The rules and regulations surrounding this are something of an assault course and I found myself jumping through many bureaucratic hoops in order to obtain one.

Maureen also highlighted that:

The cost of the taxi fare is another barrier – 14 pounds every week!

Whilst there are schemes available to reduce the cost of transport for disabled people, visually impaired people face another barrier when attempting to access these benefits: 80 per cent of all information is in print and much of it is inaccessible to visually impaired people, and 70 per cent of all websites are inaccessible to visually impaired people (RNIB, 2012). Many visually impaired people are unaware of the existence of such schemes because they cannot access information about them.

Many visually impaired participants experienced difficulties with some taxi drivers who appeared to have no awareness about visual impairment. As Maureen described:

I had to get a taxi to the choir and the taxi firm could not initially find the entrance to the school where the choir is held. He kept asking me for directions! He eventually found it and I asked if he would drive into the school and find the building for me. He was not too impressed with this request!

Cathy made the point that some taxi firms have a ring-back service which is helpful to visually impaired people. The firm will ring when the taxi is approaching and also give information about the make and colour of the taxi. This means that a visually impaired person can use any residual vision they may have to try to see which way the car is pointing when it arrives. This can save the embarrassment of getting into someone's car in the mistaken belief that it is your taxi!

Travelling by bus can also be a challenge. As Cathy discussed:

> The stop was on a main road with lots of traffic and if there was no one there to ask for assistance I had to stand at the kerbside with my hand out because I could not see the buses coming and they did not stop unless you put your hand out or there was a passenger getting off there. I can't remember how many times a bus went past me. When they did stop, I had to ask them if they went to the city centre or what number they were.

Preparation and planning for a night out also includes making arrangements to meet friends. Most visually impaired people try to anticipate problems they may face in finding friends in crowded places, as illustrated by the following quote from Cathy:

> My friends know to have their mobile phones at the ready because I ring them as the taxi is pulling up. That way they can either come to meet me at the door or they can tell me where they are. Although meeting with someone else who has a visual impairment can end up with both parties standing either side of the door wondering where the other one is! Mobile phones are a godsend to people with a visual impairment!

Some of the most difficult barriers to inclusion to overcome are attitudinal. Lack of disability or vision awareness may be one reason why non-disabled people seem to find it difficult to know how to 'go on' when faced with a visually impaired person. As noted in Simon's account of a visit to the gym, this can result in some difficult encounters for all concerned:

> I successfully navigated my way to reception and duly paid. In return, I was given a thick rubber band, with no explanation. Ok then ... Did they want their Hoover repairing? This was a supervised session in that it was specifically aimed at disabled people. Yet, there was only one member of staff on duty. Also, any disabled person has priority access to the equipment over the able bodied. So why did a fellow, able-bodied patron flatly refuse to vacate the accessible treadmill? He was quite abrupt with the staff member who completely failed to press my rights. There are other treadmills but this one has tactile controls and so I could speed it up or slow it down as I wished. The others do not have this functionality and I need constant supervision which was neither forthcoming nor available. (Simon)

Sometimes the accumulation of a number of barriers to inclusion has a multiplicative effect on the visually impaired person who is attempting to access a leisure facility. Most people have reported a temptation to give up trying in the face of so many obstacles. This was highlighted by Maureen in her account of trying to become part of a choir:

> The first barrier encountered was when we started the warm-up exercises. The choir leader did not describe or say what we should do. I suddenly became aware that

people near me seemed to be flinging their arms about, touching their toes, doing neck exercises, etc. – apparently all following the lead of the choir leader. I had no idea what they were doing! Rather than speak out in front of 45 people I just stood around and waited for them to stop! Presumably the choir leader noticed this but she has not changed her way of doing this. The problem continues of receiving the lyrics in time to learn the words before the session. Last week I received some lyrics on Monday afternoon so was unable to learn the words in time. So everyone else sang this particular piece whilst I stood there like a lemon! It was also the last thing we did before the end of the session and it sort of ruined my night.

Conclusion

There is a distinct lack of critical research engaging with visually impaired people to understand what the barriers to social and leisure activities are, and how they can be dismantled or overcome. In addition to physical, financial and personal barriers, negative attitudes and misunderstandings about visual impairment are considered to exclude people from employment, education and social activities (Pocklington Trust, 2011). This is set against a background in which participation in social and leisure activities is deemed crucial for building confidence, self-esteem and the general acquisition of skills that promote interaction and participation in the community (Raghavan et al., 2011).

The research project discussed in this chapter aims to address the existing research gap by working with visually impaired people to understand what barriers they face in their everyday lives. As the personal narratives above reveal, the challenges that visually impaired people confront when trying to access social and leisure activities are manifold. Bringing to life and understanding the barriers that exist is important, however it is not enough to stimulate change.

The visually impaired research volunteers involved in this project will go on to interview other visually impaired people to further unpack the barriers that they face in accessing social and leisure activities. As the project is emancipatory, however, it will not end there; instead it will seek to challenge and dismantle some of the barriers that are encountered.

We anticipate that 'mystery shopping' visits to a range of social and leisure activities will be completed by trained volunteer researchers. The data generated by the site visits will be analysed and used to structure interview questions for the service providers. The volunteer researchers will then go on to interview service providers and disseminate the findings of the research to all participants. To challenge the barriers, the service providers will be informed about examples of good practice and notified of areas that have been identified as opportunities for improvement.

To begin to challenge some of the barriers that are excluding visually impaired people, vision awareness training will be offered to all service providers. It is by challenging the barriers that exist that we hope to stimulate change that empowers visually impaired people who have been routinely marginalised from social and lei-sure activities and the benefits they bring.

References

Barnes, C. (2003) 'What a difference a decade makes: reflections on doing "emancipatory" disability research', *Disability & Society*, 18 (1): 3–17.

Duckett, P.D. and Pratt, R. (2011) 'The researched opinions on research: visually impaired people and visual impairment research', *Disability & Society*, 16 (6): 815–35.

Oliver, M. (1992) 'Changing the social relations of research production', *Disability, Handicap & Society*, 7 (2): 101–15.

Pocklington Trust (2011) *Older People and Sight Loss*. Information booklet. London: Pocklington Trust.

Raghavan, R., Pawson, N., Riasat, A. and Benn, D. (2011) *Access to Inclusive Play*. Bradford: Bradford Council.

Royal National Institute of Blind People (RNIB) (2012) *See it Right*. Available at: www.rnib.org.uk/professionals/accessibleinformation/pages/see_it_right.aspx (accessed 01/06/2012).

29

Disability, Sport and Exercising Bodies

Brett Smith and Anthony Papathomas

There has been growing interest in the physical activities of sport and exercise across the fields of disability studies, the sociology of sport, and sport and exercise psychology. However, these three fields have tended to progress in relative isolation when it comes to disability, sport and exercise (Smith and Perrier, in press). In this chapter, we bring together a selection of work from these fields under the following themes: elite disability sport, barriers to activity, and health and well-being. We close this partial review with some thoughts about future work.

Elite disability sport

Much has been written on this. For example, it has been highlighted that disability organised sport grew out of many people, communities, countries and organisations. This included sport organised by deaf communities in Germany in 1888 and by Sir Ludwig Guttmann and colleagues in England in 1948 for spinal cord injured people. In 1989, the International Paralympic Committee was founded to organise multi-disability competitions for a range of disabled people. Today, we have the Summer and Winter Paralympic Games, with approximately 4000 athletes from over 100 countries competing. In addition to the history of disability sport, much has been written on the classification of disabled athletes and on how disabled athletes are represented in the media (e.g. Thomas and Smith, 2009). There is work too on psychological skills training for enhancing sporting performance (e.g. Martin, 2010). How the Paralympic movement might not remedy the tragedy of disability, but rather continually reproduce the figure of the tragic disabled in order to reproduce itself has also been much talked about (e.g. Peers, 2009).

Extending the focus on elite sport, more recent work has investigated sporting members' perceptions of the Paralympics. For example, to understand perceptions, Purdue and Howe (2012) interviewed Paralympic stakeholders. These included current and former Paralympians as well as active and retired disability sport administrators. Purdue and Howe found that some stakeholders felt a need to appreciate the Paralympic Games as an elite sport competition that was unavoidably and positively flavoured by the presence of impaired bodies and disabled people. However, many other Paralympic stakeholders perceived the Paralympic Games simply as an elite sport event, in which impairment and disability should be largely ignored. Instead of placing value on seeing both the sport and the disability, they felt that the Paralympic Games should be about sport, not disability. Recent work on coaching in disability sport has found similar perceptions. Tawse et al. (2012) interviewed male, disabled wheelchair rugby coaches and one able-bodied coach. All coaches stated that rather than view their players as 'quads', they viewed them purely as athletes who should adopt an elite athlete mindset. Thus, once again, we see an attitude from sporting members in which sport dominates and disability is pushed firmly into the background.

Another topic researchers have recently focused on is technology, performance enhancement and disability – that is, the techno-doping of people with impairments in sport. The case of 'bladerunner' Oscar Pistorius in particular has been debated in relation to dominant notions of body and normality, transhumanism, Olympic and Paralympic values, and the reproduction of new inequalities and asymmetries between the performances of able-bodied and disabled athletes (e.g. Edwards, 2008). Moreover, Wolbring (2012) considered the impact on the Paralympic Games if the Paralympic athlete were to outperform the Olympic athlete due to technological or therapeutic enhancements. He argued that given what the future holds for the ability modification of humans, the prudent way forward appears to be to have one big Olympics. For Wolbring, this would 'very likely in the future also entail events where "disabled" and "non-disabled" athletes perform in the same event based on some external tools such as everyone in a wheelchair or exoskeleton' (p. 260).

Barriers to physical activity

Much progress has been made in creating opportunities for disabled people to participate in sport or exercise. For example, SCI Action Canada has developed and mobilised strategies which help Canadians living with spinal cord injury to initiate and maintain a physically active lifestyle. In England, the English Federation of Disability Sport has done much recently to improve disabled people's chances of experiencing sport and physical activity. By providing information about sports in local areas, Parasport, a British Paralympic Association initiative, has also created opportunities for disabled people to engage in sport or sports coaching if they so wish. Despite such opportunities, many disabled people remain sedentary or are largely physically inactive (Martin Ginis et al., 2010b). Why might this be the case? Many reasons are offered. These might broadly be gathered under the headings of psychological barriers, structural barriers and social relational barriers.

Psychological research has suggested that individuals may not feel motivated or confident to engage in physical activity (Martin Ginis et al., 2010a). People can feel sport and exercise isn't fun. Disabled athletes, often depicted and celebrated in the media as courageous and wanting to win at all costs (i.e. 'supercrip'), may inspire some disabled people to take up sport. For others though, such depictions can put people off sport (Smith and Sparkes, 2012). Another possible barrier to participation is that some disabled people do not see themselves as capable of engaging in sport or exercise. Social support might be limited too, making engaging in sport or exercise difficult.

Although much progress has been made in terms of enabling environments, another barrier faced when wishing to engage in sport or exercise is the socio-environment. As implied by the social model, people can be excluded and restricted from doing sport or exercising due to a lack of appropriate transport, accessible facilities and diverse equipment. Other socio-environmental barriers include weather conditions, finance to pay for membership to gyms or buy sporting equipment, concerns over personal safety when moving in public spaces, and inadequate knowledge within organisations (e.g. gyms) or among individuals (e.g. coaches) about disabled people's needs (Smith and Sparkes, 2012). A lack of health promotion information advising disabled people about how and where to be physically active is a further barrier.

As implied in the social relational model of disability (Thomas, 2007), the type of impairment, impairment effects and the ensuing direct or indirect psycho-emotional disablism can restrict being active. To illustrate, the biological effects of certain impairments, such as pain and fatigue, can pose limits on what activities can be done, when and where. Further, being stared at in a gym by strangers, having jokes made about one's impairment when playing sport at school, or being threatened on the way to one's local swimming pool can directly undermine a disabled person's psycho-emotional well-being. The individual may subsequently feel they cannot return to the gym, play sport, or wheel or walk to the swimming pool again. Thus, the impaired body and social oppression in the form of psycho-emotional disablism are further barriers to being active.

Health and well-being: Sport and exercise as medicine?

Whilst multiple barriers that restrict sporting or exercising opportunities exist, and many individuals with impairments are inactive, there are of course disabled people that do exercise and play sport. The impact of these physical activities on their lives has been under-researched and under-appreciated. What work there is has suggested there are benefits to be gained through sporting or exercise participation. These include benefits to *physical health, subjective well-being, psychological well-being* and *community.*

With regard to physical health, regularly playing sport or exercising can boost the immune system, help to maintain a healthy weight, lower high blood pressure, reduce the risk of developing heart disease, improve coordination and promote healthy blood sugar levels to prevent or control diabetes. Engaging in physical activities like sport or exercise can also help reduce pain as well as increase strength, balance and quality of sleep.

In addition to physical well-being, sport and exercise can boost subjective well-being. This kind of well-being refers to affective states coupled with life satisfaction. For example, sport and exercise participation has been shown to have a positive impact on spinal injured people's self-esteem, confidence, happiness, mood and general satisfaction with life (Martin Ginis et al., 2010a; Smith, 2013). Being active can also help people develop body-self compassion (Smith, 2013), which is an attitude or feeling of kindness and understanding towards one's body and self. It can involve affirmatively taking ownership of one's body and appreciating it rather than criticising it or perceiving it as 'flawed'.

Psychological well-being is derived from the eudaimonic tradition of positive psychology. Conceptually different from subjective well-being, this kind of well-being refers to existential engagement with life, purpose, autonomy and mastery. For example, engaging in sport and exercise following impairment can be related to finding a purpose in life (Martin Ginis et al., 2010a). Being regularly active can produce feelings of optimism and create resilience (Smith, 2013). Disabled people may experience personal growth and a sense of autonomy as a result of engaging in sport or exercise (Berger, 2009). Moreover, these activities can engender a positive impact on personal relationships.

In addition to promoting physical health, subjective well-being and psychological well-being, sport and exercise have been shown to promote a sense of community and affirmative identities. For example, for disabled young people with learning difficulties or physical impairments, residential segregated sport camps can cultivate a sense of identification with others and new understandings of one's physical potential (Goodwin et al., 2011). Additionally, Goodwin et al. found that for visually impaired youth the experience of sport in a camp enabled them to test their physical limits, acquire new skills while discarding ableistic stereotypes and set new self-defined standards and capabilities. The sports camps provided feelings of connection through a sense of belonging based on positive social interactions. Goodwin et al. (2011) also noted that emotional connections were formed as experiences of living as a person with a visual impairment were shared. The restorative qualities of the sense of community experienced allowed the athletes to communicate ideas about their cultural group identity. The young disabled people spoke of reaching out to discover a culture of common shared experiences, increased self-reliance and the social importance of newly developed peer relationships. In such ways, it seems, sport camps might engender an affirmative model of disability and impairment (Swain and French, 2000). This model encompasses positive social identities, both individual and collective, for disabled people grounded in the benefits and life experiences of being disabled and having an impairment (see Chapter 4).

Given that engaging in sport and exercise can impact positively on disabled people's health and well-being, it might be tempting to think that sport or exercise *is* medicine. Indeed, engaging in sport and exercise has recently been explicitly equated with a form of medicine. For example, regularly participating in physical activities like sport or exercise is said to be a cost-effective way to help prevent certain diseases (e.g. coronary artery disease) and aid recovery from illness (e.g. depression). Sport and exercise is widely considered vital to adopting and maintaining a healthy lifestyle. Although we do not dispute such matters, this does not mean that the physical activity–medicine relationship should escape critical scrutiny.

There is the danger that in talking about sport and exercise as 'medicine' we reconstruct disabled people simply in terms of the medical model. The limits of this model have been extensively documented. Primarily, it paints an overly negative and tragic image of disabled people. Individuals are depicted as defective and therefore disability is seen as a personal tragedy to be overcome. Disabled people should give up autonomy over their bodies and place themselves in the 'expert hands' of medicine. A related danger of the 'disability–physical activity–medicine' relationship is that it could promote a neo-liberal health role. The health role calls on the individual to be a responsible citizen who should take care of his or her own health. Thus, those disabled individuals who engage regularly in sport or exercise are the 'good' citizens. By corollary, those who do not are 'bad'.

When people are morally depicted in such a way, several dangers emerge. The health role directs attention away from society or culture and turns the focus directly on the individual and their impaired body. In this move, the largely inactive or sedentary disabled individual can be seen as lacking the inner motivation, mental toughness or resilience to engage in sport or exercise. Therefore, they, and only they, are to blame for their own health problems, for numerous so-called epidemics (e.g. obesity) and for rising costs to our health services. Yet in these ways, disabled people are stigmatised and could feel culturally illegitimate. It could be easy for their bodies to be externally seen or internally experienced as deviant, disgusting and unaccepted in wider society. By focusing solely on the individual, the health role can eclipse the significance that the environment and structural disablism have on people's capacities to fulfil an active life. Another possible danger of the health role in relation to sport or exercise is that it overlooks the dark side of these activities. Sport and exercise aren't always good for one's health or wellbeing. They can be associated with troubling conditions such as eating disorders (e.g. Papathomas and Lavallee, 2010). Finally, but by no means last, the health role risks hijacking notions of disabled people engaging in sport or exercise for the sake of it – to enjoy, and to experience their physicality in vibrant, disruptive, creative ways – by those more interested in controlling bodies for economic, disciplinary or normalising reasons. In the health role, the intrinsic value of playing sport or exercising can be eclipsed by a focus on the instrumental value of being active. This can be detrimental to a disabled person's well-being and motivation to be active across the life course.

Conclusion: Pointing a way forward

With regard to future work, one possible new direction to travel in is the critical examination of talent identification practices and how best to identify elite disability sporting talent. We also know very little about how to successfully promote physical activity in order to be 'fit for life' rather than 'fit for elite sport' among disabled people. A complementary way forward is the critical examination of different environments in which people might be physically active. These might include indoor centres designed specifically for disabled people to exercise in. Another environment yet to be critically focused on is the 'blue gym' – that is, our natural water-based environment in which people can be physically active. Furthermore, sociologists of sport, and sport and exercise psychologists, might engage more with work within disability studies. For example, rarely have sport scholars in these fields engaged with the social relational model, psycho-emotional disablism, impairment effects (Thomas, 2007) or, for example, critical psychological disability studies (Goodley, 2011). There is a dearth too of work that explores interconnections, such as those between disability, gender, race and athletic identity. The theoretical concept of intersectionality could be useful here (Valentine, 2007).

In this chapter, we have delved into some of the work on disability, sport and exercise being done within disability studies, the sociology of sport, and sport and exercise psychology. We do not want to uncritically celebrate sport or suggest all disabled people should be exercising. We do feel, however, that disability sport and exercise is at an exciting juncture. This chapter has pointed to some ways in which we might continue forward.

References

Berger, R. (2009) *Hoop Dreams on Wheels*. London: Routledge.

Edwards, S. (2008) 'Should Oscar Pistorius be excluded from the 2008 Olympic Games?', *Sports, Ethics & Philosophy*, 2: 112–25.

Goodley, D. (2011) *Disability Studies: An Interdisciplinary Introduction*. London: SAGE.

Goodwin, D., Lieberman, L., Johnston, K. and Leo, J. (2011) 'Connecting through summer camp: youth with visual impairments find a sense of community', *Adapted Physical Activity Quarterly*, 28: 40–55.

Martin, J. (2010) 'Athletes with physical disabilities', in S. Hanrahan and M. Andersen (eds), *Handbook of Applied Sport Psychology*. London: Routledge. pp. 432–40.

Martin Ginis, K.A., Jetha, A., Mack, D. and Hetz, S. (2010a) 'Physical activity and subjective well-being among people with spinal cord injury: a meta-analysis', *Spinal Cord*, 48: 65–72.

Martin Ginis, K.A., Arbour-Nicitopoulos, K.P., Latimer, A.E., Buchholz, A., Bray, S.R., Craven, B., et al. (2010b) 'Leisure-time physical activity in a population-based sample of people with spinal cord injury part II: activity types, intensities and durations', *Archives of Physical Medicine and Rehabilitation*, 91: 729–33.

Papathomas, A. and Lavallee, D. (2010) 'Athletes' experiences of disordered eating in sport', *Qualitative Research in Sport and Exercise*, 2: 354–70.

Peers, D. (2009) '(Dis)empowering paralympic histories: absent athletes and disabling discourses', *Disability & Society*, 24: 653–65.

Purdue, D. and Howe, D. (2012) 'See the sport, not the disability? Exploring the Paralympic paradox', *Qualitative Research in Sport, Exercise & Health*, 4 (2): 189–205.

Smith, B. (2013) 'Disability, sport, and men's narratives of health: a qualitative study', *Health Psychology*, 32 (1): 110–19.

Smith, B. and Perrier, M-J. (in press) 'Understanding disability, sport and exercise: models and narrative inquiry', in R. Eklund and G. Tenenbaum (eds), *Encyclopaedia of Sport and Exercise Psychology*. Champaign, IL: Human Kinetics.

Smith, B. and Sparkes, A. (2012) 'Disability, sport and physical activity: a critical review', in N. Watson, A. Roulstone and C. Thomas (eds), *Routledge Handbook of Disability Studies*. London: Routledge. pp. 336–47.

Swain, J. and French, S. (2000) 'Towards an affirmative model of disability', *Disability & Society*, 15: 569–82.

Tawse, H., Bloom, G., Sabiston, C. and Reid, G. (2012) 'The role of coaches of wheelchair rugby in the development of athletes with a spinal cord injury', *Qualitative Research in Sport, Exercise & Health*, 4 (2): 206–25.

Thomas, C. (2007) *Sociologies of Disability and Illness*. London: Palgrave.

Thomas, N. and Smith, A. (2009) *Disability, Sport, and Society*. London: Routledge.

Valentine, G. (2007) 'Theorising and researching intersectionality: a challenge for feminist geography', *The Professional Geographer*, 59: 10–21.

Wolbring, G. (2012) 'Paralympians outperforming Olympians: an increasing challenge for Olympism and the Paralympic and Olympic movement', *Sport, Ethics & Philosophy*, 6: 251–66.

30
Disability and Ageing

Ann Macfarlane

'Grow old along with me; the best is yet to be.' (Robert Browning, 1812–1889)

Introduction

'Or is the best yet to be?' Robert Browning's poetic words do not fit comfortably in the lives of older people; the more so if you are an older disabled person living alone, isolated from or without people you love, living with strangers in a residential setting or cut off from the local community. Negative media images of older people are those that reflect an older population as 'needy' and 'dependent' and experiencing poverty and ill health. The reality for many older people, particularly for those who have impairment and experience disabling barriers, is life as a struggle and plagued with concerns. For those who remain relatively healthy, media images focus attention on older people cruising, golfing and soaking up the sunshine by holidaying abroad each year, thus indicating that older people have little to complain about. An image often missing is one depicting the enormous contribution older people make to society, through volunteering, grandparent support and in the workplace.

While a plethora of new legislation and changing policies focus on healthcare, social inclusion and social justice, areas of concern include money, particularly pensions and investments, access to and the cost of transport, lack of accessible, affordable housing, personal care, employment, leisure and relationships. These areas are not dissimilar to those that have been of concern over the last 30 years for disabled people, the disabled people's movement and Centres for Independent Living. This has been a period in which disabled people have mobilised, come together and organised themselves in order to debate the issues that affect their lives, and has included a considerable percentage of older people. A major outcome of these debates has been the introduction and definition of the term 'independent living'. Independent living has empowered and enabled disabled people, organisations of disabled people and Centres for Independent Living to campaign on human and civil rights, and has focused on planning, commissioning, delivery, monitoring and evaluation of services.

More recently debates have focussed on 'Co-production'. Several definitions have been produced and this relates to strategic direction and services for people who use a range of services. Co-production is a way of creative thinking, designing, delivering, monitoring and evaluating services in an equal relationship between staff, people who use services, and their families, friends and neighbours. It is about staff and people who are in receipt of services working together in a collaborative way at the start of any project or service. It enables services to become more appropriate for those who may need support or those who are already receiving assistance.

Independent living

Independent living is defined as being in control of one's life. In practice, this means having choice over how assistance is provided, who provides it and when. People employed to provide this support are called 'personal assistants'. Personal assistants may be pivotal in supporting an older person to achieve independent living. A personal assistant is someone who works with the person on his or her terms. Independent living may change over time as disabled people make changes in their lives, as they grow up, grow older and have different experiences. As an older person ages, there is the very real possibility of becoming a disabled person, with one person in two acquiring an impairment. Experiences of impaired mobility, sight and hearing are the most common in older people.

Oliver summarises the independent living philosophy as follows:

> Central to this philosophy is the issue of personal assistance which is necessary for disabled people to participate in all of the activities of everyday life and includes work, leisure pursuits, education and personal relationships. Choice and control are key factors in this participation and disabled people must exercise both of these in making decisions about their personal assistance and the activities in which they wish to participate. (2000: 3)

This philosophy applies equally to older people who, traditionally, have been excluded from the independent living debate. A greater effort by medical professional people and people working in traditional organisations is required to put older people in touch with Centres for Independent Living. What does independent living mean for older people? Research undertaken by Clark et al. (1998) reveals that older people view remaining in their own home as marking the final boundary of their independence. Older people make a clear distinction between being 'at home' and being 'in a home' and they define assistance as help not care. Older people want a range of options that will support them to care for themselves. Services on offer to older people who qualify, following a community care assessment, are often home care and meals on wheels. In 2009, new legislation introduced 'reablement' which focuses mainly on older people being offered a six-week programme to gain or regain independence following hospital discharge (Age UK, 2012). Reablement concentrates on physical activity mainly within the home environment and excludes active integration into the local community. Traditional services have often fallen short of expectations and placed older people within a dependency model, which disempowers them. In 1996, the NHS and Community Care (Direct Payments) Act was available to people between the ages of 18 and 65 and gave local authorities the power to give cash for care for those who met the criteria of being 'willing and able' to manage a community care package. Disabled and older people lobbied government to extend the legislation to include older people and in February 2000 this expansion was achieved. A direct payment is one way to achieve independent living that provides choice and control. Following a community care assessment, an older person may choose to have the money in the form of a direct payment rather than traditional service provision. A direct payment continues to be provided for those people who qualify but a 'personal budget' is now the preferred term and extends to other provision apart from that of employing personal assistants either directly or through an agency (see Chapter 32). For example, a social care or health assessment may include money to pay for equipment, membership subscriptions, education courses and more. A non-means-tested entitlement, Access to Work, may be applied for if an older person needs support to continue in employment.

Pilot sites in a few areas are seeking to extend the option of Personal Budgets to include healthcare in a combined payment to individuals who qualify. The National Health Service, the Department of Health and Think Local, Act Personal, are undertaking further research to gain additional insights into people's thoughts on how to turn existing legislation into this transforming dual approach through a single assessment. For people who want to take even more control of their lives, this would be a welcome move and enable more people to be discharged back into their own home or to continue to live in their own home.

Not all older people are entitled to financial support through their local authority via a community care assessment and many older people do not want to engage with social services. Older people, if they require support irrespective of whether the local authority pays or the person themselves, are entitled to receive information. Government policy usually determines entitlements for older people by chronological age. The non-means-tested Attendance Allowance can be applied for when a person reaches 65, while the mobility allowance, unless applied for prior to 65, is not available for this age group. Yet impaired mobility causes huge difficulties in terms of accessing community services and activities. Voluntary sector and private sector organisations determine the age when people are defined as 'older' and all set age limits differently. This makes application for entitlements and services confusing, along with form-filling, and people may decide to go without support, insurance cover and other financial help.

The experience of life changes

Perhaps one way older people can be defined is through the concept of 'life changes'. Getting older is a time when children have become of an age and may leave home if accommodation and employment permit, when a career or paid work ends, or when leisure or sporting pursuits become too demanding and something less fatiguing is required. It is a time when older people may leave their home and move to a smaller dwelling, sheltered or residential accommodation. It might relate to losing a partner and friends or to a change in financial circumstances. Life changes relating to the older generation come within a wide time frame and may determine when a person feels 'older'. Acquiring impairment and experiencing disabling barriers, which occur irrespective of age, can certainly add to the image and feeling of becoming 'older'.

Dignity in later life

Many councils have appointed 'dignity' champions. Dignity and respect is high on the agenda of the Care Quality Commission, the regulator in health and social care and a government-funded body that undertakes inspections in hospitals and residential settings as well as in community health settings, such as GP practices, dentistry, opthalmology and podiatry. Research around dignity is being carried out by a number of voluntary and government-funded organisations that focus on older people and those who work in the field of health and social care. These include Independent Age, Age UK, the Joseph Rowntree Foundation, the Social Care Institute for Excellence and the National Institute for Clinical Excellence. Research, particularly in the field of social care and technology, highlights that older people feel the need to persevere in maintaining dignity and independence despite physical, health and relationship barriers.

The inclusion and participation of older people

Older people themselves are beginning to come together to determine their own agenda in a similar way to Centres for Independent Living. In the late 1990s, Better Government for Older People was established to ensure older people had a consultative role and were involved in the planning, delivery and monitoring of services. This process and others are influencing changes in health and social care and other crucial aspects of daily living, such as accessible transport, and this input has significantly raised the profile of older people at local level. National organisations, such as the Joseph Rowntree Foundation, Age UK and the Royal Voluntary Service actively consult and involve older people in research and in decision-making processes. However, some of these organisations are not controlled and managed by disabled and older people. There is still a long way to go in terms of older people taking control of their own agenda and obtaining the funding to ensure positive outcomes. It is only now that voluntary sector organisations and statutory bodies are beginning to recognise the 'added value' of including older people. A challenge for policy writers and decision-makers is to ensure that consultation, planning and commissioning processes include older people in the co-production of output and outcomes. The emphasis in deciding policies and strategies that relate to older people should be one of social inclusion and fair access. These policies and strategies require the development of integrated objectives between organisations, departments and community initiatives and should demonstrate best value in service planning, commissioning, provision and monitoring of services. Ignorance and misinformation remain as a result of professional people not making themselves aware of new and changing legislation that has the potential to enhance the lives of older people. When pressures mount, good practice diminishes. However, knowing and interpreting legislation for older people can bring benefits and change lives. A brief overview of this legislation will highlight its relevance for older people.

In 2001, the government's National Service Framework for Older People (DoH, 2001) focused on:

- routing out age discrimination
- person-centred care with older people treated as individuals with respect and dignity
- promoting older people's health and independence.

Routing out age discrimination in the provision of health and community care services could make a positive impact on the lives of older people. Service provision could significantly improve with the input of older people in the design, delivery, monitoring and evaluation of services. The inclusion of people with high support needs should come high on agendas.

Social care services are debarred from the use of age in their eligibility criteria and policies and the use of age to restrict available services. Commissioning strategies must be flexible enough to take account of individual needs, and eligibility criteria are not to be more stringent for older people than for other groups. An area of concern is that for some older people, who require non-residential community care services, it may mean demonstrating a higher level of need in order to qualify for a service. As past research has shown, older people often require 'a little bit of help', especially at the appropriate time, in order to continue managing their lives in their own environment. Focused assistance can prevent a fall, admission or re-admission to hospital. Age discrimination has also been applied to the cost of care with the bar set far higher for older people than for those under the age of 65. The cost of care packages must be levelled up to comply with the Fair Access to Care Services guidance issued by the Department of Health in April 2002. The guidance provides a national framework for councils to use when determining their eligibility criteria for supporting adults of any age. Councils are expected to adopt a consistent approach to define priorities for meeting needs in order to promote independence and quality of life. This includes a common understanding of risk assessment and reviews.

The National Service Framework for Older People (DoH, 2012) focuses on person-centred care and states that NHS and social care services are to treat older people as individuals and enable them to make choices about their own care. This is achieved through a single assessment process, integrated commissioning arrangements and integrated provision of services, including community equipment, podiatry and continence services. Older people are entitled to appropriate and accessible information so that they can make informed choices and decisions, whether that is for their health, domestic, social or personal care needs.

The Health Act of 1999 focuses on joint commissioning and pooled budgets with lead commissioners trained to provide an integrated approach to service provision, rather than working to organisational boundaries. Section 31 of the Health Act details partnership arrangements. GP practices were able to commission services from April 2013 alongside local Clinical Commissioning Groups comprising GPs and other professional people to determine priorities. Co-production must be high on all health and social care agendas to ensure that older disabled people receive support that will enable them to remain as independent as possible. Older people should have input into their lives that is responsive to gender, personal appearance, communication, diet, race, culture, religious and spiritual beliefs. This holistic and person-centred approach demands a fresh approach to training for care managers, social workers, doctors, nurses and other paramedical professionals who have been responsible for service provision. A continuing culture shift in the mindsets of many professional people is required and highlights the need for collaboration with older people in the co-production and design of training materials. Other issues arising from legislation and policies around older people's needs are:

- the importance of agencies making arrangements, undertaking assessments and placing the older person at the centre of the process to ensure that the person understands this process of what his or her rights are in determining outcomes. The older person will also need to know timescales around the assessment process, their right to question and complain, and the review and monitoring processes
- information gathering and sharing among the different agencies, thus avoiding older people, and those who support them, having to provide the same information to different people
- recognition of a greater prevalence of some illnesses among specific groups. Provision must be culturally appropriate and serve the needs of those for whom their first language is not English. Direct payments or personal budgets can be helpful in providing the flexibility that personal assistants can offer people with fluctuating impairments.

The latest legislation, the National Health Service and Social Care Act 2012, sets out a significant change in the way health and social care will be financed. This will occur with the establishment of clinical commissioning groups, partly controlled by general practitioners. Three key principles will be followed which are:

1 Patients to be at the centre of the National Health Service.
2 Clinical outcomes instead of health measurements.
3 Empowerment of health professionals, particularly general practitioners.

Equality of engagement with, and inclusion of, older people, irrespective of impairment, is vital to ensure social care options have equal status with those of health services.

End of life care

Integral to health and well-being is the support and care that older disabled people should expect when illness signifies that they may be near the end of life. Policies exist that focus on people being able to choose their preferred place to die and to experience support that provides dignity and care irrespective of diagnosis. The hospice movement continues to re-evaluate and refocus provision on people with diagnoses apart from cancer. Greater numbers of people continue to die in hospital despite efforts made to enable people to die at home if that is their expressed wish. To experience impairment *and* illness can make it harder to achieve a 'good death'. Although death continues to remain a taboo topic, much has been done by national organisations, including the NHS End of Life Care Programme, Dying Matters and the National Council for Palliative Care to support professional people in opening up the issue and supporting people to express their wishes.

Conclusion

As younger disabled people reap the benefits of the achievements of the disabled people's movement over the past 30 years, so older disabled people will begin to see improvements now they are coming together to debate the way forward. Disabled people can benefit from technology and the next ten years will see further advances and create higher expectations. Expectations in other areas will increase, such as more accessible public and private transport, particularly for those in residential settings and people who cannot leave their home unaided. Disabled people want the right to inclusive mainstream services, good quality information, personal assistance, direct payments and personal budgets that may include healthcare. This list is not exhaustive and indicates the pressure placed on commissioners and providers responsible for effecting and achieving change. The National Institute for Clinical Excellence and the Social Care Institute for Excellence are two key national organisations tasked with raising health and social care standards and providing evidenced-based materials to support the delivery of good practice. As the population grows in number and age, the cost of high-quality appropriate services needs to become quickly affordable. Andrew Dilnot, in his 2011 research 'Fairer Funding for All', addressed the cost of health and social care, and the debate continues as to how these costs will be met and by whom.

As older people engage with key independent living principles placed at the forefront of development and planning together with ever-expanding and continuing development of technology, Robert Browning's philosophical approach alluded to at the beginning may have a ring of truth: 'Grow old along with me; the best is yet to be.' Undoubtedly, it will not be without a struggle.

References

Age UK (2012) *Intermediate Care and Re-ablement*. Factsheet. London: Age UK.

Clark, H., Dyer, S. and Horwood, J. (1998) *That Bit of Help: The High Value of Low Level Services for Older People*. Bristol: Policy Press and Joseph Rowntree Foundation.

Department of Health (DoH) (2001) *The National Service Framework for Older People*. London: DoH.

Department of Health (DoH) (2002) *Fair Access to Care Services: Policy Guidance*. London: DoH.

Department of Health (DoH) (2012) *The National Service Framework for Older People*. London: DoH.

Dilnot, A. (2011) *Fairer Funding for All: The Commission's Recommendations to Government*. London: DoH Commission on Funding of Care and Support.

Oliver, M. (2000) *Three Year Review*. London: National Centre for Independent Living.

Royal Voluntary Service (2013) *Shaping Our Age: The Route to Twentieth Century Wellbeing*. Brunel University, de Montfort University, Royal Voluntary Service.

31

Disabled People, Work and Welfare

Alan Roulstone

Background

The relationship between disabled people and work has exercised many social science writers and many disabled people's organisations globally (Roulstone and Barnes, 2005). Seemingly intractable barriers to work, alongside growing economic recession, have added increased urgency to these analyses. Disabled people have traditionally been seen by many employers as 'unfit' for work, or only suited to certain often stereotyped forms of employment. More recently, economic crises have led some states to redefine who is fit for work, regardless of whether there are paid work opportunities (ENIL, 2012). Scope for new jeopardies is very real where disabled people are forced off disability benefits into mainstream benefit systems, but in the absence of any real employment opportunities. On top of the established cultural prejudices towards disabled people are new risks of disabled people being presented as an economic stigma, one which has previously only been pervasive at times of major conflict, unrest and of course most notably during the holocaust (Burleigh, 1994).

This chapter will look at the global position of disabled people and work to ensure readers get a broad picture of disabled people and work. It will however use the UK as a focus in highlighting some common facets of exclusion from paid work for many disabled people globally and as a reference point from which very different experiences can be gauged. It will argue that a key factor in the exclusion of disabled people has been the historical shift towards seeing work as synonymous with paid employment. Typical of many 'advanced' economies, the employment position of disabled people in the UK is very stark. In 2011, the employment rate of disabled people was 48.8 per cent, compared with 77.5 per cent of non-disabled people (LFS, 2011). A more fine-grained analysis shows impairment-specific data and yet greater exclusion. For example, figures are yet more concerning for people with learning disabilities or mental health issues. The employment rate for people with mental health problems was only 20 per cent in 2009 (LFS, 2009). Emerson and Hatton noted that in 2008 only 8 per cent of working-age people with learning disabilities were in paid work (Emerson and Hatton, 2008). These figures broadly reflect those of 'advanced' economies (OECD, 2003).

Work or welfare for disabled people?

Strong British anti-welfare discourses have developed since 1997 which aim to redefine just who counts as disabled, who is too 'disabled' to work and those who should be reasonably expected to undertake or seek paid employment. The UK Coalition government has used both sympathetic and harsh discourses to highlight the problem of 'worklessness' amongst disabled people (HMG and DWP, 2010). Current discussions of 'wasted lives' sit alongside unprecedentedly harsh media portrayals of some disabled people as malingering (Garthwaite, 2011). The current government position is that too many disabled people have been written off by disincentives to enter paid work and benefits that reinforce this 'perverse' incentive to remain outside of work (DWP, 2011). These ideas can be seen to sit alongside anti-discrimination (AD) principles that say employers must be open to the employment of those previously excluded from the contemporary workplace. Overall however, the limited impact of an AD approach and the continued growth in out-of-work benefits during the late 2000s amongst sick and disabled claimants (Anyadike-Danes and McVicar, 2008), have increased government frustration. Contemporary debates and solutions are by their nature short-term, while attempts to reduce headline figures for disability and out-of-work benefits have been largely ineffective. The years 1995–2011 have witnessed a dizzying array of employment schemes targeted at disabled people – the National Disability Development Initiative (NDDI), New Deal for Disabled People (NDDP), Pathways to Work, Workstep and now the proposed Work Programme and Work Choice. To date, few of these activities have proved effective beyond higher success rates for more flexible and generously funded programmes. However, these have not substantially altered the broad employment gap. Major research on employer attitudes points to continued attitude barriers despite legislative and educational initiatives (Roberts et al., 2004). Attempts to use anti-discrimination legislation (ADL) to increase access to the labour market via reasonable adjustment ideas and non-discriminatory clauses (Lawson, 2008), whilst providing a small number of keynote successes, has not proven of major value in increasing paid work objectives. Indeed in the USA, ADL has sat alongside a reduction in disabled people's employment.

Disability and employment in 'advanced societies'

Across all 'advanced' OECD countries, disabled people are less likely to be in work and to receive vocational training and support. Those with more significant impairments and more limited educational attainments are the least likely to obtain paid work (OECD, 2003). We also know that most of the programmes in advanced OECD countries are largely not that effective, such as financial incentives for employing disabled people, tax credits and benefit withdrawal sanctions against disabled people perceived to be closer to the labour market. Disabled people are more likely to be supported into paid work where they are already close to the labour market. In other words, these disabled people may well have entered work without such interventions, and the effect of a programme is often more apparent than real. The most effective national welfare schemes supporting disabled people are those that afford more flexible build-up of hours and provide protected re/entry and exit from paid work where periods of illness supervene, where wider benefit claw-backs are least severe on re-entering paid work and where flexible and adjusted working are well supported by fiscal and local disability support measures. Countries with active labour market policies and high tax–spend rations in public services are also the most successful in supporting disabled people into paid work (Roulstone and Barnes, 2005). Overall, however, there is very limited evidence that employment programmes, ADL and workplace adjustments have made any great difference to disabled people (OECD, 2003). For those in paid work, they have often gained that work despite, not because of, state or market interventions. The best way to sum up the paradox of limited positive impacts of employment programmes, ADL and reasonable adjustments is that they can be seen as ameliorating but not challenging the paramount economic-social system that equates work with paid contractual employment.

There is therefore a compelling argument for reflecting on the longer-run structural exclusion of disabled individuals if the barriers to paid employment are to be addressed in a meaningful and enduring way. A failure to reappraise these historical developments and a contemporary comprehension of diverse forms of productive activity will arguably ensure policy failure and continued stigmatisation of many disabled people (Prideaux et al., 2009). By way of explanation, the following will explore the diversity of economic activity that preceded advanced economic systems (both capitalist and communist), and which offer some clues as to how contemporary economic and social contributions could be opened up for scrutiny in a way that values and validates a broader range of activities.

Work and productive activity before 'advanced' economic systems

Disabled people and their 'productive' contribution has been the 'spectre at the feast' from early capitalist industrialisation across Europe (Abberley, 1999; Barnes, 2000). The rise of industrial capitalism, one whose apotheosis is symbolised in the factory system of the late 1800s, attempts to control key aspects of work by disaggregation, deskilling and the calculation of constituent work elements all helped forge the links between work and a corresponding monetary value (Taylor, 2003). Although not inherently inimical to all disabled people's specific productive capacity, many disabled people were in time essentially 'designed out' of productive activity where norms of effort, stamina, strength, awareness of danger (good eyesight, for example) and endurance became increasingly pervasive (Finkelstein, 1980; Gleeson, 1999). Although industrialisation and capitalisation were haphazard and never conformed neatly to industrial ideologies, what might be called the 'negative serendipity' associated with the factory system had a profound impact on those with non-standard bodies or minds (Roulstone, 2002). This pattern was not unique to capitalist industrialisation and was a feature of state socialist countries suggesting complex dynamics (Littler, 1984).

McClelland is useful here in stating that 'traditional culture is characterised generally by norms of diffuseness, particularism, affectivity and ascription, whereas industrial culture leans heavily towards norms of specificity, universalism, neutrality and performance' (McClelland, 1961). Nothing here suggests that pre-industrial societies and economies were preferable or somehow less challenging. A general consensus amongst otherwise diverse commentators on disability is that disabled people have faced cultural and at times physical exclusion and ridicule (Stiker, 1999). In pre-industrial societies, productive norms and expectations were diffuse and not tied to impersonal financial contracts. With industrialisation, work becomes synonymous with paid contractual exchanges of labour for externally determined reward. In time, political citizenship begins to be definable as those individuals who are able to sell their labour and have a marketable brain or body. Alongside the development of market economies, market rates for fixed quantities of paid work, and the public contractual underpinnings of paid work, was the corresponding definition of other forms of economic activity such as domestic labour as 'informal' and correspondingly downgraded activities. Economic and structural barriers in time began to overlay established cultural negativity towards some disabled people, ensuring that disabled people would only begin to re-engage in a limited way during the two world wars (Borsay, 2005; Humphries and Gordon, 1992). Disabled people were more likely to be welcome at times of labour shortage, leading some commentators to describe them as a 'reserve army of labour' (Grover and Piggott, 2005).

Work, disability and the majority world

Beyond historical awareness that much work was not synonymous with paid employment, even a cursory look at contemporary low-resource countries shows this still to be the case. Globally, disabled people face disproportionate barriers to economic livelihood. If we look at all OECD countries (OECD, 2003), we can see that disabled people are only half as likely to be in paid work as their non-disabled counterparts. Disabling barriers to paid work are not simply an issue in certain countries or even continents. In both 'advanced' economies and largely poor rural majority world contexts, disabled people are disadvantaged in both accessing and sustaining work and other forms of economic activity. The work situation of disabled people in the majority world, whilst diverse, is largely very challenging, with most countries that collect reliable statistics suggesting that for the most part people deemed disabled are not likely to be in work (Mitra and Sambamoorthi, 2006). One major problem with many evaluations of disabled people, work and employment is the attempt to transpose western notions of work as employment into majority world contexts. These arguments tend to assume that employment (as paid work) and work are the same thing. This is a very important distinction as in much of the majority world work is a broad spectrum of non-contractual economic activity which can range from barter, small commodity production, hawking, provisioning (from wasteland and tips) and begging to wider exchanges of labour which include goods, services and promissory activity which are not based on contractual arrangements. In this way, an attempt to graft minority world perspectives onto majority world contexts can be hugely problematical. Somewhat ironically, however, the very haphazard nature of work in the majority world does afford or demand forms of economic activity. Disabled people take their place in the population begging, hawking, scavenging and doing small commodity. Where progressive charities are active and where microfinance is available, disabled people have been aided to set up small workshops, cooperative and local manufacture and trading activity.

Conclusion

It is tempting to describe those disabled people who are not undertaking paid work as 'unproductive'. If we broaden the lens to include those disabled people doing 'informal' economic activity or adding to their communities but not with financial reward, then we get a very different picture of their productivity and social value. The work of Prideaux and colleagues in the British context provides one small example of how this redefinition would change any objective appraisal of disabled people's social value (Prideaux et al., 2009). They note that disabled people may be employers of personal assistants (PAs), provide civic contributions, act as unpaid voluntary workers (especially those who cannot get access to paid work) and are often engaged in family 'care' roles. In a way parallel to domestic labour debates, they note how disabled people are often forced to remain in the 'informal' or 'support-based' economy, but offer a range of unacknowledged social contributions. Perhaps most stark is the assertion that carrying out employment functions, activities highly valorised in modern society, disabled employers of PAs are still treated in policy terms as dependent on social welfare and care services. It is notable that as disability and poverty are closely correlated in modern society, disabled people also put a higher proportion of their income into their local economy in buying non-discretionary items such as a food and household consumables.

The rise of the neo-liberal notion of the 'big society' somewhat ironically exhorted local communities to give something back. These unpaid activities would, to an extent, substitute for an overgrown local state which fostered dependency. Working-age disabled people have been making just such contributions, many of which have gone unacknowledged. For example, each time an access improvement results from disabled people's local access group activity, the whole community arguably benefits from this enhanced public space.

There is a clear need, in the absence of enabling and sustained paid work, to reflect again on the economic contributions of disabled people, both the multiplier effect of their spending and their contribution to the development of a skill set (for themselves as employers and for PAs), and on the often unpaid voluntary work contributions that they make in the absence of paid work. We need further critical evaluation of the value of disabled people's activities outside of paid work if we are to develop an equitable policy platform fit for the twenty-first century. We know that 8.1 million people were deemed economically inactive in 2010. Given that sufficient quantities of good quality paid work are not available for large tracts of the UK population, it would be better to reframe our understandings of work and welfare to recognise the full economic and social contributions that many disabled people make in contemporary society (Abberley, 1999). A good universal income and the social crediting of the contributions of those historically unable to access paid work is an urgent consideration across developed countries (De Wispelaere and Stirton, 2004). In a majority world context, good quality alternatives to paid work might be better investments for disabled people. The causes of impairment, such as landmines and avoidable disease, ought to be major priorities. For those countries struggling to develop economically, advice and support from the minority world are also important.

The key paradox at the heart of the disability and work equation is that of an economic and social system that, having designed out many disabled people from the paramount system of work as paid employment, now expends much energy in how it can design them back into the very system that excluded them without challenging paramount constructions of productive value. A fundamental review of the nature of work itself and the reward of wider forms of productive and socially useful activity are needed if disabled people are to be accepted as fully fledged and valued citizens.

References

Abberley, P. (1999) The Significance of Work for the Citizenship of Disabled People. Paper presented at University College Dublin, 15 April.

Anyadike-Danes, M. and McVicar, D. (2008) 'Has the boom in Incapacity Benefit claimant numbers passed its peak?', *Fiscal Studies*, 29 (4): 415–34.

Barnes, C. (2000) 'A working social model? Disability, work and disability politics in the 21st century', *Critical Social Policy*, 20(4): 441–57.

Borsay, A. (2005) *Disability and Social Policy in Britain since 1750*. Basingstoke: Palgrave.

Burleigh, M. (1994) *Death and Deliverance: Euthanasia in Germany 1900–1945*. Cambridge: Cambridge University Press.

De Wispelaere, J. and Stirton, L. (2004) *The Many Faces of Universal Basic Income*. Boston: Political Quarterly Publishing. Available at: www.usbig.net/pdf/manyfacesofubi.pdf [accessed 13/07/12].

DWP (2011) RR 821 *Work Programme Evaluation: Findings from the First Phase of Qualitative Research on Programme Delivery*. London: TSO.

Emerson, E. and Hatton, C. (2008) People with Learning Difficulties in England. CeDR Research Report, May. Available at: www.lancs.ac.uk/staff/emersone/FASSWeb/Emerson_08_PWLDinEngland.pdf [accessed 13/07/12].

ENIL (2012) Report on the Hearing at the European Parliament of the Impact of Austerity on Independent Living in Europe. Brussels: ENIL. Available at: www.onafhankelijkleven.be/upload/EOL/Publicaties/English%20def/Report28Feb2012_ENIL_Hearing%20in%20the%20European%20Parliament_Report.pdf [accessed 13/07/12].

Finkelstein, V. (1980) *Attitudes and Disabled People*. New York: World Rehabilitation Monograph.

Garthwaite, K. (2011) 'The language of shirkers and scroungers? Talking about illness, disability and coalition welfare reform', *Disability & Society*, 26 (3): 369–72.

Gleeson, B. (1999) *Geographies of Disability*. London: Routledge.

Grover, C. and Piggott, L. (2005) 'Disabled people, the reserve army of labour and welfare reform', *Disability & Society*, 20 (7): 705–17.

Her Majesty's Government (HMG) and Department for Work and Pensions (DWP) (2010) *The Coalition: Our Programme for Government*. London: TSO.

Humphries, S. and Gordon, P. (1992) *Out of Sight: The Experience of Disability 1900–1950*. Plymouth: Northcote House.

Lawson, A. (2008) *Disability and Equality Law in Britain: The Role of Reasonable Adjustments*. Oxford: Hart.

LFS (2009) *Labour Force Survey: Quarter 1 Survey*. London: TSO.

LFS (2011) *Labour Force Survey: Quarter 1 Survey*. London: TSO.

Littler, C. (1984) *Labour Process in Soviet-type Economies*. London: SAGE.

McClelland, D.C. (1961) *The Achieving Society*. New York: Oxford University Press.

Mitra, S. and Sambamoorthi, U. (2006) 'Unemployment of persons with disabilities: evidence from a national sample survey', *Economic & Political Weekly*, 41 (3): 199–203.

OECD (2003) *Transforming Disability into Ability*. Paris: OECD.

Prideaux, S., Roulstone, A., Harris, J. and Barnes, C. (2009) 'Disabled people and self directed support schemes: re-conceptualising work and welfare in the 21st century', *Disability & Society*, 24 (5): 557–69.

Roberts, S., Heaver, C., Hill, K., Rennison, J., Stafford, B., Howat, N., et al. (2004) *Disability in the Workplace: Employers and Service Providers' Responses to the Disability Discrimination Act in 2003 and Preparation for 2004 Changes*. London: DWP.

Roulstone, A. (2002) 'Disabling pasts, enabling futures: how does the changing nature of capitalism impact on the disabled worker and jobseeker?', *Disability & Society*, 17 (6): 627–42.

Roulstone, A. and Barnes, C. (2005) *Working Futures: Disabled People and Social Inclusion*. Bristol: Policy Press.

Stiker, H. (1999) *A History of Disability*. Ann Arbor: University of Michigan Press.

Taylor, F. W (2003) *The Principles of Scientific Management*. London: Routledge.

Part 4

In Charge of Support and Help

32

Care: Controlling and Personalising Services

Sarah Woodin

Most disabled people receive assistance with daily living from family members. However, the value of paid assistance that is under the control of service users, for disabled people and their families, has been conclusively shown in recent years. The disabled people's movement has questioned the value of the concept of 'care', emphasising instead the importance of support for control and decision-making in daily life. Direct payments, personal budgets and personal assistance developed from the early initiatives of the disabled people's movement (Barnes, 1993), and the policy of personalisation broadly supports these developments. It emphasises an individual perspective rather than a 'one size fits all' approach typical of services such as day centres or residential homes. This chapter describes how services have developed in recent decades and concludes by discussing some current issues.

Care

The term 'care' is used to convey a wide range of meanings and these include caring *about* other people, indicating concern, love and affection, and caring *for* people, often used to describe work that ensures another's well-being (Beresford, 2008). Caring, in both senses of the word, is a common experience for almost everyone at different points in their lives. Often the two forms of 'care' go together, in that we help others because we are concerned about their well-being, but this is not always the case.

Even though 'care' is a very familiar common-sense idea, it presents particular problems for disabled people as it is used in public policy. This is because the way the term is used often attributes negative qualities to disabled people. As Beresford (2008) points out, even though 'care' is often thought to be a good thing in society, and very necessary for children, few of us like the idea that we might be 'cared for' as adults and in our old age. This is because being 'cared for' implies dependency and helplessness and a lack of control over daily living decisions – things that are taken for granted for adults. Generally then, receiving 'care' is something to be avoided where possible.

No one, disabled or non-disabled, can survive completely independently and a complex set of social relationships is involved in all daily activities. However, some of these are called care and some are not, depending on who is involved. For example, if a manager has help from a personal assistant at work, this is often seen as a status symbol rather than a need for assistance or care, even if the work involves organising activities for another person. Furthermore, disabled people often have less access to daily support and assistance in the course of everyday life than do non-disabled people: help is not given to all people equally, both interpersonally and by social institutions. So, for example, men get more help than women and non-disabled people get more help than disabled people, this being due to attitudes, expectations, different opportunities and environmental design. These inequalities may reflect a lack of affective equality: some people are also cared *about* more or less than others (Lynch et al., 2009).

Feminist scholars, including some disabled feminists, have found the concept of care to be a useful one because it describes the unpaid work that women, including disabled women, typically do within households and recognises that it has affective aspects. Informal 'care' has its roots in everyday relationships and women have traditionally kept homes running and looked after children. Being able to do this effectively often requires kinship and friendship relationships that are based on reciprocity: the expectation that there will be a more or less equal balance in favours done for one another in families or between friends, even if this is over the long term. If the balance of favours is not equal, the person who is not able to reciprocate is disadvantaged socially (Rae, 1993; Morris, 2001). Caring *for* others therefore may involve unequal relationships and there is plenty of evidence of the corrosive effect of a lack of reciprocity on personal relationships, for both parties involved (Galvin, 2004; Thomas, 1999). This presents a major problem for many disabled people who receive a great deal of care assistance from family members.

Reasons why 'care' is needed are usually said to be due to impairment. However, it is also important to bear in mind that the need for assistance is also related to social conditions and the existence of social and environmental barriers (Finkelstein, 1998). By way of example, a disabled person who is said to need a 'carer' in order to cast her vote at the ballot box, might not need this assistance at all if the polling station and its procedures were made accessible. Another distinction in the concept of *caring for* may be drawn between the informal 'care' that is part of interpersonal relationships, described above, and that which is paid for. Stereotypes of disabled people as dependent and in need of specialist 'care' and intervention are still prevalent, and may be used to justify the existence of for-profit enterprises and a charity sector that depends on disabled people for a living (Albrecht, 1992; Wolfensberger, 1988).

Because of these issues, disability studies authors have often used alternative terms, such as help (Shakespeare, 2000), or, more widely, assistance, in preference to care. Some of the ways that new services have been developed in line with this are described next.

Independent living and personal assistance

The concept of independent living is an alternative to care and has been central to the campaigns of disabled people's organisations. Disabled people mobilised to further their political and civil rights from the 1960s onwards (Hunt, 1966), and between 1981 and 1993 the number of organisations of disabled people grew from 16 to over 80 in the UK (Davis and Mullender, 1993). Campaigning, led by the British Council of Organisations of Disabled People (now replaced by the UK Disabled People's Council), focused on access issues, legislative change and independent living (Pridmore, 2005; Priestley, 2003). Personal assistance services were and still are a key focus for action within a broader framework.

There are a variety of definitions of independent living but all are concerned with choice, control, freedom and equality (Hasler, 2003). It has also been termed inclusive or interdependent living, to more clearly distinguish the term from doing things on one's own or without assistance.

> 'Independent Living' means that disabled people want the same opportunities and the same choices in everyday life that their non-disabled brothers and sisters, neighbours and friends take for granted ... Most importantly, just like everyone else, disabled people need to be in charge of their own lives, need to think and speak for themselves without interference from others. (Ratzka, 1996: 1)

For some disabled people, personal assistance is essential for independent living and direct payments are the key to paying for it. Disabled people's organisations in many countries took inspiration from the Berkeley Center for Independent Living's first personal assistant (PA) support scheme in California, and the European Network for Independent Living (ENIL) has campaigned for a right to user-controlled personal assistance since 1989 (ENIL, 1989).

Direct payments

In the UK, direct payments are sums of money paid by local authorities, following assessments, to eligible disabled people to purchase assistance needed for daily living. Typically, they allow the employment of personal assistants, who are accountable to the service user rather than the service system, but the money may also be spent on equipment or other relevant services.

The first direct payments in the UK were made to a small group of disabled people in Hampshire in the early 1980s, enabling them to leave the institutions they were living in. This was a 'third party' arrangement, with the money paid into a voluntary sector trust, because it was then illegal for payments (rather than services) to be made directly to service users. Following many years of campaigning by disabled people, the Community Care (Direct Payments) Act 1996 finally reversed the National Assistance Act 1948, permitting local authorities to make direct payments to those eligible (Glasby and Littlechild, 2002). With cost a concern to governments, an important study by Zarb and Nadash (1994) demonstrated that direct payments were no more expensive than directly provided services. When implemented, direct payments were 'bolted on' to already existing community care measures: cash payments were equivalent to the cost of the service that they would have received under community care assessments.

Initially, payments were restricted to adults with physical impairments under 65, deemed 'willing and able' to manage the payments, primarily due to concerns about demand. As direct payments were seen to be successful, with substantial improvements in many disabled people's quality of life (Priestley et al., 2009), eligibility was widened to include more groups: older people, children aged 16–18, carers and parents of disabled children.

However, consistent evidence emerged of the widespread omission of people with learning difficulties and those with mental health conditions. Local authorities consistently judged that these groups were not able to manage direct payments and constituted too much of a 'risk'. Patchy implementation remained, even after it became mandatory for social workers to offer the option of direct payments to eligible applicants, and the 'willing and able' clause was removed in 2009. Overall, local authorities have been considered to be unsupportive of direct payments and there is some evidence that many social workers have not understood them or agreed with them (Ellis, 2007).

Individual and personal budgets

Attempts to widen access for people with learning difficulties were led by *In Control*, a social enterprise that worked primarily with local authorities to change structures and systems, also aiming to influence national government. Efforts largely focused on making changes from the top down, independently of the disabled people's movement. *In Control* advocated providing money to each individual based on a 'resource allocation system', although this has been used less in recent years due to the bureaucracy it generated (Duffy, 2011). Service providers investigated whether it was possible to pool money from several sources (such as the Department of Health and the Department of Work and Pensions) into one pot controlled by the service user: an individual budget. Pilot programmes to merge some pools of funding were set up but ran into difficulties with administrative complexity (Glendinning et al., 2008). Beyond the possibility of merging aspects of health and social care, these have not been subsequently pursued and personal budgets have only been used for social care finances.

The key initiative implemented was the introduction of personal budgets, mainly aimed at people with learning difficulties but also other service users. While similar to direct payments, personal budgets allow some variation in terms of management of the funding. A number of options besides taking full responsibility for managing money are possible, including paying third-party organisations (such as a private agency or voluntary organisation) for management services, setting up trust funds or asking a local authority to manage the money on the recipient's behalf. These options aimed to make it possible for more people with learning difficulties to gain control over funds because of the removal of the requirement to manage payments without support. They also aimed to save money (Leadbetter et al., 2008).

Notable successes were reported in the early days of implementation, when the more enthusiastic councils reported innovative ways of putting disabled people in charge of their own assistance. However, there are indications that local authorities have become much more restrictive in recent years and that progress has once again slowed (Duffy, 2011).

Personalisation

Both direct payments and personal budgets have received cross-party support in the UK. Current social policy in relation to disabled people may be summed up by the term 'personalisation' and a drive towards 'self-directed support'. However, personalisation is not neatly defined – the meaning has shifted over time and it is used to mean different things by different groups of people. Leadbetter (2004) first introduced the term during the New Labour regime, suggesting a continuum of five possible meanings, ranging from an increased orientation towards service users as customers, to co-producing solutions to social problems with service users:

> by putting users at the heart of services, enabling them to become participants in the design and delivery, services will be more effective by mobilising millions of people as co-producers of the public goods they value. (Leadbetter, 2004: 19)

While broadly in line with independent living, therefore, personalisation has drifted away from an emphasis on independent living, involvement and partnership, and towards a concern with reforming services through direct payments and personal budgets.

In the UK, institutions, community care services and direct payments/personal budgets exist side by side (Woodin et al., 2009). In 2011, one third of all eligible service users were receiving a personal budget or direct payment and, of these, 44 per cent were direct payments and 56 per cent budgets that were managed by other people (Jerome, 2011). For England, the Association of Directors of Social Services (ADSS, 2012) reported an increase of 38 per cent in the number of people receiving personal budgets between 2010–11 and 2012, with 52.8 per cent of eligible service users in receipt at March 2012. Clearly, this represents a considerable increase in numbers. This being said, a mechanistic approach to implementation and a watering down of the degree of control have been reported, especially where budget management is retained by local authorities (Hatton and Waters, 2011). With pressure from national government for all service users to receive budgets, there may be a tendency for local authorities to rename what they are already doing, personalisation.

The trends discussed in this chapter are also apparent in other European countries. Despite variations in western capitalist welfare states (Esping Andersen, 1990), the replacement of institutions by community services and greater individualisation of support services are apparent in most EU countries (Evans, 2003). Townsley et al.'s (2010) review of progress for the Academic Network of European Disability Experts (ANED) project also points out that while most European countries have policies supporting independent living, implementation is patchy and people with learning difficulties are still likely to be left out of important legal safeguards (such as the recognition of the right to make decisions). ENIL and others have criticised the use of European Union funding by some countries to pay for the maintenance of institutions, and while Townsley et al. (2010) describe positive developments, only three countries in their study reported having no institutions. Even in these, there were indications that larger group homes were being re-opened.

Conclusion: Progress and issues

Austerity measures in western welfare states are also affecting the balance between informal care provided by families and that provided by the welfare state. While the benefits of direct payments and personal budgets have been well established, the majority of disabled people do not receive them and instead receive informal assistance from family and friends if it is needed. In England, there are indications that this trend is increasing, with the number of people receiving social care services decreasing by 7.7 per cent between March 2011 and 2012 (ADSS, 2012), despite rising demand for public services overall. Over the same time period, the number of carers in receipt of personal budgets rose by 15 per cent, with just under half being one-off payments. The state is pushing responsibility for providing assistance back into the home and it does not appear likely that this will change dramatically while the welfare state continues to shrink (see Jolly, undated for European examples). At the same time, these developments take place in a wider economic and social context where there are a range of views about the value and significance of personalised support (Oliver and Barnes, 2012), as well as the degree to which disabled people are entitled to it.

There is little doubt that for many disabled people access to personal assistance has truly been groundbreaking and a revolution in service provision. At the same time, they are an individual, and therefore limited, solution to a wider social problem concerning the social creation of dependency.

References

Albrecht, G. (1992) *The Disability Business: Rehabilitation in America*. London: SAGE.

Association of Directors of Social Services (ADSS) (2012) *Personal Budgets Survey, March 2012: Results*. London: ADSS.

Barnes, C. (ed.) (1993) *Making Our Own Choices: Independent Living, Personal Assistance and Disabled People*. Nottingham: Barnes and Humby.

Beresford, P. (2008) *What Future for Care?* York: Joseph Rowntree Foundation.

Davis, K. and Mullender, A. (1993) *Ten Turbulent Years: A Review of the Work of the Derbyshire Coalition of Disabled People*. Nottingham: The Centre for Social Action.

Duffy, S. (2011) A Fair Society and the Limits of Personalisation. Available at: www.centreforwelfarereform.org/uploads/attachment/261/a-fair-society-and-the-limits-of-personalisation.pdf [accessed 21/05/11].

Ellis, K. (2007) 'Direct payments and social work practice: the significance of "street-level bureaucracy" in determining eligibility', *British Journal of Social Work*, 37 (3): 405–22.

ENIL (1989) The Strasbourg Resolutions. Available at: www.independentliving.org/ [accessed 26/06/12].

Esping Andersen, G. (1990) *The Three Worlds of Welfare Capitalism*. Cambridge: Polity.

Evans, J. (2003) Disabled People in Europe are Demanding the Right to Independent Living. Paper presented at Paris Disability Expo, 27 March. Available at: www.leeds.ac.uk/disability-studies/archiveuk/evans/ [accessed 16/06/12].

Finkelstein, V. (1998) Re-thinking Care in a Society Providing Equal Opportunities for All. A discussion paper. Available at: www.leeds.ac.uk/disability-studies/archiveuk/finkelstein/finkelstein2.pdf [accessed 19/05/12].

Galvin, R. (2004) 'Challenging the need for gratitude: comparisons between paid and unpaid care for disabled people', *Journal of Sociology*, 40 (2): 137–55.

Glasby, J. and Littlechild, R. (2002) *Social Work and Direct Payments*. Bristol: Policy Press.

Glendinning, C., Challis, D., Fernandez, J., Jacobs, S., Jones, K., Knapp, M., et al. (2008) Evaluation of the Individual Budgets Pilot Programme: Final Report. Available at: http://php.york.ac.uk/inst/spru/profiles/cg.php#pubs [accessed 24/06/12].

Hasler, F. (2003) 'Philosophy of independent living', in J. Alonso and G. Vidal (eds), *The Independent Living Movement: International Experiences*. Santa Barbara, CA: Independent Living Institute. Available at: www.independentliving.org/docs6/hasler2003.html [accessed 22/4/13].

Hatton, C. and Waters, J. (2011) The National Personal Budget Survey. Available at: www.thinklocalactpersonal.org.uk/ [accessed 26/06/12].

Hunt, P. (1966) 'A critical condition', in P. Hunt (ed.), *Stigma*. London: Geoffrey Chapman.

Jerome, J. (2011) Putting People First: Third Year Progress. Available at: www.thinklocalactpersonal.org.uk/_library/Resources/Personalisation/Personalisation_advice/2011/ADASS_Personal_Budgets_Survey_March_2011_-_Summary_of_Results_9.6.11_3.pdf [accessed 20/05/12].

Jolly, D. (undated) Personal Assistance and Independent Living: Article 19 of the UN Convention on the Rights of Persons with Disabilities. Available at: www.leeds.ac.uk/disability-studies/archiveuk/ [accessed 23/06/12].

Leadbetter, C. (2004) Personalisation through Participation: A New Script for Public Services. Available at: www.demos.co.uk/publications/personalisation [accessed 20/05/12].

Leadbetter, C., Bartlett, J. and Gallagher, N. (2008) *Making it Personal*. London: Demos.

Lynch, K., Baker, J. and Lyons, M. (2009) *Affective Equality: Love, Care and Injustice.* Basingstoke: Palgrave Macmillan.

Morris, J. (2001) 'Impairment and disability: constructing an ethics of care that promotes human rights', *Hypatia*, 16 (4): 1–16.

Oliver, M. and Barnes, C. (2012) *The New Politics of Disablement.* Basingstoke: Palgrave Macmillan.

Pridmore, A. (2005) *Fighting Talk.* London: British Council of Disabled People.

Priestley, M., Woodin, S., Matthews, B. and Hemingway, L. (2009) *Choice and Control/ Access to Goods and Services: A Rapid Evidence Assessment (REA) of Disability Research.* London: Office for Disability Issues.

Rae, A. (1993) 'Equal opportunities, independent living and personal assistance', in C. Barnes (ed.), *Making Our Own Choices: Independent Living, Personal Assistance and Disabled People.* Nottingham: Barnes and Humby. pp. 47–50.

Ratzka, A. (1996) Introduction to Direct Payments for Personal Assistance. Available at: www.independentliving.org/docs5/IntroDirectPayments.html [accessed 23/06/12].

Shakespeare, T. (2000) *Help: Imagining Welfare.* Birmingham: Venture Press.

Thomas, C. (1999) *Female Forms: Experiencing and Understanding Disability.* Buckingham: Open University Press.

Townsley, R., Ward, L., Abbott, D. and Williams, V. (2010) The Implementation of Policies Supporting Independent Living for Disabled People in Europe: Synthesis Report. Available at: www.disability-europe.net/theme/independent-living [accessed 22/05/12].

Wolfensberger, W. (1988) 'Human service policies: the rhetoric versus the reality', in L. Barton (ed.), *Disability and Dependency.* Brighton: Falmer Press. pp. 23–40.

Woodin, S., Priestley, M. and Prideaux, S. (2009) ANED Report on the Implementation of Policies Supporting Independent Living for Disabled People: United Kingdom, Academic Network of European Disability Experts. Available at: www.disability-europe.net [accessed 16/06/12].

Zarb, G. and Nadash, P. (1994) *Cashing in on Independence: Comparing the Costs and Benefits of Cash and Services.* Sommercotes: Bailey & Sons.

33

Counselling and Disabled People: Help or Hindrance?

Donna Reeve

Introduction

In recent years, more and more people have been turning to counselling to help resolve personal difficulties in their lives. Disabled people also want access to counselling which meets their perceived needs (McKenzie, 1992) – whether they want to look at marriage problems, childhood traumas, stress or bereavement, or issues associated with disability/disablism or impairment. However, some writers have acknowledged that disabled people have been generally avoided as a client group by psychotherapists and counsellors and that there is a legacy of prejudiced attitudes, with an associated dire need to undertake more consciousness-raising, training and research (McLeod, 2009). The introduction of disability discrimination legislation in 2004 obliged counselling agencies to make their services more accessible to disabled people. While many disabled people do experience counselling as helpful and enabling, others find counsellors who do not understand the complexity of the lived experience of disability.

In this chapter, I discuss some of the particular problems which can undermine the counselling experience of disabled clients, showing how and why the counselling relationship can end up being more of a hindrance to personal growth and self-fulfilment, than a help. As well as identifying some of the potential pitfalls, I suggest changes which could remove some of the barriers that can cause disabled people to give up on counselling as having anything useful to offer them.

Counselling theory: The dominance of individual models

The avoidance of disabled people as a client group is reflected in the relatively small number of pages in the counselling literature devoted to understanding personal responses to disability. Swain et al. (2003) argue that there has been little engagement with the social model of disability and instead various individual models of disability predominate. For example, the tragedy model of disability underpins a common assumption that there will be a process of psychological adjustment as the individual comes to terms with their impairment. In order to overcome their perceived loss, disabled people are expected to grieve and go through a process of mourning akin to that of bereavement, expressing feelings of anger and denial before they can become psychologically whole again (Lenny, 1993). These 'loss models' arise from the imagination of non-disabled people about what it must be like to experience impairment, assuming that becoming disabled must be psychologically devastating (Oliver, 1996). This contradicts reports of disabled people themselves, who instead locate the source of emotional distress in the failure of the environment to take account of their needs (Oliver, 1995). These loss models have been criticised for failing to take into account the socially constructed nature of disability, although they may have limited use for understanding individual responses to *impairment* (Reeve, 2000).

Counselling responses that are based on individual models of disability are disempowering because they reinforce the notion that disability is an individual problem caused by impairment, rather than recognising the role that society plays in creating and maintaining this form of social oppression. It is important that the emotional reactions of a disabled client to the experiences of exclusion and discrimination – such as justifiable frustration and anger – are not pathologised (Olkin, 1999). This failing is exemplified by Wilson (2003), who, after discarding the social model in two pages, instead draws on object relations theory to conclude that those with congenital impairments perceive 'that they must be the result of bad intercourse' (Wilson, 2003: 100).

As well as using models which predict the way that people are expected to adjust to disability, counsellors also work within different theoretical frameworks; most commonly used are the first-wave counselling approaches which include psychodynamic, cognitive-behavioural and person-centred approaches. Whilst all of these focus on the individual rather than society, person-centred counselling would appear to offer the least intrusive approach with its lack of assumptions about how people respond to disability (Lenny, 1993). However, Swain et al. (2003) point out that one pitfall of person-centred approaches, which deliberately resist labelling people or groups, is that they end up producing 'a de-politicising of disablement. The oppression of disabled people is disavowed' (Swain et al., 2003: 143).

Despite the suggestion by the loss models that disabled people need counselling to deal with disability (and that disability is going to be the only issue they want to talk about), there is relatively little literature about working with this particular client group. Whilst there are some books which provide practical information about working with disabled people (such as Brearley and Birchley, 1994), there are fewer books which treat disability as a form of social oppression rather than an individual problem (see, for example, Corker, 1995; Olkin, 1999). This dearth has ramifications for counselling training and practice which I will now discuss in more detail.

Disability: A missing element of counselling training

Although there has been a substantial rise in the number of counsellors being trained, the number of disabled counsellors and counselling students remains low (Withers, 1996). The high cost of training courses, coupled with inaccessible teaching rooms and course materials, results in the exclusion of many disabled people who have the potential to train as counsellors. The increasing need for such courses to become accredited and recognised academically can exclude even more disabled students when entry requirements stipulate a first degree. Courses require students to undertake skills practice within counselling agencies and many also expect students to have received counselling themselves. The inaccessibility of many counselling venues, together with the high cost of receiving personal counselling, further compounds the barriers faced by disabled people who want to become counsellors. The scarcity of disabled students on counselling courses means that disability is not present 'in the room' in the same way that gender, sexuality and ethnicity often are. Many disabled people who train as counsellors have to deal with reactions of pity, anger and embarrassment from prejudiced tutors and fellow students (Withers, 1996).

A major difficulty for many counselling courses is that they are expected to cover a lot of counselling theory and practice within a relatively short space of time. Consequently, there is little teaching time devoted to issues around diversity – maybe two days in a two-year part-time diploma course – and Disability Equality Training is generally absent from these courses. The general lack of social model approaches within the counselling literature, coupled with little or no teaching of disability as a diversity issue alongside gender, ethnicity and sexuality, mean that the prejudices and stereotypes which abound in society around disability are not exposed and challenged within counselling courses (Reeve, 2000). This can have adverse effects on future counselling relationships if the counsellor is unaware of their own prejudicial attitudes towards disabled clients (Parkinson, 2006).

Counselling services: Inaccessible or 'elsewhere'

It can be very difficult for disabled people to find accessible counselling services. Voluntary-sector counselling agencies operate on a shoestring budget and are often sited in old buildings with poor access. Consequently, disabled clients who cannot access the available counselling rooms may be offered counselling by telephone or in a different place; one agency counselled clients with mobility impairments in a local church because their usual counselling rooms were located up a flight of stairs with no available lift. Private counsellors do not provide a viable alternative because they are expensive and very few homes in the UK are wheelchair-accessible. This experience of exclusion from services that non-disabled people take for granted, can be a source of indirect psycho-emotional disablism (see Chapter 13) because of the way that it serves to remind disabled clients that they are different and 'out of place'. This form of psycho-emotional disablism can be further compounded by counsellors who fail to treat their disabled clients with forethought and respect – for example, by failing to move furniture out of the way before a client who is a wheelchair user arrives for their counselling session.

The low number of disabled counsellors within counselling practice contributes to the failure of counselling agencies to bear in mind the access needs of potential disabled clients. Some agencies believe that disabled people do not want counselling because they never see disabled clients – being situated in an inaccessible building or failing to produce information about the counselling service in accessible formats may contribute to this misconception! Another myth is that disabled people are counselled 'somewhere else' by experts who have the perceived specialist counselling skills needed to work with this client group. In reality, there are a few counselling agencies which specialise in working with disabled clients, but these are not available to the vast majority of disabled people. This myth defends a counsellor against having to look at their own fears and vulnerabilities about illness, disability or death. Other counsellors feel de-skilled and out of their depth when working with disabled clients because counselling cannot 'fix' disability or impairment.

The way forward

Although it is fair to say that counselling services are gradually improving for disabled people – helped by disability discrimination legislation that has increased the visibility of disabled people in society – I would suggest that there are four areas which would benefit from continued improvement.

First, it is vital that Disability Equality Training becomes a mandatory part of all counselling courses so that students (and tutors) learn about the social model of disability and understand how disability is socially constructed rather than being caused by a person's impairment. The training also needs to include a discussion about psycho-emotional disablism, social practices and processes which undermine the emotional well-being of people with impairments (see Chapter 13). Counsellors need to be more aware of the emotional consequences of living with prejudice, exclusion and discrimination and how this can impact on the self-esteem and self-worth of their disabled client, often in the form of internalised oppression (see also Watermeyer and Swartz, 2008). Not only would this training enable students to realise the extent of disablism within all aspects of social life, but it would directly challenge many of their own prejudices and stereotypes about disabled people. Unfortunately, some students (and counsellors) are reluctant to look at their own prejudices around disability because they already 'unconditionally accept all people' (Reeve, 2000). It would also be useful to introduce students to disability culture, helping them appreciate the diversity of disability experience (Marks, 2002).

Second, it is important that disabled people are not viewed as a client group to be counselled 'somewhere else' and instead that all counsellors are trained to be able to work with disability-related issues if and when they arise. Whilst it would improve the degree of client choice if more trained disabled counsellors were available within the counselling profession, it is not *necessary* for disabled clients to be counselled by disabled counsellors. Disabled people are not just people with impairments, they are also parents, siblings, children, workers and friends; as such they are subject to the same range of emotions and difficulties as non-disabled people and should have access to the same choice of counselling services if they want them. More importantly, as anyone can become disabled or be affected by disability in the family, disability issues are likely to be present in some form or other in much of the work done by mainstream agencies. For example, counsellors working within alcohol and drug agencies may see clients who have become disabled through substance misuse or who are drinking because of the stresses of caring for a disabled family member. Disability may or may not be the presenting issue, but counsellors need to be aware of the effects disablism can have on the lives of their clients and their families.

Third, counselling agencies must conform to the Equality Act 2010 which means making 'reasonable adjustments' to make their services accessible to both disabled and non-disabled people. This includes supplying information in accessible formats and where premises cannot be made accessible, alternative counselling provision through telephone counselling or home visits must be made. There are issues about safety, neutrality and privacy when seeing a client in their own home but these should not be used as an excuse to refuse counselling services to disabled clients. If British Sign Language (BSL) provision is available, then counsellors who are not fluent in BSL will need to adapt to the particular challenges of working with a third person in the room when counselling a Deaf client. Counsellors need to be flexible about the parameters of counselling sessions when working with disabled clients because impairment effects may impact on the frequency, timing and length of counselling sessions (Olkin, 1999). External factors such as the availability of community transport may influence when a disabled client can attend as well as their punctuality.

Finally, working with disabled clients not only challenges where and for how long counselling sessions take place, it also questions the usefulness of first-wave counselling approaches which pay little attention to issues of power both within the counselling relationship and outside the counselling room (McLeod, 2009). One solution to this would be to make person-centred counselling more relevant for disabled clients by making the conditions of worth better contextualised to take account of history and culture (Johnson, 2011). Alternatively, second-wave counselling approaches could be considered which explicitly work with issues of power and diversity and recognise the potential danger for oppressive counselling practice. Therefore, systemic, feminist, multicultural and narrative approaches to counselling might be very helpful as a starting point when working with disabled people because they 'incorporate the socio-political into the therapeutic' (Olkin, 1999: 300). These anti-oppressive approaches would meld seamlessly with a social model viewpoint of disability (Swain et al., 2003) because of the shared goals of emancipation and empowerment.

Conclusion

Whilst many disabled people do experience counselling which is supportive and empowering, others face inaccessible counselling rooms, inappropriate counselling models and prejudiced counsellors – these factors can result in counselling which instead is an oppressive, disabling experience. The introduction of disability discrimination legislation has improved *physical access* to counselling services for disabled people, although much work still needs to be done in improving counsellor training, practice and theory to improve the quality of the counselling *relationship*.

Current counselling theory is still based largely on the experiences of non-disabled people, which means that individual model interpretations of disability predominate, which at best produce emasculated non-politicised understandings of disablism (Swain et al., 2003). As well as recognising the many different ways that disabled people deal emotionally with the experience of disablism, it would be beneficial to move towards more socially aware forms of counselling which recognise the impact of the world 'out there' on the counselling room 'in here'.

Counsellor training must include a social model approach to disability, educating students about both structural and psycho-emotional disablism and the potential impact on the emotional well-being of disabled clients. Counsellors also need to consider their own prejudices and assumptions about disabled people if they themselves are not to become part of an oppressive culture (Corker, 1995). Disabled people have a right to the same range and quality of counselling services as other client groups in society, and the Equality Act 2010 must be implemented by counselling agencies in order to make their services available to disabled people. However, change does not stop with the provision of ramps and large-print information; it needs to permeate policy and practice within counselling agencies at all levels.

References

Brearley, G. and Birchley, P. (1994) *Counselling in Disability and Illness* (2nd edn). London: Mosby.

Corker, M. (1995) *Counselling: The Deaf Challenge*. London: Jessica Kingsley.

Johnson, C. (2011) 'Disabling barriers in the person-centered counseling relationship', *Person-Centered & Experiential Psychotherapies*, 10 (4): 260–73.

Lenny, J. (1993) 'Do disabled people need counselling?', in J. Swain, V. Finkelstein, S. French and M. Oliver (eds), *Disabling Barriers – Enabling Environments*. London: SAGE, in association with the Open University. pp. 233–40.

Marks, D. (2002) 'Some concluding notes: healing the split between psyche and social – constructions and experiences of disability', *Disability Studies Quarterly*, 22 (3): 49–56.

McKenzie, A. (1992) *Counselling for People Disabled through Injury*. York: Joseph Rowntree Foundation.

McLeod, J. (2009) *An Introduction to Counselling* (4th edn). Maidenhead: Open University Press.

Oliver, J. (1995) 'Counselling disabled people: a counsellor's perspective', *Disability & Society*, 10 (3): 261–79.

Oliver, M. (1996) 'A sociology of disability or a disablist sociology', in L. Barton (ed.), *Disability and Society: Emerging Issues and Insights*. Harlow: Longman. pp. 18–42.

Olkin, R. (1999) *What Psychotherapists Should Know About Disability*. New York: The Guilford Press.

Parkinson, G. (2006) 'Counsellors' attitudes towards Disability Equality Training (DET)', *British Journal of Guidance & Counselling*, 34 (1): 93–105.

Priestley, M. (2003) *Disability: A Life Course Approach*. Cambridge: Polity Press.

Reeve, D. (2000) 'Oppression within the counselling room', *Disability & Society*, 15 (4): 669–82.

Swain, J., Griffiths, C. and Heyman, B. (2003) 'Towards a social model approach to counselling disabled clients', *British Journal of Guidance & Counselling*, 31 (1): 137–52.

Watermeyer, B. and Swartz, L. (2008) 'Conceptualising the psycho-emotional aspects of disability and impairment: the distortion of personal and psychic boundaries', *Disability & Society*, 23 (6): 599–610.

Wilson, S. (2003) *Disability, Counselling and Psychotherapy: Challenges and Opportunities*. Basingstoke: Palgrave Macmillan.

Withers, S. (1996) 'The experience of counselling', in G. Hales (ed.), *Beyond Disability: Towards an Enabling Society*. London: SAGE and the Open University Press. pp. 96–104.

34

Developments in Mental Health Policy and Practice: Service User Critiques

Peter Beresford

Introduction

If anything, the pace of change in mental health policy and services has accelerated in recent years. However, for many service users and people experiencing madness and distress, the system shows little improvement; indeed there are suggestions that problems with the psychiatric system are getting worse. For example, a 2012 report from the London School of Economics argued that only 25 per cent of people in need get help, referring to the 'scandalous' scale of the NHS's neglect of mental health problems (Boseley, 2012; CEP Mental Health Policy Group, 2012). There are few areas of health and welfare activity as contradictory, ambiguous and politicised as modern mental health policy. To make sense of it, it is necessary to examine its formal arrangements, its stated aims and some of the inconsistencies between them and the reality that service users experience.

Three big changes, representing a break from the past, have shaped mental health policy and practice over the last 30 or so years, and look like shaping it for the foreseeable future. The first was the closure of most of the old big Victorian institutions and the move to 'care in the community'. The second was the emergence of the mental health service users/survivors movement. The third and most recent involved efforts to drive mental health service users off benefits and into employment. All have fundamental implications for both policy and practice and service users.

Care in the community

The ending of the old 'asylums' and the closure of hospital beds was linked to a move to a new philosophy – 'care in the community', based on people being able to stay in their own homes, live in a 'neighbourhood' and have suitable support to do so. Care in the community was associated with the expansion of a wide range of 'community-based' services, including day centres/hospitals, supported housing, non-residential support workers, training and employment opportunities. The community care reforms of the early 1990s were introduced by Conservative governments committed to an increased emphasis on private provision in health and welfare and the reduction of state intervention and expenditure (Rogers and Pilgrim, 2001). Their policies were based on a market approach and emphasised 'consumer choice' and involvement. Their argument was that the use of public services, including health and welfare services, should be seen in the same way as the consumption of any other goods or services. Here was the meeting point of government with the other key new development: the emergence of the mental health service users/survivors movement.

The developing service user/survivor movement

Building on new official opportunities for user involvement, service user organisations expanded dramatically during the 1990s. A large and growing number (albeit a small proportion overall) of mental health service users/survivors have become involved in service user groups and organisations at local, regional, national and international levels. The mental health service user/survivor movement is concerned not only with self-help and mutual support, but also with collective action to reform the service system and make wider changes. There are now black and minority ethnic organisations as well as organisations for people hearing voices, with eating distress and who self-harm. Service users have also exerted some influence on traditional charitable mental health organisations (Campbell, 1996, 2009).

While both government policy and the survivor movement have placed an emphasis on 'partnership' and 'involvement', they have often meant different things by them. The state and service system has predominantly been concerned with a managerialist/consumerist approach to user involvement based on consultation and information gathering, comparable to the market research of commercial companies. Service users have been more interested in a democratic approach to involvement that challenges existing inequalities of power and offers service users an increased role in decision-making over both their individual and collective experience of mental health and other services. The focus of government interest in user involvement has been on improving the operational efficiency of the service system; that of the survivor movement has been on improving the quality of people's lives. These are significantly different, sometimes conflicting goals.

Service users and 'dangerousness'

Despite the hopes that many service users and workers invested in care in the community, successive governments failed to fund it adequately or implement it properly. Funds gained from the closure of long-stay psychiatric hospitals were not used to develop community-based mental health services, but instead diverted to other areas of healthcare. Poor agency and service coordination, communication and integration created additional problems (Coppick and Hopton, 2000). The reality for many service users was being left without adequate or appropriate support, sometimes without a roof over their heads or in poor quality and unsuitable accommodation, but this was not the issue that became the news story. Instead, the tabloid press attacked care in the community as defective in principle and accused it of leading to an increase in killings of members of the public by mental health service users. While this was contradicted by the evidence (Taylor and Gunn, 1999), media preoccupation with violence rapidly had the effect of politicising mental health policy. Where the tabloids led, politicians seemed prepared to follow. There has been a consistency in this policy thrust since just before the 1997 general election, with politicians and governments seeking to increase the compulsory powers that can be imposed upon mental health service users, to extend these beyond the hospital and, in the case of people categorised as having 'severe dangerous personality disorder', prior to the commission of or conviction for any offence. Service users have increasingly been framed in terms of dangerousness and negative risk, restrictions have increasingly been imposed on their rights and increasing numbers have been restricted in secure and forensic services (*Daily Telegraph*, 1998; Kemshall, 2009). Thus, three government concerns have dominated government mental health policy through to the second decade of the twenty-first century:

- a view of mental health service users as dangerous
- the need to give top priority to 'public safety'
- the achievement of this by emphasising control and compulsory 'treatment'.

Service users as dependent

More recently, an additional pressure has been imposed on mental health service users. This has been the pressure for them to get off benefits and into paid employment. It can be seen as part of broader policies directed at disabled and long-term sick people. The Labour government first associated itself with this policy goal, with its slogan of getting 'a million people off incapacity benefits', regarding unemployment as the key criterion of social exclusion (Levitas, 1998). More recently, Coalition welfare reform has sought to reduce the number of disabled people and people with long-term conditions receiving benefits, both by reducing access to such benefits and developing harsh and arbitrary review procedures.

This has had particularly negative effects on mental health service users, as their impairments are not as well recognised or understood as those of people with physical and sensory impairments. While this has been done in the name of reducing the 'public deficit', it has also been strongly associated with the government's anti-state agenda and its regressive approach to social policy (Davison and Rutherford, 2012). Coupled with hostile and stigmatising political and media campaigns against 'benefit scroungers', it has massively increased anxiety and insecurity among mental health service users (Strathclyde Centre for Disability Research and Glasgow Media Unit, 2011; Beresford and Andrews, 2012; Diary of a Benefit Scrounger et al., 2012). It has been accompanied by 'disinvestment' from support services, like day centres, and a shift to ideas of 'reablement' and provision to get people into paid work, however appropriate and possible this may or may not be.

Policy pointing in two directions

Ideas of 'empowerment', 'involvement' and 'well-being' lie at the heart of government mental health policy and pronouncements. The question, however, for both policy makers and service users is whether you can have a successful and supportive policy driven by what appear to be contradictory goals and values, both to compel and empower service users, and to involve, control and stigmatise them. Policy and philosophy are both ambiguous and contradictory (Newnes et al., 2001). Service users and their organisations have rightly feared that the focus of policy would increasingly be on controlling people seen as a threat, rather than on ensuring support for the many more who need it but are not seen to pose any danger. The barriers facing mental health service users are already substantial (Sayce, 2000). There are strong links between poverty, social deprivation and mental health service use. People with mental health problems are identified as having the highest rate of unemployment among disabled people (Mind/ BBC, 2000). It can only be expected that with increasing stigmatisation, these barriers will increase.

The problems of provision

Acute (hospital) services, particularly in the big cities, are associated with poor conditions. They are frequently unsafe for women service users, who are still placed in mixed wards. Mental health service users report problems accessing adequate, appropriate and reliable support services. They are much more likely to be offered neuroleptic drugs than the 'talking' and 'complementary' therapies which service users experience more positively. Some groups of black and minority ethnic service users still face particular discrimination and poor support in the service system. The low status of mental health service users and services means that there are continuing problems of funding, staff recruitment and retention. While the integration of health and social care in mental health was envisaged as a route to improved services and service coordination, service users have real concerns that it will undermine social understandings of their distress and reinforce traditional (unhelpful) medicalised individual understandings of their situation and experience. This is also reflected in government interest in and emphasis on the idea of 'recovery', which is explicitly based on a medical understanding of madness and distress. Service users are understandably concerned that the only services they may access are those provided through extended compulsory powers of mental health legislation, based on the chemical and mechanical approaches about which service users have particular worries and fears.

Since the 1990s, different approaches have been developed to try and ensure that service users receive a careful assessment of their needs and a suitable plan for their support, both of which they are meant to be involved in shaping. Multidisciplinary community mental health teams have also developed to increase the involvement of service users and to work in a more holistic and coordinated way. However, service users often report little real involvement in their treatment and so far have had little effective involvement in the development of policy and practice at a broader level. While it has been a central focus of their activities, mental health service users and their organisations have so far had very limited success in reforming the service system (Campbell, 2009).

Different ways of understanding

Service users and their organisations have increasingly been arguing for different ways of understanding and responding to their situation, because existing 'treatment' can often be worse than their original distress. A survey of people with mental distress carried out by the Mental Health Foundation found that different things helped different people at different times. Neuroleptic drugs did not work for everyone. They affected people differently, were not enough on their own and were often prescribed without information about their unwanted effects. People wanted to have a holistic approach to their support, which took account of all aspects of their life, including the material, emotional and spiritual. They wanted their own expertise about themselves to be valued and to have choices in the 'treatment' they were offered (Faulkner, 1997). The user-led Strategies for Living project found that some of the supports and activities that people find most helpful are acceptance, shared experience, emotional support, finding meaning and purpose, feeling secure and safe, pleasure, relaxation and having a reason for living (Faulkner and Layzell, 2000).

Mental health service users place an increasing emphasis on user-led, non-medicalised alternatives to provide the kind of support they want. These include complementary therapies, peer support and personal survival strategies. This has also encouraged service users/survivors to campaign for and develop their own non-medicalised user-led crisis and out-of-hours services, including safe houses and refuges, helplines staffed by survivors, peer counselling and advocacy schemes, and so on. These are valued by service users, but still only exist on a small scale. Mental health service user/survivor organisations have also developed their own advance directives and crisis card schemes so that individuals can specify in advance what they want to happen and who they want contacted if they have a bad time and don't feel able to take control (Beresford, 2010).

Mental health service user/survivor organisations are now paying more attention to combating the discrimination they face and adopting the kind of rights-based approach to securing support and countering prejudice which the broader disabled people's movement pioneered. This has been encouraged unintentionally by government attempts to increase compulsory provisions for 'treatment' and increasingly hostile welfare reform policies, which have led to more campaigning and direct action by service users/survivors. Mental health service users/survivors are paying increasing attention to safeguarding their rights and have begun to develop stronger links with the disabled people's movement. They have looked at how they can use the Equalities Act 2010 and Human Rights Act 1998 to safeguard their rights.

Many mental health service users/survivors are eligible for 'personal budgets' and 'direct payments' which can put them in control of the support they receive (see Chapter 32). So far, relatively few mental health service users/survivors are getting direct payments, but the numbers and interest have grown. They offer a valuable way of getting the kind of non-medicalised support that many service users/survivors value. They offer a practical basis for preventive support. Many mental health service users/survivors are keen to get back into employment, but they continue to face major obstacles. Government emphasis on employment as an obligation, rather than a right, poor conditions in the labour market, and the continuing failure of the benefits system to enable people to move flexibly in and out of work as their changing situation demands, all make this unnecessarily difficult. Evidence is already growing, however, that where the contribution of service users/survivors is valued and supported, they have much to offer (Snow, 2002).

Some mental health service users/survivors reject the idea of 'mental illness' as damaging and stigmatising. For others, it is the only model for understanding their situation that they have been offered. Service users/survivors are now, however, showing a much greater interest in social approaches to understanding and responding to distress. Many also see medicalised individual models as inherently damaging in effect (Beresford et al., 2009).

The survivor movement has not yet developed a *social model* of madness and distress that might challenge medicalised individual models of 'mental health' which still predominate and require service users to prove mental 'incapacity' to get benefits or support (Beresford et al., 2002). However, discussions about such an equivalent of the social model of disability have now begun. Such a model perhaps offers one of the most hopeful bases for transforming attitudes towards, and services for, mental health service users/survivors. Like the social model of disability before it, it may offer service users a way of understanding their experience in relation to the barriers and discrimination they face and highlight more clearly the priorities and strategies that will most effectively overcome them.

References

Beresford, P. (2010) *A Straight Talking Guide to Being a Mental Health Service User*. Ross-on-Wye: PCCS Books.

Beresford, P. and Andrews, E. (2012) Caring for Our Future: What Service Users Say. A programme paper, March, Joseph Rowntree Foundation. Available at: www.jrf.org.uk/publications/caring-our-future-what-service-users-say

Beresford, P., Harrison, C. and Wilson, A. (2002) 'Mental health, service users and disability: implications for future strategies', *Policy and Politics*, 30 (3): 387–96.

Beresford, P., Nettle, M. and Perring, R. (2009) *Towards a Social Model of Madness and Distress? Exploring What Service Users Say*, 22 November. York: Joseph Rowntree Foundation.

Boseley, S. (2012) 'Scandal of mental illness: only 25% of people in need get help', *The Guardian*, 18 June, p. 7.

Campbell, P. (1996) 'The history of the user movement in the United Kingdom', in T. Heller, J. Reynolds, R. Gomm, R. Muston and S. Pattison (eds), *Mental Health Matters: A Reader*. London: Macmillan. pp. 18–25.

Campbell, P. (2009) 'The service user/survivor movement', in J. Reynolds, R. Muston, T. Heller, J. Leach, M. McCormick, M. Wallcraft and M. Walsh (eds), *Mental Health Still Matters*. Basingstoke: Palgrave. pp. 46–52.

CEP Mental Health Policy Group (2012) How Mental Illness Loses Out in the NHS. Centre for Economic Performance's Mental Health Policy Group, London, LSE, June.

Coppick, V. and Hopton, J. (2000) *Critical Perspectives on Mental Health*. London: Routledge.

Daily Telegraph (1998) 'Care in the community is scrapped', 17 January, p. 1.

Davison, S. and Rutherford, J. (eds) (2012) 'Welfare reform: the dread of things to come', in *Soundings On*. London: Lawrence and Wishart.

Diary of a Benefit Scrounger, Campbell, S.J., Anon, M.E., Marsh, S., Franklin, K., Gaffney, D., Anon, Dixon, M., James, L. and Barnett-Cormack, S. (2012) Responsible Reform: A Report on the Proposed Changes to Disability Living Allowance. London: Spartacus. Available at: http://wearespartacus.org.uk/spartacus-report/ [accessed 19/09/12].

Faulkner, A. (1997) *Knowing Our Own Minds: A Survey of How People in Emotional Distress Take Control of Their Lives*. London: Mental Health Foundation.

Faulkner, A. and Layzell, S. (2000) *Strategies for Living: A Report of User-Led Research into People's Strategies for Living with Mental Distress*. London: Mental Health Foundation.

Kemshall, H. (2009) 'Mental health, mental disorder, risk and public protection', in J. Reynolds, R. Muston, T. Heller, J. Leach, M. McCormick, M. Wallcraft and M. Walsh (eds), *Mental Health Still Matters*. Basingstoke: Palgrave. pp. 147–59.

Levitas, R. (1998) *The Inclusive Society? Social Exclusion and New Labour*. Basingstoke: Macmillan.

Mind/BBC (2000) *Mental Health Factfile*, January. London: Mind.

Newnes, C., Holmes G. and Dunn, C. (eds) (2001) *This is Madness Too*. Ross-on-Wye: PCCS Books.

Rogers, A. and Pilgrim, D. (2001) *Mental Health Policy in Britain* (2nd edn). Basingstoke: Palgrave Macmillan.

Sayce, L. (2000) *From Psychiatric Patient to Citizen: Overcoming Discrimination and Social Exclusion*. Basingstoke: Macmillan.

Snow, R. (2002) *Stronger than Ever: Report of the First National Conference of Survivor Workers UK*. Stockport: Asylum Press.

Strathclyde Centre for Disability Research and Glasgow Media Unit (2011) *Bad News for Disabled People: How the Newspapers are Reporting Disability*. Glasgow: University of Glasgow.

Taylor, P. and Gunn, J. (1999) 'Homicides by people with mental illness: myth and reality', *British Journal of Psychiatry*, 174: 9–14.

35

The Global Economy of 'Care'

Maria Berghs

Disabled people have generally been critical of notions of 'care' pointing to a legacy of institutionalisation and dehumanising care, medical paternalism and the failures of adequate provision of alternatives, such as community care or even independent living. Feminists, too, have pointed to the dangers of essentialism in not only linking care to a specific gender but also the rising global inequalities that structure much paid and unpaid caring work. In an increasingly globalised world, the provision of care has also become a transnational commodity which is gradually becoming more market-driven. Globalisation or a process of increasing economic, political, social, cultural and technological interconnectedness now affects all forms of care.

The business of providing healthcare, social care or other services for disabled people is now being exported economically, politically, socially, culturally and technologically to other parts of the world, contributing to a growing internationalisation of care (Holden, 2002). Under the guise of offering more consumer 'control' and 'choice' to individual service users, what we are witnessing is the neoliberal privatisation, commercialisation and dismantling of services that disabled people use, both in Europe and in a more global context. Instead of a system that allows service users to demand and protect their rights, with respect to how care is commissioned, the commodification of care shows that those individual rights are being eroded. This chapter will illustrate this, beginning with the marketisation of care.

The commodification of care

The way that the global economy of care is structured in an international context is understood through the increasing importance of transnational international organisations and the global flow of capital and services. All countries have to decide how to structure and pay for health and social care and which economic model to use. Depending on what the political background of a state is, a liberal, conservative, communist or socialist model can be enacted with some sort of welfare provision. However, in an increasingly globalised world, most countries do not have a choice about adopting neo-liberal economic policies and this has a big impact on the fragmentation and privatisation of health and social care services.

After the Second World War in 1945, the Bretton Woods institutions were established by 44 countries to regulate the global monetary system and financial markets. These institutions included the International Monetary Fund (IMF) and the International Bank for Reconstruction and Development. The IMF was responsible for lending money internationally and regulating the financial markets. The International Bank for Reconstruction and Development was in charge of loans to aid the reconstruction of European countries after the war. The International Bank for Reconstruction and Development later become the World Bank Group (WBG). The WBG is a group of five organisations that have a broad mandate which ranges from reducing poverty to providing technical assistance and services.

The IMF later developed to monitor the world's economy, loan money to any country facing financial difficulties and also give low- and middle-income countries technical financial assistance. Low- and middle-income countries are classified by these institutions in terms of a country's gross national income or as developing economies (World Bank, 2012). WBG policy is to work with very low-income countries all over the world; those whose governments are fragile and have been affected by conflict, Arab countries undergoing transition, middle-income countries, and also to provide multilateral trade and services.

The IMF and WBG have a history of working together, such as in terms of the 1980s' structural adjustment policies which set out certain conditions for loaning money. These conditions have now been reframed in Poverty Reduction Strategy Papers (PRSPs) to ensure greater ownership by countries. PRSPs are nationally and internationally agreed plans to reduce poverty in a country and they are also monitored under an established time frame. In 1947, the General Agreement on Trade and Tariffs (GATT) was also established to work with the IMF and WBG. GATT is an international multilateral agreement that was designed to regulate global trade. In 1995, GATT was further developed to become an institution, the World Trade Organisation (WTO), not only ensuring the regulation of goods but also services. Under a General Agreement on Trade in Services (1995), expanded in 2000, services have become part of multinational trade negotiations. Over 188 countries are members of these institutions and committed to neo-liberal free trade agreements, privatisation of state services, deregulation of the labour market and global public–private partnerships (PPPs).

In order for a country to gain access to global capital to implement economic reforms, rebuild after a conflict or protect against market shocks, they have to go to the world's bankers, the IMF or the WBG. The IMF, WBG and WTO are also members of the United Nations (UN) system and work closely with other international institutional bodies. The global agenda determining how health and social care are organised is set through international legislation by the UN and defined in universal terminology and policy. This is often directed by the World Health Organization (WHO) and other institutional bodies dealing with such services. An example is the

UN legislation on the Convention on the Rights of Persons with Disabilities (CRPD) where 'Persons with Disabilities' is defined according to WHO terminology. Other examples, impacting health and social care, are the UN's Millennium Development Goals (MDGs) – eight internationally agreed goals which range from ending poverty, combating infectious diseases, improving maternal and child health to promoting access to education by 2015. Despite a global understanding that to tackle poverty, attention needs to be paid to the differing inequalities that face disabled people, they are not mentioned in the MDGs. It remains to be seen if they will be included post-2015. However, there are commitments to mainstream or include disabled people and their issues in development aid and policy by international institutions. The WHO and the UN also work closely with national governments setting health and social care policy.

Delimiting health and social care services

In the European context, health and social care services used to be seen as distinct sectors, one focusing on combating illness and the other on improving quality of life. Healthcare was provided mainly in clinical settings or in the community by health-care professionals. In contrast, social care services were provided by local authorities, voluntary or charitable organisations. Social care services can be for both children and adults. Depending on a given country's social policy, they can range widely from provision of social services, care in homes, long-term care facilities and day services for disabled people to information and support for carers. The multi-faceted nature of social care services illustrates a rise in demand for such services.

Both health and social care provision are currently managed by local government authorities, as well as the independently operated private and voluntary sector. They are increasingly being integrated due to European Union (EU) and international policy but with mixed results. Leichsenring (2012: e7) argues that this is due to: (1) 'long-term care for older persons'; (2) 'marketisation'; (3) 'lack of managerial knowledge'; (4) a 'shortage of care workers'; and (5) a 'downsizing of social care services'. There is thus a consolidation of the limited services provided and a widespread move towards the valorisation of health over social care.

Financial demands and lack of resources mean an increasing focus on prevention of disease and disability, over cure and duty of care. This has entailed that health and social care services have had to be contracted out to third parties, often multinational and commercial in nature, or taken up by the community. This focus is not incidental but in line with the recent WHO emphasis on public health within community settings (i.e. WHO and UNICEF, 2012). However, limited integration can open up the debate between institutionalisation and care in the community. In a time of austerity, where government budgets are being cut, social care services are often the first to be affected and independent living or care in a community cannot be ensured. Periods of financial crisis usually go hand in hand with an increase in socio-economic problems. A protracted period of austerity strains communities and families' abilities to cope and depletes their resources. Media coverage on increases in poverty in Southern and Eastern Europe illustrate a renewed reliance on voluntary, charity and religious organisations and social care institutions.

Thus, the current financial crisis calls into question the ability of local governments and the EU to achieve the UN CRPD or even all MDGs. European Disabled People's Organisations (DPOs) are warning that commitments to the CRPD are being flouted. ENIL (2011) has found that austerity measures and cuts in EU structural funds are disproportionately affecting disabled people and leading to social exclusion. While privatisation and integration of health and social care is not new, austerity measures can accelerate the speed of privatisation. If we examine the UK in particular, a clearer picture is given of what integration means. The UK's Coalition government, in order to reduce the public deficit, is reviewing funding for health and social care and implementing policy changes.

A Vision for Adult Social Care: Capable Communities and Active Citizens (Department of Health, 2010) outlines the personalisation and privatisation of adult social care. Additionally, there is a move towards integrating care across health and social care, such as in mental health services. This is enacted in the Health and Social Care Act 2012, outlining the reforms bringing together both health and social care. Many of these reforms are economic, and target not only social care services but also who can access them. Studies that ask service users about social care paint a bleak picture of the devastating consequences of spending cuts and a lack of engagement with service users (Beresford and Andrews, 2012). Current evidence states: 'the reduction in social care budgets and increased demand is resulting in local authorities tightening their eligibility criteria for people to receive state-funded community care' (Care Quality Commission, 2011: 5).

Pollock et al. (2012: e1729) note that the Act had a framework limiting the duty of care of the National Health Service (NHS), effectively paving the way for 'transition from tax financed healthcare to the mixed financing model of the United States'. This gives greater powers to clinical commissioning groups (with strong involvement from general practitioners) and local authorities to delegate health and social care services to global commercial companies. In line with the current Coalition government's idea of the 'big society', individual service users are also expected to engage with the voluntary sector, the NHS, local government authorities and/or independent companies who offer health and social care services, to 'personalise' their care. However, what this means in practice is that social care services are fragmented, delimited and exclusionary – since they have to make a profit.

The provision of care seems to be shifting back to individuals, families and local communities, disproportionally affecting certain groups of people such as the elderly, single parents, women, disabled people and those living in deprived areas and from ethnic minorities. Ultimately, the powers and responsibility of the state to care are being diluted, and Whitfield (2001: 84) argues that its role has become that of 'enabling' and 'facilitating' rather than interventionist. The same thing is happening in an international context where the voluntary sector is becoming increasingly responsible for the provision of services that the government cannot or will not provide.

NGO-isation and corporatisation care

If we take a concrete case-study example from Africa, we can see the impact of institutional polices on health and social care. Examining the aid history of the West African country Sierra Leone, after its ten-year civil war ended in 2002, a trend is noted towards multilateral development aid to donors over bilateral aid to the government, with medical care getting funding before any social care services could be developed (Berghs, 2012).

Sierra Leone, defined as low-income and a fragile recovering state, took out loans from the IMF and WBG in order to rebuild. It was required to write PRSPs and within those papers there is mention of poverty reduction work linked to disabled people and the promotion of their human rights. The country has also ratified UN legislation on the CRPD and now has a Disability Act but there is very little enforcement of either national or international legislation protecting disabled people. Indigenous understandings of impairment and disability are ignored in favour of WHO terminology and policy objectives set out in western terms. Donors tackle issues linked to public health concerns with huge private philanthropic investment, such as HIV/AIDs, that do not reflect local realities. Additionally, public health concerns, stories and imagery of disabled people are commodified. This aids charitable funding for donors, the disability business and financial rebuilding of the economy.

The Sierra Leonean state does not have the resources to implement a fully functioning healthcare system or social care, thus in order to reach part of the MDGs, donors have had to go into partnership with voluntary, religious and other non-governmental organisations (NGOs) who can provide the infrastructure, procurement, technical training and social care services that are missing. An additional development is that many multinational companies will provide either infrastructural support, health or social care services but at an economic cost to the state, in terms of the expectation of access to resources, such as land or minerals. Most of these organisations are not Sierra Leonean but are international and have transnational funding. They face no regulation of service provision nor do any partnerships between health and social care services and the private sector. There are no strong trade unions; nor is there any protection of workers or service users.

Additionally, there is no welfare system or minimum wage and most people cannot afford private social insurance contributions. Instead, people rely on minimal state services and access the voluntary sector, extended family or community to provide services or pay user fees in an impoverished context. Service funding is often not secure, transparent or mainstreamed towards disabled people and long-term planning is not possible. In practice, this means that disabled people fall back on the segregated specialised services, vocational schools and charitable institutions that existed in the past, as well as new services that certain NGOs provide.

The process of service provision and care is largely top-down and lacking true partnership, although it claims to have service users' human rights as a guiding universal principle. The focus on the prevention of poverty as an MDG goal linked to disabled people has also involved a charitable approach to aid viewing disabled people as vulnerable. This ignores the heterogeneity of impairment and historicity of how disability is created. The critical ability of disabled people to question this status quo is also silenced as DPO funding is tied to accepting certain frameworks of aid linked to disability. A commodification and colonialisation of health and social care is being imported. The effects of the above on disabled people are profound, as people learn to take on a mentality of 'victimhood' as dependency is enforced (Berghs and Dos Santos-Zingale, 2011). Using discourses of rights, and revalorising their cultural resources, disabled people are trying to fight against such victimisation but it remains to be seen how the financial crisis will affect the provision of care to this group of people and whether it will ever be on their own terms.

Conclusion: The future of global care

In this chapter, using examples from a European and an African context, it has been shown how it is now the large international organisations and voluntary sector that will have to provide both health and social care. Demand for both services is expected to rise worldwide. There will also be problems in ensuring the sustainability of many community and voluntary organisations whose funding will be affected by budget cuts and the global recession. While multinationals may fill in the gaps in some places, they will increasingly require payment for their services, meaning necessary PPPs.

In such a way, a consumer model is required as service users or local authorities are expected to contribute towards services so a profit is made. Neo-liberalism delimits the state's intervention in places such as Eastern and Southern Europe as well as the BRIC countries (Brazil, Russia, India and China). There we see outcomes of rapid urbanisation, hunger for new resources and the capitalist model of consumption contributing to rising inequalities between people, social injustice and environmental degradation.

This is in line with IMF, WBG and WTO policies linked to the neo-liberalisation of economies, privatisation of services and proliferation of the global economy. Development agencies such as the UK's Department of International Development and the Asian Development Bank now promote PPP as integral to aid, outlining a bigger trend of all donor agencies, such as the UN, becoming increasingly corporatised in terms of demanding aid effectiveness, value for money, budget monitoring, as well as profit, in order for services to remain sustainable in the long term.

In terms of funding health and social care, priority has been given to healthcare because of the possibility of measuring outcomes statistically and getting that value for money which is not always evident in social care. However, implementing the PPP model undercuts ideas of equity and social justice in terms of access to healthcare. In response to this, the WHO is now actively promoting a Commission on Social Determinates of Health which seeks to investigate the links between economic and social causes of health inequalities and how to reduce those. In such an approach, a lot of attention is placed on primary care services, prevention of impairment and the good health of new generations rather than on the duty of care and rights of existing service users. The socio-political context, violence, historicity and racism behind many health inequalities in a global context are ignored as well as the need for care linked to social justice.

When funding is cut to the voluntary sector and state services are not financially equipped to deal with caring for service users, care becomes a burden that is often borne by the family and disproportionally by the female gender. Instead of understanding care in terms of a moral responsibility to enable access, both in a local and global context, neo-liberalism has led to widening inequalities. These inequalities lead not only to disabling barriers in accessing health and social care, but also a violation of human rights.

References

Beresford, P. and Andrews, E. (2012) *Caring for Our Future: What Services Users Say*. York: Joseph Rowntree Foundation.

Berghs, M. (2012) *War and Embodied Memory: Becoming Disabled in Sierra Leone*. Aldershot: Ashgate.

Berghs, M. and Dos Santos-Zingale, M. (2011) 'A comparative analysis: everyday experiences of disability in Sierra Leone', *Africa Today*, 58 (2): 18–40.

Care Quality Commission (2011) *State of Care Report 2010/11*. London: Care Quality Commission.

Department of Health (2010) *A Vision for Adult Social Care: Capable Communities and Active Citizens*. London: Department of Health, Social Care Policy.

European Network on Independent Living (ENIL) (2011) *ENIL Proposal for a Resolution of the European Parliament on the Effect of Cuts in Public Spending on Persons with Disabilities in the European Union*. Background note, September. Valencia: ENIL.

Holden, C. (2002) 'The internationalization of long term care provision: economics and strategy', *Global Social Policy*, 2 (1): 47–67.

Leichsenring, K. (2012) 'Integrated care for older people in Europe: latest trends and perceptions', *International Journal of Integrated Care*, 12: e7.

Pollock, A.M., Price, D. and Roderick, P. (2012) 'Health and Social Care Bill 2011: a legal basis for charging and providing fewer health services to people in England', *British Medical Journal*, 344: e1729.

Whitfield, D. (2001) *Public Services or Corporate Welfare: Rethinking the Nation State in the Global Economy*. London: Pluto Press.

WHO and UNICEF (2012) *WHO/UNICEF Joint Statement Integrated Community Case Management (iCCM)*. Geneva: WHO and UNICEF.

World Bank (WB) (2012) *How We Classify Countries*. Washington, DC: World Bank.

Part 5

Looking to the Future for Disabled People

36
Disability and Social Inclusion in the Information Society

Sally French and John Swain

Introduction

Over 30 years ago, Finkelstein (1980) welcomed the beginning of the third of what he identified as separate historical phases. Without going into detail, phase two saw the onset of the industrial revolution and capitalism in the nineteenth century in Western Europe and North America. This was an era of the enforced dependency and exclusion of disabled people. Disabled people were often debarred from paid employment due to the nature of work and they were also often segregated from mainstream society, most obviously through placement in large-scale institutions. If phase two was a time of the disablement of people with impairments, 'phase three heralds the elimination of disability' (1980: 8). Phase three is the emergence of post-industrial society, referred to by various terms including postmodern and, most relevant to this chapter, the information society. The central feature is the developing technology which, for Finkelstein, would enable 'the most severely physically impaired people to operate environmental controls which can enable them to live relatively independently in the community' (1980: 11).

The years since Finkelstein put forward these ideas have been years of dramatic change. Technology has developed so rapidly and been taken up so extensively that any list will be out of date almost before it is published, but must include: the computer, the Internet, emails, mobile phones, texting, blogging, iPhones, iPods, iPads, Twitter, Facebook and digital radio and television. In western societies, and increasingly globally, technology is ubiquitous and it is hardly possible to walk down a street without seeing someone plugged-in in some way, receiving and sending messages.

The purpose of this chapter is to consider whether the processes of change to an information society that began to emerge in the last quarter of the twentieth century are associated with the inclusion of people with impairments, as consistent with Finkelstein's views, or whether they are generating a process of exclusion in other forms. To facilitate the writing of this chapter, and to complement the literature and relevant research, we conducted three interviews with blind people about their particular experiences with technology and accessing information.

The information society

What, then, is the information society? Perhaps not surprisingly, this is not an easy question to answer. To start with, there are numerous closely related concepts such as the post-industrial society, post-fordism, postmodern society, knowledge society, information revolution and network society. Webster (2006) recognised five types of definitions of the information society which pinpoint different central criteria: technological, occupational, economic, spatial and cultural. Analysing what has changed in the move from an industrial society to an information society is indeed complex but the following points seem to recur throughout the literature:

1 Change is reverberating throughout society. It is economic, political and cultural.
2 Change is therefore inherent to all aspects of people's lifestyles: work, leisure, relationships, beliefs, identity, and so on. It has transformed how we live.
3 Since the 1970s, a transformation from industrial society to information society has happened on a global scale.

The information society is one in which the creation, distribution, diffusion, use, integration and manipulation of information is a significant economic, political and cultural activity (Castells, 2009).

As we saw above, for Finkelstein this emerging historical phase would be one of radical change for disabled people. His ideas have been challenged, however, from within disability studies. In his seminal work, Oliver (1990) argued that Finkelstein's historical model was both 'over-simplistic and over-optimistic' (p. 29). In his review of the literature, Sapey came to the following conclusion:

> The question I am interested in is whether these changes in the economic sphere have in any way changed the nature of disability and at the moment it would appear from the evidence that rather than liberating disabled people, new technologies have created forms of work and welfare that may be more exclusionary than those of the industrial era. (2004: 278) (see Chapter 23)

Before we look in some detail at the possibilities for disabled people, let's look a little further at general changes in the post-industrial information society. It is a subject which of course requires volumes, particularly as it needs a global perspective. Here, we shall return to Webster's five criteria mentioned above for a brief word about each. Turning to developing technology first, to a certain extent we hardly need academics to verify that change has taken and is taking place. It is there in our homes and at work on the streets. For instance, overall Internet usage has seen tremendous growth. From 2000 to 2009, the number of Internet users rose globally from 394 million to 1.858 billion (www. internetworldstats.com/stats.htm, 28 April 2012). The revolution is rolling at such a speed it is impossible to select significant landmarks, but certainly the spread of computer communication technologies has been crucial (email, texting, online information exchange, and so on), particularly as these have taken off on iPhones and iPads (see Chapter 24).

For many sociologists, it is the changes in the nature, meaning and organisation of work which are central in defining the information society. The number of employees producing human services and information is seen as the indicator for the informational character of a post-industrial society. Bell (1976) explained this as follows:

> A post-industrial society is based on services ... What counts is not raw muscle power, or energy, but information ... A post-industrial society is one in which the majority of those employed are not involved in the production of tangible goods. (p. 127)

This has implications for education, including the need for a system of mass higher education and, given the speed of development, the necessity of re-skilling.

Information and technology are clearly central to the economy, with the possibility of shifting money at the push of a button becoming possible for everyone with online and now mobile phone banking, but this only provides the means. What matters is ownership and control and, with it, power. Crucial here are growing economic inequalities, globally between the majority and minority worlds, and also between rich and poor within nations. For example, the richest 2 per cent of the world's population owns about half of the global household wealth, while the bottom 50 per cent of the population owns about 1 per cent of the wealth (UNDP, 2007).

Space is another clear characteristic of the information society, with technology that connects different locations in towns, countries and indeed around the world. Constraints of distance and time, given the speed of flow of information, have been radically relieved. Finally, living in a smaller world, there is now a torrent of culture. Again, the evidence is there surrounding us – television all day with multiple channels, radio, music and films to download, and so on, and being regularly added to (such as recently by Kindle). With the global media market we have seen the domination of transnational corporations including Disney, News Corporation and General Electric (Held, 2004).

There are considerable debates around this whole area, but we can only mention one of particular relevance to this chapter. There has not been an equal access to, ownership and use of technology. If we look globally, for example, while there is about 75 per cent of the population of the minority world on the Internet, in the majority world it is only about 20 per cent (www.internetworldstats.com/stats.htm, 28 April 2012). We shall return to this 'digital divide' later.

Towards exclusion and inclusion

We turn, then, to the lives and experiences of disabled people, drawing first on the three interviews we conducted. All were positive about the effects of technology on their lives and, as is evident in the following quotes, across a variety of activities:

> Anybody, whether they're blind or sighted can get in touch with me by email and I can read it. I can send emails to them and my visual impairment doesn't impede contact with people because it will come to them in a visual format and it will come to me in a Braille format or speech. (Mary)

> I've been able to help my children with their homework. I've got two kids. I can look up the subjects they're learning and find the answers. I can also organise things such as holidays. It's the best thing. It's given me more independence. I can book my own flights abroad. I can look at all the fares from different airlines. (Jagdish)

> I find it's lovely having emails especially from my friends abroad, my pen friend in America, my two pen friends in Russia and my nephew in Australia. My nephew used Scipe [sic] one Christmas and I think that's absolutely wonderful. (Jane)

Jane also finds the Internet useful in maintaining her hobbies:

> I look things up on Google which is good. I found a lot of information about crocheting and knitting because I do a lot of that. I've found addresses of people who supply thread and wool for my crafts which is very useful.

This echoes the findings of, amongst others, Harris (2010). She researched disabled people's views and experiences of the use of technology in the home. She generally found that 'disabled people engage enthusiastically with advanced technologies and appreciate the increased independence that access to such devices can bring' (p. 436). She also found that this reflected the views of disabled people irrespective of their impairment.

The interviewees talked about the importance of technology in their work. Indeed, Jagdish's work involves training disabled people to use computers. He has become something of an expert:

> Now I can take apart any computer and re-build it, I can deal with any problem. Now, without the computer I would be lost. I never used a computer in my sighted days. The only thing I used was a typewriter and that was it. I do everything now, PowerPoint, spreadsheets, Word processing, just about everything.

Mary spoke of the control new technology gave her over her work:

> I worked as a typist for nearly 30 years using an ordinary typewriter and quite honestly it was stressful. The computer took an awful lot of stress out of it

because you could make corrections and you were in charge of your own work and were independent. I was working for the Inland Revenue.

Roulstone (1998) conducted the first large-scale study in the UK which was directed at investigating disabled people's experiences in relation to paid employment, as workers and job-seekers. He found that: 'The majority of participants felt that new technology had in some way begun to enhance their employment as disabled workers' (p. 126).

The benefits his participants mentioned included being able to compete on equal terms, making working from home possible and enhancing communication. Nevertheless, there has not been a substantial improvement in the numbers of disabled people in employment in the information society (Stanley, 2005).

In their review of 'digital disability', Goggin and Newell (2003) observed that there is a large array of websites, information, newsgroups, discussion lists and groups, and chat rooms on the Internet concerned with disability. In recent years, this has been added to in unknown numbers by blogging, Twitter, Facebook and YouTube. Whatever the numbers are, it seems likely that the number of disabled people included and participating is growing. A variety of disabled people embrace the online world. There is a thriving online world for people who identify culturally as being Deaf. There is also an active, energetic online world of blind and visually impaired people.

The Internet has also fostered the disabled people's movement, particularly the international movement, through the formation of the online disability community. The Internet has become a key site for the sharing of common experiences and the shaping of shared values between disabled people. The discussion of disablism, and the shared and differing experiences of oppression and discrimination, is one of the constitutive parts of the online disability community. The formation of communities of interest, on email discussion lists, web-based chat rooms, Internet messaging, websites, online magazines and journals, and so on, furthers the possibilities for disability cultures and the disability arts movement, with numerous examples of film-making, expressive writing, music and art by disabled people.

Guo et al. (2005) investigated the growing online disability community in China. They found that the Internet provided 'both a forum for discussion and a vehicle for new social relations unlike that found in the real world where issues of accessibility and discrimination constrain social participation' (p. 64). One of their research participants expressed this expansion of social networks very eloquently:

The Internet has greatly extended my social network. It is exciting and interesting to know various people across the country. With the Internet, disabled people have their wings. When on the Web, I feel like an angel freely flying. (p. 59)

Goggin and Newell (2003) found that some disabled people claim the Internet removes their disability, which is an interesting finding in the light of Finkelstein's model. Nevertheless this is, of course, not the full picture. Our interviewees talked of two problems that are regularly referred to by disabled people. The first is prohibitive cost, particularly for assistive technology, that is specialist devices designed specifically to assist disabled people. Mary told us: 'The software I have is called Keysoft and it comes from a company called Humanware. The only drawback is that it is very expensive but it does give you accessibility that you wouldn't have otherwise.'

Assistive devices can be problematic for a number of reasons as well as cost. Harris (2010) found that her participants sought to use mainstream rather than specialist assistive devices. Söderström and Ytterhus (2010) investigated the views of visually impaired young people concerning the use of assistive technologies from the world of information and communication technology (ICT). They found that the use of ICT was generally associated with competence, belonging and independence but the use of ICT assistive technologies symbolised quite the contrary view of restriction, difference and dependency, for these young people. Control of the application of technology in the home was the key for Harris's participants.

Second, in terms of the Internet and other sources of information, lack of access is a recurring problem:

Sally: Do you find that some websites are more accessible than others?

Mary: Some of them are quite difficult. The London Borough of Sutton website is being revamped but until recently it's been really hard to get into. Lots of images which obviously don't come up in Braille or speech.

The lack of accessible information has been a consistent finding in disability research. Hemingway (2011) found that information and advice on housing tend to be lacking for disabled people, particularly people with sensory impairments, creating substantial barriers in disabled people's housing choices and opportunities. Lobel also found that of '1,000 UK websites covering Government, business, entertainment and e-commerce ... 81 per cent failed prevailing web access guidelines' (2004: 45).

Finally, we return to what can be called the 'digital divide', that is the divide between Internet users and non-users. It is associated with factors such as education, the availability of Internet knowledge and economic status. Reporting from their research in six countries in Africa and Asia supplemented by evidence from the Disability Awareness in Action (DAA) archives, Dube et al. (2006) state that 'the Internet can provide an inexpensive and generally effective means to promote the inclusion and participation of disabled people' (p. 110). They then point out that the converse is equally true and the denial of access to the Internet, for whatever reason, further excludes disabled people from the mainstream. This 'disability divide' has increasingly become a crucial issue in the struggle for inclusion of disabled people (Jaeger, 2011).

Conclusion

To conclude, we will return to Finkelstein's proposition concerning the elimination of disability in the third historical phase, the information society. Is it over-optimistic? There are numerous indications that it is, particularly if paid employment remains the touchstone of inclusion. Nevertheless, it also seems undeniable that, for many disabled people, the technological age has brought greater control over the environment, enhanced independent living and inclusion. On the other hand, new technology is deepening the digital divide furthered by growing economic inequality. Perhaps, then, the safest conclusion which embraces Finkelstein's optimism for phase three is that it holds substantial possibilities for the elimination of disability and the inclusion of disabled people.

References

Bell, D. (1976) *The Coming of Post-industrial Society*. New York: Basic Books.

Castells, M. (2009) *The Rise of the Network Society: Information Age – Economy, Society, and Culture v. 1* (Information Age Series) (2nd edn). London: Wiley-Blackwell.

Dube, T., Hurst, R., Light, R. and Malinga, J. (2006) 'Promoting inclusion? Disabled people, legislation and public policy', in B. Albert (ed.), *In or Out of the Mainstream: Lessons from Research on Disability and Development Cooperation*. Leeds: The Disability Press. pp. 104–18.

Finkelstein, V. (1980) *Attitudes and Disabled People: Issues for Discussion*. New York: World Rehabilitation Fund.

Goggin, G. and Newell, C. (2003) *Digital Disability: The Social Construction of Disability in New Media*. Lanham, MD: Rowman & Littlefield.

Guo, B., Bricout, J.C. and Huang, J. (2005) 'A common open space or a digital divide? A social model perspective on the online disability community in China', *Disability & Society*, 20 (1): 49–66.

Harris, J. (2010) 'The use, role and application of advanced technology in the lives of disabled people in the UK', *Disability & Society*, 25 (4): 427–39.

Held, D. (2004) *A Globalizing World? Culture, Economics, Politics: Culture, Economics and Politics (Understanding Social Change)* (2nd edn). London: Routledge.

Hemingway, L. (2011) *Disabled People and Housing: Choices, Opportunities and Barriers*. Bristol: Policy Press.

Jaeger, P.T. (2011) *Disability and the Internet: Confronting a Digital Divide (Disability in Society)*. Boulder, CO: Lynne Rienner.

Lobel, A. (2004) 'Spreading the net', *Money Marketing*, 30 September. Available at: www.moneymarketing.co.uk/analysis/spreading-the-net/50775.article

Oliver, M. (1990) *The Politics of Disablement*. Basingstoke: Macmillan.

Roulstone, A. (1998) *Enabling Technology: Disabled People, Work and New Technology*. Buckingham: Open University Press.

Sapey, B. (2004) 'Disability and social exclusion in the information society', in J. Swain, S. French, C. Barnes and C. Thomas (eds), *Disabling Barriers – Enabling Environments* (2nd edn). London: SAGE, pp. 273–8.

Söderström, S. and Ytterhus, B. (2010) 'The use and non-use of assistive technologies from the world of information and communication technology by visually impaired young people: a walk on the tightrope of peer inclusion', *Disability & Society*, 25 (3): 303–15.

Stanley, K. (2005) 'The missing millions: the challenges of employing more disabled people', in A. Roulstone and C. Barnes (eds), *Working Futures? Disabled People: Policy and Social Inclusion*. Bristol: Policy Press. pp. 28–41.

United Nations Development Program (UNDP) (2007) *Human Development Report 2007*. New York: Oxford University Press.

Webster, F. (2006) *Theories of the Information Society* (3rd edn). London: Routledge.

37

Designing Inclusive Environments and the Significance of Universal Design

Rob Imrie

Introduction

> Design is only one part of the solution to a more inclusive world in which all people have equal opportunity for independence, autonomy and participation. But design matters. (Institute for Human Centered Design, 2011: 1)

In November 2010, a disability strategy was adopted by the European Parliament supporting the rights of disabled people to full and equal participation in society (European Commission, 2010). This followed on from Article 9 of the United Nations (2007) Convention on the Rights of Persons with Disabilities, which recognises the oppressive and unjust position of disabled people in society. It notes that governments must ensure that disabled people have 'access, on an equal basis with others, to the physical environment, to transportation, to information and communications ... and to other facilities and services open or provided to the public, both in urban and in rural areas'. This observation is based on the understanding that minimum standards of access are a pre-requisite for living independently and participating fully in all aspects of life. Article 9 provides a point of reference for other organisations, such as the European Union. It identifies the need for a mix of actions, including legal redress, to ensure that social justice for disabled people becomes enshrined in the activities and actions of providers of goods and services.

These observations are a response to the failures of decades of voluntary schemes and 'soft measures', and the realisation that disabled people's lives continue to be characterised by a palpable lack of access to goods and services. Disabled people are second-class citizens who, more often than not, are placed in contexts of dependence by socio-attitudinal values and practices that render much of the designed environment unusable or only accessible with third-party assistance. The problems for disabled people are well documented, and range from the inability of wheelchair users to use kitchen tabletops and work surfaces because they are placed too high for them to reach, to vision-impaired people experiencing difficulties in navigating around places because of the lack of legible signage sensitised to the needs of people with sight loss. In these instances, people with different impairments may experience disadvantage, and be prevented from an autonomy of action partly because design conceptions, in relation to artefacts ranging from laptops to doors, chairs and public transit systems, rarely conceive of impairment, disease and illness as part of everyday habitation or being.

The unjust nature of unequal access to, and lack of usability of, much of the designed environment, has not gone unchallenged, and viewpoints have emerged that promote the possibility of designed environments sensitised to the manifold complexities of the body (Pullin, 2009). The most significant is universal design (UD), defined by Ron Mace (1988: 1) as promoting 'the design of products and environments to be usable by all people, to the greatest extent possible, without the need for adaptation or specialized design' (see also Sanford, 2012). Since Mace's formative pronouncement, UD has become increasingly prominent and it is advocated by some national and international government, and non-governmental, organisations, including private corporations. Not only is UD seen as a solution to the problems posed to disabled people by poor design, it is also presented as 'design for all' and responsive, potentially, to any person's needs, irrespective of their bodily comportment and performance.

In the rest of the chapter, I assess UD and its significance in addressing the needs of disabled people in gaining access to, and being able to use, the many artefacts that comprise the designed environment. In doing so, I divide the chapter into three parts. First, I outline what UD is, and describe its development and evolution. Second, I evaluate the underlying principles of UD, and question how far they are able to form the basis of equitable or non-disabling design. I suggest that while UD is the basis of a progressive, forward-looking, social movement, it is not necessarily the panacea that some claim it to be in redressing the problems posed to disabled people by poorly designed environments. Third, I conclude by noting that there is much more to be done in developing the conceptual basis and practical applicability of UD. Greater scrutiny of the principles and practices of UD may enhance its value in seeking to overcome disablism by design (see also Imrie, 2012).

The popularisation of universal design

From the design of material artefacts, such as crockery, cutlery and light fittings, to the crafting of interior spaces in dwellings and public buildings, the character of people's everyday functioning is entwined with the quality of the designed environment (see Bardzell, 2009; Ewart and Luck, 2012). Quality of/in design can be defined, in part, as the usefulness of material artefacts, or the extent to which they facilitate people's capabilities to function in ways that they choose (Nussbaum, 2003; Sen, 1985). The notion of usefulness describes the basis of UD, that is, 'to make our built environment, products, and systems as enabling as possible' (Steinfeld and Maisel, 2012: 3). UD is a reaction to, and critique of, conventional design discourse that rarely considers users' interactions with(in) the material world. Rather, design discourse is characterised more by a focus on aesthetics, and the style, beauty and fitness of the designed environment, and less on the social responsibility of designers and the moral content of design (Owens, 2009; Tisdale, 1966).

A consequence is designers' preoccupation with the form not the function of artefacts, and the sidelining of issues relating to how well the designed environment performs in relation to people's needs. The latter are poorly defined and articulated in design discourse, characterised by a reductive conception of the human body that fails to identify the manifold ways in which bodies interact with different material objects (Bloomer and Moore, 1977; Imrie, 2003; Pallasmaa, 1996; Pullin, 2009). This is compounded by broader economic forces shaping the standardisation of products, creating design-types as part of an economy of design (see Holder, 1990; Papanek, 1971; Stone, 1983). The outcome is the (re)production of designed environments that are not necessarily sensitised to bodily variations, or to the almost constant changes in people's bodies over the life course. This may disable rather than enable people's ease of use of products, buildings and places, and restrict their independence and opportunities to self-express.

Proponents of UD regard much of the designed environment as hostile to people's ability to use material artefacts with ease, and as characterised by its inflexibility to respond to corporeal variations. Their starting point is the importance of sensitising design to the capabilities of the human body, in ways whereby anyone, irrespective of how their body performs, is able to gain access to, and make use of, the artefacts that comprise the designed environment. In this respect, UD is not aimed at any specific group, population cohort or type. Rather, the underlying feature of UD is its universal applicability or the 'design of places, things, information, communication and policy to be usable by the widest range of people operating in the widest range of situations without special or separate design' (Institute for Human Centered Design, 2011: 1; see also Mace, 1988). These broader sentiments have been codified into seven principles that conceive of the body as neither fixed nor static but as fluid and ever changing. As described by the Center for Universal Design (2011), these principles are:

Principle 1: *Equitable Use.*
The design is useful and marketable to people with diverse abilities.

Principle 2: *Flexibility in Use.*
The design accommodates a wide range of individual preferences and abilities.

Principle 3: *Simple and Intuitive Use.*

Use of the design is easy to understand, regardless of the user's experience, knowledge, language skills or current concentration level.

Principle 4: *Perceptible Information.*

The design communicates necessary information effectively to the user, regardless of ambient conditions or the user's sensory abilities.

Principle 5: *Tolerance for Error.*

The design minimises hazards and the adverse consequences of accidental or unintended actions.

Principle 6: *Low Physical Effort.*

The design can be used efficiently and comfortably and with a minimum of fatigue.

Principle 7: *Size and Space for Approach and Use.*

Appropriate size and space is provided for approach, reach, manipulation, and use regardless of user's body size, posture or mobility.

Government policies have yet to embrace, whole-heartedly, the principles of universal design. Instead, access legislation and directives, such as Part M of the building regulations in the UK, and the Americans with Disabilities Act 1990 in the USA, are favoured. The legislation compensates disabled people for the difficulties they experience in using the designed environment by providing specialised design, and creating bespoke products responsive to particular types of impairment. Proponents of UD are critical of this approach because they feel it draws attention to a person's impairment with the potential for stigma and social exclusion (Steinfeld, 1994). Instead, UD seeks to integrate the accommodation of impairment with the basic concept of the design, by sensitising the environment to the broadest possible range of bodily shapes, dimensions and movements. The objective is to draw attention away from people's impairment as a source or site of difference to minimise the possibilities of social ostracism.

Such views underpin UD's support for equitable use or the development of design that does not disadvantage any group of users (Sanford, 2012; Steinfeld and Maisel, 2012). A reduction in energy usage is one of the core principles or, as Steinfeld (1994) notes, people need an environment that eliminates unnecessary expenditure of effort. As Steinfeld (1994: 2) amplifies: 'this can be achieved by organising space and designing devices to simplify the task of using them ... useless movements should be eliminated'. Likewise, the illegibility of the built environment, and related products, is a constraint on their use and UD seeks to simplify environments by the use of colour and texture contrasts (see Ware, 2004, 2008). While Steinfeld (1994: 3) acknowledges that not all products and places will be usable by all people from the beginning, an objective of UD is to promote the flexibility, adaptability and interchangeability of fittings and fixtures to enable the greatest numbers of people to interact with them.

This reflects the development of UD, from its formative, idealistic understanding that design solutions were possible that could cater for all possible scenarios, to one whereby, as Vanderheiden (1996: 1) suggests, 'it is not possible, however, to create a product which is usable by everyone or under all circumstances' (see also Imrie, 2012). Proponents of UD accept, broadly, this viewpoint but note that the process of UD 'involves continuous improvement … towards the ultimate goal of full inclusion' (Steinfeld and Maisel, 2012: 29). This retains the, perhaps utopian, thinking that design solutions, responsive to all needs, can be attained. In this vein, some commentators, such as Steinfeld and Tauke (2003), support a progressive, linear understanding of human change, in which the processes shaping UD are, inevitably, part of a progression to an inclusive society. They suggest that the process of designing universally 'reflects a constant evolutionary process leading to more and more inclusion over time' (Steinfeld and Tauke, 2003: 1).

The definition of UD is also undergoing challenge, and refinement, in relation to how far designers can respond, practically, to the diverse nature of impairment, and the manifold interactions between bodies and material objects. Whereas the formative definition of UD appeared to discount any design that drew attention to impairment, by virtue of the use of specialised, assistive devices, recent enunciations recognise that there is a role for using technologies and techniques that are orientated, specifically, to meeting the needs of people with particular types of impairment. This view is reflected in the United Nations (2007) definition of UD, which states that 'universal design shall not exclude assistive devices for particular groups of persons with disabilities where this is needed' (United Nations, 2007). This highlights an unresolved tension in the UD movement, that is, how far can the universalisation of design co-exist with the recognition of bodily differences, and the need to respond to specific needs within a particularistic framework?

An evaluation of universal design

While UD appears to offer possibilities for liberating disabled people from disabling design, some commentators express reservations about how far its principles and practices are able to challenge, effectively, the embedded nature of discrimination by design in society (Imrie, 2012; Tobias, 2003; Ward et al., 2012). UD is, primarily, a technical approach to what are, predominantly, social and cultural issues that require, first and foremost, a political response based on systemic changes to those values and practices implicated in the (re)production of poorly designed environments (Imrie, 2012; Tobias, 2003). Yet, there is little evidence of the UD movement politicising the subject matter of design, or articulating an ethical-political philosophy that can guide such endeavours. Beyond some general observations about social justice, it is not clear what the ethical critique of society is that proponents of UD are propagating, nor how they envisage effective change to disabling design will take place (see Steinfeld and Maisel, 2012: 40–2).

The UD movement is characterised by a political conservatism that seeks to encourage voluntary uptake by organisations of design standards, codes and guidance. While this might be regarded as a pragmatic, realistic approach to crafting inclusive design, the evidence suggests that most corporate, and other, organisations pay lip service to issues of equity and access in relation to the designed environment, usually by providing a minimal response to the needs of disabled people (Imrie, 2006; Imrie and Hall, 2001; Ward et al., 2012). Ward et al.'s (2012: 410) research, based on interviews with house builders in Brisbane, Australia, generated responses such as 'it will only work voluntarily if they make money out of it' and 'the developer's not going to do it unless ... [he] gets all his money back'. Such responses indicate that only where a clear, demonstrable market demand, and profit to be made, are evident will organisations rise above minimum standards, and often in ways whereby what is provided does not depart from the provision of standardised design-types.

This reflects the social and technical relations of the design and development industry, underpinned by an economic rationale that does not prioritise, first and foremost, use value or the usefulness of the designed environment. This runs counter to the ethos of UD, yet there is little evidence of the UD movement seeking to develop a critique of the market model. If market mechanisms are unable to respond to corporeal diversity, it is incumbent on proponents of UD to suggest alternative ways of providing for bodily diversity outside of the mentalities of a cost calculus. This is not, as yet, evident, and part of the problem relates to lack of clarity about what, precisely, UD is requiring from designers. Further development of UD is required, including clarification of what the term 'universal' means and may entail in practice. How far does UD preclude the possibilities of particularistic responses to the needs of people with specific impairments? Or, conversely, does it require, as core to its realisation, a re-orientation of the socio-technical systems of design towards diversity and difference?[1]

Advocates of UD note that the key to developing and implementing such systems is technology, and writings about UD are dominated, disproportionately, by evaluations of technique and technological process. This emphasis is important, yet some commentators, such as Tobias (2003: 1), question the technological utopianism of UD, or the movement's 'uncritical belief in the benefits of technology'. For Tobias (2003), the realisation of benefits requires the UD movement to assert less the independent nature and power of technology per se, and, instead, to adopt a non-deterministic standpoint that conceives of technology as a socio-cultural construction, embodied and shaped by values, human intentionality and actions. Technology, in and of itself, is limited in its effects, and an illustration is a recent case of London bus drivers refusing to pick up wheelchair users, despite having the technological means, i.e. electronic ramped access, to do so (see Bellisario, 2012). Here, the technology was rendered irrelevant by the disabling socio-cultural attitudes of a cohort of bus drivers.

The UD movement also claims to be committed to a user-led design process that draws on the diverse experiences of people in interacting with the designed environment. However, there is a lack of clarity about how, practically, knowledge of the diverse design needs of people can be generated and designed into the UD process. Despite proponents of UD claiming that users are, or ought to be, more than passive recipients of expert opinion, there is little evidence of dissolution of the social relations of 'design authority', or the dominance of professional design-ers as the main agents (see Cohn et al., 2010). Most writings about UD see users in conventional terms, as consumers of a service, and only active in its production through market-based testing or exercises similar to those carried out by large private corporations prior to developing their latest products. A typical view is enunciated by two leading advocates of UD, Salmen and Ostroff (1997: 6), who suggest that 'designers must involve the future users, the customers of the design, through universal design reviews'.

This retains intact the hierarchical social relations of design, in which, in the writ-ings about UD, 'the user' is usually presented as a vague, subservient figure, described in ways that do little to reveal the subject's 'own interpretation of their condition' (Sayer, 2011: 250). This is compounded by the bypassing of direct, experiential data by recourse, in some instances, to stakeholder representation, or, as Salmen and Ostroff (1997: 6) suggest, 'designers must listen to and hear from perceptive spokespeople who can articulate the needs and responses of people of all stages of life'. Too often, such representations do not capture, or convey, the complexities of people's lives, and, in Sayer's (2011: 140) terms, they may fail 'to recognise humans as needy and vulnerable social beings'. Rather, the user is usually categorised in one-dimensional terms, as a rational, economically calculating agent, prone to acting in ways that can be 'pre-known', that is, an automaton more or less bereft of emotions, feelings and desires, and without subjectivity.

UD has universal, cross-cultural relevance but only if it is sensitive to, and seeks to work with, socio-cultural variations. For some, UD has ethnocentric overtones, by propagating western, Enlightenment values that conceive of UD as a process of linear progression and a stage-by-stage evolution to a better society. In making these claims, UD may be naturalising and normalising particular socio-cultural charac-teristics, or what Bauman (1993: 14) notes is the tendency for modern societies to practise 'moral parochialism under the guise of promoting universal ethics'. Such feelings are influenced by the perception that UD is, largely, an American export, shaped by values of consumerism and voluntarism as the basis for the development and delivery of design. That other countries may differ in their value-bases, socio-cultural dispositions and attitudes to how design for all ought to be attained, is not well reflected in the literature about UD. This is surely a significant gap that needs to be redressed as part of a process to develop a design that is sensitive to local social and cultural traditions.

Conclusion: Towards a research agenda

UD is a significant social movement that has the potential to liberate disabled people from disabling design and, in doing so, to contribute to broader objectives relating to the eradication of disablism in society. There is still much to be done to identify and evaluate the theoretical concepts shaping UD discourse, and to assess their impact in challenging, and changing, mainstream approaches to design and develop-ment (for an amplification of this point, see Imrie, 2012). This requires further evaluation of the socio-institutional development of UD. The growth of the UD movement, evidenced by major conferences on the topic, new networks of scholarly interchanges and adoption of UD principles by major corporate organisations, requires explanation. In and of itself, UD is a subject worthy of sociological investigation. To date, there has been no such investigation, and there is little knowledge of the genesis and development of UD and the role of key actors, and their organisations, in shaping its core concepts, values and practices.

Likewise, there is little assessment of the development and diffusion of the principles and practices of UD, in what ways states intercede with, and are influenced by, UD discourse, and, more broadly, how UD may become institutionalised as a particular domain of expertise and arena of policy and practice. Integral to the shaping of UD in practice is its governance, and there is a lack of understanding of what UD is or ought to be, and often conflicting and contradictory advice contained in design standards and guidance. Anecdotal evidence suggests that professionals do not always know what advice or guidance to use, or in what combinations. A key focus for future research should be how far, and in what ways, different (statutory and non-statutory) instruments are used and/or combined, and with what effects in delivering UD in the designed environment. This ought to include, amongst other things, evaluations of both voluntary and legal mechanisms, and evidence-based assessments of how far market mechanisms are able to deliver good quality design and be in the vanguard of crafting a universally designed future.

Acknowledgement

My thanks to Sarah Fielder who read a couple of earlier drafts of the chapter and provided relevant comments that have enabled me to clarify some of the arguments.

Note

1 To pose the universal and the particular in this way may be a misnomer, given that they are indissoluble or two sides of the same coin (see Bickenbach, 2009). As Sayer (2011: 99) suggests, universalism does not imply a uniformity of response, and 'we can note similarities without denying difference'.

References

Bardzell, S. (2009) 'Enchanted artifacts: social productivity and identity in virtual material ecologies', *Artifact*, 123–36.
Bauman, Z. (1993) *Postmodern Ethics*. Oxford: Blackwell.
Bellisario, R. (2012) 'Refused access: fighting for the right to travel on the buses', *The Guardian*, 10 July.

Bickenbach, J. (2009) 'Disability, culture and the UN convention', *Disability and Rehabilitation*, 31 (14): 1111–24.

Bloomer, K. and Moore, C. (1977) *Body, Memory, and Architecture*. New Haven, CT: Yale University Press.

Center for Universal Design (2011) The Principle of Universal Design. Available at: www.ncsu. edu/project/design-projects/udi/center-for-universal-design/the-principles-of-universal-design/

Cohn, M., Kerridge, T., Light, A., Lindtner, S. and Ratto, M. (2010) Tracing Design(ed) Authority: A Workshop on Critical Modes of Making. Proceedings of the 8th ACM Conference on Designing Interactive Systems, New York.

European Commission (EC) (2010) *European Disability Strategy 2010–2020: A Renewed Commitment to a Barrier-Free Europe*. Brussels: EC.

Ewart, I. and Luck, R. (2012) 'Portals to the world: technological extensions to the boundaries of the home', *Interiors: Design, Architecture, Culture*, 3 (1–2): 7–22.

Holder, J. (1990) 'Design in everyday things: promoting modernism in Britain, 1912–1944', in P. Greenhalgh (ed.), *Modernism in Design*. London: Reaktion Books. pp. 123–44.

Imrie, R. (2003) 'Architects' conceptions of the human body', *Environment and Planning D: Society and Space*, 21 (1): 47–65.

Imrie, R. (2006) *Accessible Housing: Quality, Disability and Design*. London: Routledge.

Imrie, R. (2012) 'Universalism, universal design and equitable access to the built environment', *Disability and Rehabilitation*, 34 (10): 873–82.

Imrie, R. and Hall, P. (2001) *Inclusive Design: Designing and Developing Accessible Environments*. London: Routledge.

Institute for Human Centered Design (2011) State of the Art. Available at: http://humancentereddesign.org/universal-design/state-art [accessed 20/07/12].

Mace, R. (1988) *Universal Design: Housing for the Lifespan of all People*. Rockville, MD: US Department of Housing and Urban Development.

Nussbaum, M. (2003) 'Capabilities as fundamental entitlements: SEN and social justice', *Feminist Economics*, 9 (2/3): 33–59.

Owens, K. (2009) 'Design and art: the aesthetic turn', *Journal of Visual Literacy*, 27 (2): 139–54.

Pallasmaa, J. (1996) *The Eyes of the Skin: Architecture and the Senses*. London: Academy Editions.

Papanek, V. (1971) *Design for the Real World: Human Ecology and Social Change*. New York: Pantheon Books.

Pullin, G. (2009) *Design Meets Disability*. Cambridge, MA: MIT Press.

Salmen, J. and Ostroff, E. (1997) 'Universal design and accessible design', in D. Watson (ed.), *Time-saver Standards for Architectural Design Data: The Reference of Architectural Fundamentals*. New York: McGraw Hill. pp. 1–8.

Sanford, J. (2012) *Universal Design as a Rehabilitation Strategy*. New York: Springer.

Sayer, A. (2011) *Why Things Matter to People: Social Sciences, Values, and Ethical Life*. Cambridge: Cambridge University Press.

Sen, A. (1985) *Commodities and Capabilities*. Oxford: Oxford University Press.

Steinfeld, E. (1994) The Concept of Universal Design. Unpublished paper presented at the Sixth Ibero-American Conference on Accessibility. Centre for Independent Living, Rio de Janeiro, 19 June.

Steinfeld, E. and Maisel, J. (2012) *Universal Design: Creating Inclusive Environments*. Hoboken, NJ: Wiley & Sons.

Steinfeld, E. and Tauke, B. (2003) Reflection and Critique on Universal Design. Paper presented at the Proceedings of the American Collegiate Schools of Architecture annual meeting, Louisville, KY.

Stone, P. (1983) *Building Economy: Design, Production and Organisation – A Synoptic View.* Elmsford, NY: Pergamon Press.

Tisdale, S. (1966) 'Is there such a thing as irresponsible art?', *Cardozo Studies in Law and Literature*, 8 (2): 253–7.

Tobias, J. (2003) 'Universal design: is it really about design?', *Information Technology and Disabilities* (ejournal), 9 (2). Available at: http://people.rit.edu/easi/itd/itdv09n2/tobias.htm

United Nations (UN) (2007) *Convention on the Rights of Persons with Disabilities.* New York: United Nations. Available at: www.un.org/disabilities/default.asp?id=269.

Vanderheiden, G. (1996) Universal Design: What it is and what it isn't. Available at: http://trace.wisc.edu/docs/whats_ud/whats_ud.htm (accessed 09/07/12).

Ward, M., Franz, J. and Adkins, B. (2012) 'Inclusive housing in Australia: a voluntary response', *World Academy of Science, Engineering and Technology*, 67: 405–12.

Ware, C. (2004) *Information Visualisation: Perception for Design.* Burlington, MA: Elsevier.

Ware, C. (2008) *Visual Thinking for Design.* Burlington, MA: Elsevier.

38

Genetics, Disability and Bioethics

Alice Maynard

Introduction

Developments in genetic technology are moving fast and society's use of genetics has increased exponentially in the past 10 years or so, though understanding has not perhaps increased at the same rate. This raises a wide range of bioethical issues. The impact on disabled people of how these are debated and resolved cannot be underestimated and we must therefore be present in the debate.

Many are extremely optimistic about the future for disabled people, anticipating therapies that will ameliorate impairment effects and perhaps even cures for impairments. Others are deeply pessimistic, citing eugenics[1] and drawing parallels with programmes that sought to eradicate disability by eradicating disabled people, such as sterilisation programmes across many countries, some of which endured into this century.

Some disabled people believe they suffer from their impairment or the effects of their impairment. Some, even those who embrace their impairment as part of their identity, may consider that they suffer from impairment effects and would prefer not to experience them (Crow, 1996). For them, the prospect of removing impairments or alleviating impairment effects offers hope. It causes problems, however, for those disabled people who believe it is oppressive and discriminatory to say that they suffer. For them, addressing the impairment is to oppress further and to destroy the diversity in humanity (Disabled People's International, 2000). Because of this dichotomy in the way that people view their impairment, the very opportunities that some people see will be barriers to others.

Arguably, the developments themselves are neutral; it is the way in which they are used within society that has a positive or negative impact on disabled people. The possibilities opened up by a greater understanding of the way in which our bodies work are immense. Insight into the nature of our impairments, the kinds of impairments and conditions we might acquire in later life, the characteristics that our children might have – all of this potentially enables us to plan and manage our lives more effectively.

We have known about the inheritance of personal traits and used this knowledge in selective breeding of animals, for instance, since before records began. The 'science' of genetics as such began with Gregor Mendel in the mid-nineteenth century. He observed the way in which characteristics of plants were systematically handed down from one generation to another. Our understanding of genetics progressed from there, through the linking of DNA to genetic inheritance in the 1940s and 1950s, through James Watson and Francis Crick's double helix model of DNA in the 1950s, to the sequencing of the human genome in 2000. It is really the discovery of DNA and its role in shaping our minds and bodies that is significant for disabled people.

Using DNA in practice

DNA profiling (or finger-printing) uses the 0.1 per cent variation in the genetic code between individuals to draw up a complex barcode that can easily be compared. This part of the genetic code is often called 'junk' DNA, as it is not believed to have a functional role in shaping who we are. Profiling is extensively used in forensic work and is a highly effective method of identification. It can tell us about likely familial relationships. The closer the relationship, the more accurate it is, and it is commonly used for paternity testing. Profiling is not generally understood to provide information about health, racial origins or other DNA determined factors, although ongoing work suggests that 'junk' DNA may not be junk after all (Fletcher, 2010).

Research into conditions such as cystic fibrosis and muscular dystrophy initially focused on identifying the particular gene causing the condition. Identifying the relevant gene means we can determine if an embryo or fetus will go on to develop the condition or not, which is important for techniques such as pre-implantation genetic diagnosis (PGD – see below). Not all conditions are single gene conditions that can be identified in this way – many are polygenic conditions resulting from the interaction between a number of different genes or between genes and environmental factors.

The ability to sequence an individual's exome (the coding regions of our genome) or the whole genome (the complete sequence of DNA information) can tell us a huge amount about our bodies, including conditions that we are susceptible to developing such as cancer or multiple sclerosis. Improvements in computing power and laboratory techniques mean sequencing is now much cheaper and thus more widely available.

Some genetic techniques

A range of different techniques can be used to understand or manipulate someone's genetic make-up. There is a wealth of information available on the Internet, but a few of the techniques are outlined here to illuminate the discussion:

- PGD tests embryos to see whether they carry a particular genetic trait, in order to avoid implanting an affected embryo into the mother's womb.
- Prenatal screening identifies whether a fetus carries one of a range of genetic traits. A non-invasive screening technique recently developed – cell-free fetal DNA testing – tests the baby's DNA in the pregnant mother's blood.
- Mitochondrial donation (or transfer) bypasses a condition passed down from the mother by substituting the mitochondrial material from another egg during IVF treatment.
- Gene therapy replaces one ('faulty') gene with a different ('working') version of the gene or prevents a gene from 'faulty' functioning by 'switching it off'.

What constitutes genetic information?

By its nature, much of our genetic information is publicly available. Our phenotype – our eye colour, the shape of our nose, how quickly we age, etc. – gives information about the nature of our genotype. Impairments that are recognisable from physical attributes also reveal information about genotype.

An area where the sensitivity of genetic information is critical is in the provision of insurance. Insurers seek to minimise risk, whereas the insured seek to protect against negative future events. DNA testing for specific conditions, although not foolproof, has the potential to reduce risk for insurers, who can better predict the likelihood that someone will develop a condition that will cost them money. Arguably, though, it undermines the very rationale for insurance – pooling our resources to protect ourselves against future uncertainties – by rendering more certain those uncertainties. In the UK, there is a moratorium on the use of DNA test results in insurance, with the single exception of Huntington's disease for life insurance policies worth more than £500,000. But DNA test results are not the only genetic information insurance companies use. Family history, in the same way as phenotype, gives rich information about genetic inheritance. It does not provide unequivocal information, but nor (with a few exceptions) does DNA testing, which is indicative rather than predictive.

Medicine, genetics and disability

Oliver (1990) describes how, in the nineteenth century, the rise of western medicine led to the medicalisation of disability. The enthusiasm for the germ theory of illness and disease created an erroneous perception that all disability could be cured once the (disease) cause had been found. In the latter half of the twentieth century, disabled people developed, in contrast, a model of disability as a social construct. Impairment may be a medical condition, but disability results from the barriers society creates, unnecessarily, which prevent disabled people from participating fully. Although a social perspective on disability is now more widely accepted, disabled people still experience the limitations imposed by the medical approach in almost all areas of life. In the twenty-first century, we see the rise of genomic technology. Increasingly, our genes are understood to hold the key to our identity. As we explore cause and effect in genetic inheritance, we are in danger of making the same mistakes about disability as those made when germ theory first took hold. There is significant enthusiasm for 'finding the gene for' a whole range of impairments (e.g. Starr, 2010; Jayakody, 2011), given that, if the gene can be isolated, it can be eradicated or treated. The question of whether and why we necessarily want to do this should, however, be asked.

Barriers to access

In a discussion of the 'new' science and its implications for disabled people, it is important not to forget that, within the context of genetic services, the 'old' barriers to access for disabled people still remain. Physical, information and communication, and organisational barriers disempower in the very environment where people need to feel powerful enough to make significant decisions about their lives and the lives of those they love.

Language used in relation to genetic difference is often negative. Within the scientific community, terms may have precise meanings, but they take on different connotations in the public domain. For instance, genetic mutation is a specific scientific term for change but, in common parlance, mutation is not positive – indeed it is somewhat sinister. We talk of people being 'at risk' of having a child with a genetic condition, of 'breaking the news' – always associated with bad news – to (prospective) parents that their child has an impairment, of genetic 'disorders' and 'diseases', and of 'faulty' or 'defective' genes.

Health services, the main providers of genetic services, are large, bureaucratic and heavily regulated. They embed systems and practices that create significant barriers for disabled people and are not amenable to removal – often no one person has authority to make the decision to accommodate a disabled person's needs.

Attitudes

As disabled people, we experience significant discrimination and negative attitudes from the public and health professionals alike. And we often come with our own internalised oppression (Mason, 1990: Chapter 13), making it harder to reject negative attitudes. Whilst environmental, information and system barriers are frustrating, challenging and may deny a disabled person access to the opportunities presented by genetic developments, it is in the attitudes of everyone involved – health professionals, friends and relations and society at large – that the most intransigent barriers lurk, often hidden or denied.

Attitudes towards disabled people are complex and coloured by social, historical and religious factors. Stereotypes such as disabled people as tragic objects of pity or something to be feared – even cursed by God – presuppose that no one would wish to be disabled and that any disabled person would want to be cured, to be normal. These stereotypes lead people to believe that any contribution genetic developments can make to 'normality' must be welcome. They promote the view that no one would want to bring into the world someone who was going to suffer the personal tragedy of disability, so being able to identify and eliminate impaired fetuses, or even prevent the tragedy before conception, must be the right thing to do.

These attitudes are so prevalent within society that no one, including disabled people themselves, can expect to be free of them. For someone who has a child with an impairment and has not encountered disability before, the initial 'shock' is like a bereavement: there is grief for the child they were going to have but 'lost' (Birkett, 2011). This is the backdrop against which decisions about the appropriate use of genetic developments and research into new techniques is taking place, and it sometimes feels unbalanced to disabled people.

The balance of power

Disabled people are under-employed in the medical professions. For instance, only 7 per cent of UK National Health Service staff declare as disabled and the percentage declines as the grade of the job increases (Department of Health, 2011). Education programmes do not routinely include disability issues. Disabled people will remain recipients of health interventions rather than become active participants if they are not seen on both sides of the consulting couch. This calls into question professional judgements about the quality and value of disabled people's lives, and the nature of suffering. Disabled adults' judgements based on personal experience can diverge from professionals' about the current or future quality of life of babies and young children. Who decides whether a life is worth living or not (Sokol, 2006)? This is an important question given professionals' inexperience of living with disability and the prevalence of stereotypes.

Economics

An economic argument is often put forward for the use of genetic techniques. Some consider it morally wrong to bring a child into the world who, it is surmised, will place a greater economic burden on society than a child without an impairment. There is evidence that the way disabled people are portrayed in the media is as scroungers, draining the meagre resources of the state and failing to make an economic contribution (Strathclyde Centre for Disability Research and Glasgow Media Group, 2012). This bolsters the economic argument. Furthermore, we are all constantly exhorted to be healthier to avoid being a burden on society, economically or physically. As disability and ill health are commonly conflated in discussions around genetics as elsewhere, this puts pressure on disabled people not to refuse genetic treatments that would enable them to improve their health.

Prevention and pre-emption

For some disabled people, genetic techniques that prevent babies being born with their condition are unsettling, as they themselves might not have been born had the techniques been in use at the time. Few of us object, however, to improving road safety to prevent spinal injury. Is this qualitatively different from using genetic techniques to prevent the birth of a child with an impairment? Many disabled people feel that preventing the birth of a child with an impairment sends a negative message that such lives are not worth living. This is known as an expressivist objection, and bioethicists debate its legitimacy. Although disabled people do not wish to be defined as their impairments (he's Downs, she's an arthritic), many of us see our impairments as a crucial part of our social identity – we would not be the same people without them. Edwards (2004) does not consider that this is enough of a reason for rejecting genetic techniques for reducing impairment. Rather, an individual should be able to weigh up the harms or benefits to themselves and their families against the harms perceived by disabled people and make their own decisions. In this context, it is important to note that, in the UK, whereas people may make their own decisions about *not* having a disabled child including when in receipt of interventions such as PGD, they are not free to make such a decision about *having* a disabled child, as the Human Fertilisation and Embryology Act 2008 specifically precludes it.

One term taken for granted in much of the discourse around genetic developments is 'serious'. 'Serious condition' is often used, undefined, in discussion as if its meaning were understood clearly by all parties. Professionals come with their own cultural and experiential perspectives, and without a clear definition these perspectives will colour their judgement. The prevailing approach is that seriousness must be determined on a case-by-case basis. The Human Fertilisation and Embryology Authority has, however, 'fast-tracked' for PGD certain conditions that have been previously approved. These two approaches seem contradictory: fast-tracking conditions for PGD suggests that they are 'serious' *regardless of* the 'case', i.e. the extent to which the person would be affected or the personal circumstances of the family.

Conclusion

Genetic developments are moving extremely fast. They offer us the potential to conquer more of and explain more about the unknowns in our world. But we often treat them in isolation, rather than recognising the sophisticated social and cultural context in which they take place. We may not understand the impact that many of the changes we propose will have and that has a tendency to polarise views: we believe it will all be good or fear it will all be bad. The science will continue to develop, the number of techniques available will increase, and the more we use techniques the more we will become comfortable with the concepts, for good or ill. Whatever we believe, it can only be beneficial to discuss the issues openly, to recognise how genetic developments fit into the whole social system and to try to define more closely some of the concepts we use so readily, such as 'serious': 'Free and open debate is the lifeblood of medical ethics – without it medical ethics becomes a dogmatic system devoid of intellectual life' (Holm and Harris, 2004: 519).

That free and open debate must involve disabled people, whether we are for or against genetic developments. Without our views in that debate, developments that may benefit society may be ignored or overlooked whilst those that may cause significant harm may flourish.

Acknowledgement

My thanks go to Professor Anneke Lucassen and Professor Frances Flinter for their helpful reviews.

Note

1 Eugenics is a term first used by Francis Galton (1907: 17), which he defined as: 'the science of improving stock, which is by no means confined to question of judicious mating, but which [...] takes cognisance of all influences that [...] give the more suitable races or strains of blood, a better chance of prevailing speedily over the less suitable'.

References

Birkett, D. (2011) 'Rebekah Brooks's phone call to Gordon Brown is unforgiveable', *The Guardian*, 12 July. Available at: www.guardian.co.uk/commentisfree/2011/jul/12/rebekah-brooks-gordon-brown-phone-call (accessed 05/06/12).

Crow, L. (1996) 'Including all of our lives: renewing the social model of disability', in C. Barnes and G. Mercer (eds), *Exploring the Divide: Illness and Disability*. Leeds: The Disability Press. pp. 55–72.

Department of Health (2011) Equality Information and Equality Analysis. Available at: www.dh.gov.uk/health/files/2012/01/Download-Department-of-Health-Equality-Information-and-Equality-Analysis-pdf-66K.pdf (accessed 05/06/12).

Disabled People's International (2000) Disabled People Speak on the New Genetics. Available at: www.mindfully.org/GE/Disabled-People-Speak.htm (accessed 29/07/12).

Edwards, S. (2004) 'Disability, identity and the "expressivist objection"', *Journal of Medical Ethics*, 30: 418–20.

Fletcher, W. (2010) '"Junk" DNA makes us unique, study finds', *Bionews*, 29 March. Available at: www.bionews.org.uk/page_57456.asp (accessed 16/05/12).

Galton, F. (1907) *Inquiries into Human Faculty and its Development* (2nd edn). London: J.M. Dent & Co.

Holm, S. and Harris, J. (2004) 'Free speech, democracy, and eugenics', *Journal of Medical Ethics*, 30: 519.

Jayakody, S. (2011) '"Language learning genes" uncovered', *Bionews*, 21 February. Available at: www.bionews.org.uk/page_89310.asp (accessed 06/06/12).

Mason, M. (1990) Internalised Oppression. Available at: www.leeds.ac.uk/disability-studies/archiveuk/Mason,%20Michelene/mason.pdf (accessed 06/06/12).

Oliver, M. (1990) *The Politics of Disablement*. Basingstoke: Macmillan.

Sokol, D. (2006) 'Baby MB: a medical ethicist's view', BBC News Magazine, 15 March. Available at: http://news.bbc.co.uk/1/hi/magazine/4809908.stm (accessed 04/06/12).

Starr, S. (2010) 'Rare genetic variants found to play role in development of autism', *Bionews*, 14 June. Available at: www.bionews.org.uk/page_64413.asp (accessed 06/06/12).

Strathclyde Centre for Disability Research and Glasgow Media Group (2012) Bad News for Disabled People: How Newspapers are Reporting Disability. Inclusion London. Available at: www.inclusionlondon.co.uk/disabled-and-deaf-people-and-media-representation (accessed 06/06/12).

39

Disability, Death and Dying: A Rights-Based Discussion of the Ultimate Barrier Facing Disabled People

Bill Armer

Building on the statement of UPIAS (1976: 3), that '[d]isability is something imposed on top of our impairments', there is a cogent argument that 'disability' is neither more nor less than life-long institutionalised discrimination against people who have a physical or intellectual endowment judged by their host culture to be 'abnormal' or 'substandard' (e.g. Barnes, 1991). It may seem that not only are disabled people in general forced to live in a way that is different to 'the non-disabled', but that often responsibility for the most intimate human decisions of all, whether and how to live or die, is denied them. From a disability studies perspective, some might view this as the ultimate act of dispowerment to be visited upon a disabled person, others more simply as the logical culmination of a lifetime of imposed discrimination. From other perspectives, this may well be seen as perfectly right and proper.

For example, eugenicists have, for over a century, sought to establish criteria on which to decide who is 'worthy of life' and, of course, who is not (Armer, 2005). Philosophically, it may be thought that to attempt to assign a relative value to human life is to dis-value it. Pragmatically, the very real effects on the self-esteem of disabled people who live with conditions thought appropriate for euthanasia (or indeed for assisted dying) should not be ignored.

Because this volume is themed around the enablement of disabled people to overcome 'disabling barriers', in this chapter I will confine my arguments to the case wherein disabled people are fully aware of their circumstances, or have made a 'living will' clearly expressing their future wishes. In doing this, I do not seek to deny or belittle the fact that there is an extremely important debate with which I will not then fully engage: whether or not society should have the right to impose death upon non-consenting or non-aware people (including babies). I merely make the point that, in the absence of consent or awareness, I believe that a disabled person cannot meaningfully be said to have been 'enabled'.

This chapter is structured into two main parts – the first examining cases where disabled people or others purporting to speak on their behalf have claimed a 'right to die', and the second considering arguments by disabled people and others insisting on a 'right to live' – with a brief postscript. Although at face value the 'right to die/to live' positions may appear to be mutually exclusive, both arguments, I claim, imply a deeper right: that to self-determination, or autonomy, for disabled people.

A right to die?

Crown Counsel in the Diane Pretty case, which sought to clarify the law on assisted suicide, made a relevant and thought-provoking point: '[a] philosopher might say that death is the corollary to life, but the lawyer must answer that the right to die is the antithesis of the right to life' (Capon, 2012: unpaginated).

There is a fundamental legal flaw in the appeal to 'rights' here. Neither the United Nations Universal Declaration of Human Rights (UDHR) nor the Convention on the Rights of Persons with Disabilities (CRPD) confer any 'right to die'. In Europe, the same applies to the European Convention on Human Rights (ECHR). To the contrary, the UDHR, CRPD and ECHR all contain 'right to life' clauses which may be (and in the case of the ECHR has been) taken to preclude any right to demand death.

Despite the fact that disabled people have a deep vested interest in this topic, which is usually portrayed as seeking to 'help' them, Not Dead Yet UK (NDYUK) states that the debate did not originate within the disabled people's movement and it 'does not have our support' (NDYUK, 2010: 2). The basic overt argument in favour of assisted dying has changed little, if at all, in over a century. It is that a 'good death' (which is what 'euthanasia' means), and more recently a 'dignified' one, should be a right for all. The underlying premise is that many people may die in great pain or squalor. Quite possibly, this was the case in 1906 when, in the USA, the first attempt to pass a Bill legalising euthanasia was made in Ohio (Death with Dignity National Center, undated), or even in 1936 which saw the first attempt to pass such legislation in the UK. The most obvious point to make here is that medicine, including pain relief and palliative care, has made tremendous progress in the intervening years. The arguments for assisted suicide/euthanasia have not.

Coincidentally or not, the 1930s saw the high-water mark of the British eugenics movement, whilst eugenics movements were active in the USA before 1906 (Armer, 2005: 141). The 1930s UK campaign to introduce euthanasia was led by the Voluntary Euthanasia Legalisation Society (VELS), leading members of which had close links with the British Eugenics Society. VELS has undergone a series of name changes, including the recent Voluntary Euthanasia Society, and is at present known as Dignity in Dying.

The facts that medicine has progressed very significantly and that early 'right to die' campaigners had links to eugenics, do not dispose of the 'rights' element of the debate:

I am asking for my right to choose when and how to die to be respected ... [W]hy should I be denied ... the right to die of my own choosing when able bodied people have that right and only my disability prevents me from exercising [it]? (Nicklinson v MoJ 2012)

These words form part of the Statement of Facts made by Tony Nicklinson in his 2012 UK High Court action seeking judicial sanction to be assisted in committing suicide. The Judge found that two of the three legs of the application were legally arguable and Nicklinson, who had Locked-in Syndrome, was granted a full hearing in which to argue his case further. The Court ultimately found against Nicklinson on a point of constitutional principle:

It is not for the court to decide whether the law about assisted dying should be changed and, if so, what safeguards should be put in place. (*The Independent* online edition, 23 August 2012)

'Dignity' is an important consideration for many people, disabled or not, and is raised by Nicklinson (v MoJ 2012). It is also central to the argument of Terry Pratchett (2010: unpaginated) who, diagnosed with Alzheimer's, notes that dementias:

place a huge care burden on the country ... We then have to consider the quality of whatever care there may be, not just for dementia, but for all long-term conditions. I will not go into the horror stories, but it appears that care is a lottery.

Pratchett (2010) makes the point that he is a wealthy man able to purchase care on the open market. Even so, he has little faith in the quality of such care and fears living without dignity. This point is important, for it leads us to question just how much true autonomy would be allowed disabled people should they be empowered to decide to die. Put in its most brutal simplicity, the fear of a painful and sordid death is a powerful incentive to seek assisted dying and must often override philosophical considerations about 'rights'.

Indeed, both Nicklinson (v MoJ 2012) and Pratchett (2010) make reference to fears about the potential manner of their dying, and similar points were raised by both Diane Pretty and Debbie Purdy in their respective UK legal actions. Pretty lost her argument about a right to die (House of Lords, 2005; Verkaik, 2002), whilst Purdy made some progress in that the Director of Public Prosecutions issued clarifications as to his understanding of the UK law on assisted suicide, which were later 'welcomed' by the House of Commons (Hansard, 2012), and are seen by some as being a liberalising move (Lifenews.com, 2012: unpaginated).

A right to live

Inclusion Scotland, an organisation of disabled people, provides an informative signpost: '[t]he focus must shift from assisted dying to the ... concept of Assisted Living. That is the valuing of all lives irrespective of impairment and the provision of high quality palliative care' (cited by The Christian Institute, 2010: unpaginated).

The collective response to the 'right to die' proponents from disabled people and their organisations, allowing for individual dissenters, is a two-pronged defence. On the one hand, and perhaps the most widely championed, is a 'slippery slope' argument that a 'right' to die would quickly become a 'duty'. Indeed, with his comment about the 'huge care burden', Pratchett (2010) appears to be already heading in that direction.

The 'slippery slope' argument has been flagged up by Reichel, a medical doctor involved in bioethics, who first draws attention to the fact that the 'early death' of a disabled person 'can save money', before concluding that: '[t]hose who believe legal assisted suicide will assure their "choice" are naive' (Reichel, 2009: unpaginated).

The second prong is that any widespread acceptance that people with named impairments could or should seek death has profound psychological effects on people in similar situations:

> we are living now in a world [which] ... says the quality of life of ... these people is not worth living (The Life Resources Charitable Trust, undated); our lives are seen as inferior to those of non-disabled people ... legalising euthanasia or even assisted suicide would place disabled people in potential danger. (Campbell, 2006: 1)

From Canada, the view of an organisation of disabled people is that society's generally negative stereotypes of disabled people, assumed loss of 'quality of life' and perceived burdens brought by impairment to individuals and society combine to 'increase the vulnerability of people with disabilities' to pressures to end their lives in a so-called voluntary manner (Council of Canadians with Disabilities, 2010). This position is supported by the (UK) Disability Rights Commission in a submission made in relation to the failed 2005 attempt (Joffe Bill) to legalise 'assisted suicide' in the UK: '[t]he likely effect of assisted dying legislation is that many disabled people would experience further negative assumptions about their position in society' (Disability Rights Commission, 2005: 4).

The thrust of both these prongs of argument is that there is a grave danger that many disabled people would come under increasing societal pressure to 'volunteer' to die. Were that to become the case, there would be serious and unquantifiable questions about just how voluntary such a decision could be said to be. Far from adding to the autonomy of disabled people, as many proponents of a 'right to die' argue, their opponents hold that such a right could actually further constrain the autonomy of disabled people.

There is another aspect to the debate which not only denies any notion of a 'right to die', but also makes continuing to live a duty. This is bound up with the religious underpinnings of diverse cultures around the world and, as such, has great if some-times hidden influence. Culture, and with it our sense of right and wrong (and our laws), is often informed by a dominant religion.

The three major monotheistic religions of the world – Judaism, Christianity and Islam (in chronological order) – contain similar prohibitions to the killing of either oneself or another, on the grounds that life and death are entirely in the gift of God (Allah). Thus, in Judaism we have the unequivocal injunction: 'Thou shalt not kill' (Exodus 20: 13). This leads to the position whereby 'Judaism regards the taking of one's [own] life as abhorrent and tantamount to murder' (Breitowitz, undated). In addition to the Commandment from Exodus cited above, the Catechism of the Roman Catholic Church (undated) is clear that: '[w]e are stewards … of the life God has entrusted to us. It is not ours to dispose of.' The Anglican Movement is less unified than is Roman Catholicism, and there is some dissent, but the authoritative view of the Archbishop of Canterbury is that neither suicide, assisted or not, nor euthanasia is in keeping with Anglican doctrine (Lifesitenews, 2005). In Islam, 'Muslims are against euthanasia' (Aramesh and Shadi, 2007: 37), partly on the authority of the Holy Qur'an (3: 145): 'no person can ever die except by Allah's leave and at an appointed term'. This is understood to extend to committing or assisting suicide.

Buddhism and Hinduism take a different view on suicide and euthanasia, but the general thrust of both is that difficult, painful or challenging situations are part of a process of learning and evolving spread over a number of lifetimes (incarnations). To deliberately avoid a situation by suicide is to prolong that process, and to assist the suicide of another is to be a party to interfering with the ordained scheme of things. In Buddhist teachings, 'there's no room for euthanasia or assisted suicide' (Bhikkhu, 2010: unpaginated), whilst in Hinduism 'euthanasia … will cause the soul and body to be separated at an unnatural time' (BBC, 2009: unpaginated). Both religions posit serious spiritual ill-effects for all parties concerned.

Conclusion: Rights, duties and desires – whither now?

I have outlined the bare details of the 'rights-based' arguments for and against granting disabled people assistance in ending their own lives. We have seen the 'slippery slope' argument that a right to die for disabled people may become a duty to do so, and it may well appear to many that there is much truth in this. However, it might also be the case that a similar argument exists regarding the right to live leading to a danger of disabled people feeling pressured into unwillingly accepting a duty to live. The argument from rights has its dangers on either side.

It may be that this 'rights' argument, whilst important, is misdirected. Although this is not the place for profound sociological theory, the work of the sociologist Emile Durkheim (1951) is relevant here. He describes, amongst other categories, cases of 'anomic' suicide where the prime motivation is a feeling of a lack of integration into society, and 'altruistic' suicide which is committed for the benefit of others. Briefly, for Durkheim, someone who feels tightly embraced by society is unlikely to be suicidal, whilst another who feels burdensome to others, or to society in general, is.

For so long as society portrays disabled people as living 'tragic lives' which impose extra costs on society, many disabled people will view themselves as being apart from, rather than a part of, their host society. In the terms of Durkheim (1951), they may become anomic. Alternatively, if they feel they are a burden on society, they may feel an altruistic duty to die. Either way, they are at especial risk of becoming suicidal, but the root cause lies with society not the individual.

I began this chapter with UPIAS (1976) and end with Durkheim (1951) which brings me full circle. The social model of disability holds that whilst impairment is an attribute of the individual, disability is the result of society's action or inaction towards impairment. The way to combat disability is to change society, not the individual. Societal and cultural attitudes have to shift, or rather be shifted, so that disabled people become fully integrated and win full equality within their host societies. Indeed, the expressions 'host society' and 'disabled people' would become redundant.

Durkheim (1951) teaches us that people who are fully integrated into society are far less likely to seek suicide. The implementation of the social model of disability in practice rather than theory may well render the debate about assisted dying largely redundant: if disabled people had a genuine right to both an equal standard of living and sense of social worth on the one hand, and equal access to suicide on the other, would they feel the need to exercise the latter right? The fact is that people who feel secure in society rarely seek premature death.

References

Aramesh, K. and Shadi, H. (2007) 'Euthanasia: an Islamic ethical perspective', *Iranian Journal of Allergy, Asthma and Immunology*, 6 February (Suppl. 5): 35–8. Available at: www.iaari.hbi.ir/journal/archive/articles/v6s5ar3.pdf (accessed 05/07/2011).

Armer, W.G. (2005) In the Shadow of Genetics. Unpublished PhD thesis, University of Leeds. Available at: www.disability-archive.leeds.ac.uk/authors_list.asp?AuthorID=28&author_name= Armer%2C+William+George+%28Bill%29 (accessed 10/04/12).

Barnes, C. (1991) *Disabled People in Britain and Discrimination: A Case for Anti-discrimination Legislation*. London: Hurst and Co. Chapter 1. Available at: www.leeds.ac.uk/ disability-studies/archiveuk/Barnes/disabled%20people%20and%20discrim%20ch1.pdf (accessed 14/06/12).

BBC (2009) Euthanasia, Assisted Dying, and Suicide. Available at: www.bbc.co.uk/religion/religions/ hinduism/hinduethics/euthanasia.shtml (accessed 02/07/11).

Bhikkhu, T. (2010) 'Educating compassion', *Access to Insight*, 5 June. Available at: www.accesstoinsight.org/lib/authors/thanissaro/compassion.html (accessed 26/06/11).

Breitowitz, Y. (undated) Physician: Assisted Suicide – A Halachic Approach. *Jewish Law Articles*. Available at: www.jlaw.com/articles/suicide.html (accessed 02/07/11).

Campbell, J. (2006) Assisted Dying: A Question of Choice? Paper presented to the Centre for Disability Studies, School of Sociology and Social Policy, University of Leeds, 15 November. Available at: www.disability-archive.leeds.ac.uk/authors_list.asp?Author ID=23&author_name=Campbell%2C+Jane (accessed 05/04/12).

Capon, F. (2012) The Proposed Change to the Law on Assisted Dying: Light at the End of the Tunnel? 21 February. Available at: http://felicitycapon.com/2012/02/21/the-proposed-change-to-the-law-on-assisted-dying-light-at-the-end-of-the-tunnel/ (accessed 09/04/12).

Council of Canadians with Disabilities (2010) Canadians with Disabilities: We Are Not Dead Yet, 16 June. Available at: www.ccdonline.ca/en/humanrights/endoflife/euthanasia/Canadians-with-disabilities-we-are-not-dead-yet (accessed 05/07/11).

Death with Dignity National Center (undated) Chronology of Assisted Dying. Available at: www.deathwithdignity.org/historyfacts/chronology/ (accessed 05/07/11).

Disability Rights Commission (2005) Assisted Dying Policy Statement, October. Available at: www.epolitix.com/.../AssistedDyingPolicyStatementOct05FINAL.pdf (accessed 06/07/11).

Durkheim, E. (1951) *Suicide*. New York: The Free Press.

Hansard (2012) Official Reports of Proceedings of the House, 27 March. Available at: www.publications.parliament.uk/pa/cm/cmtoday/cmdebate/c_05.htm

House of Lords (2005) Assisted Dying for the Terminally Ill Bill. First Report (Session 2004–05). Available at: www.publications.parliament.uk/pa/ld200405/ldselect/ldasdy/86/ 8602.htm (accessed 05/07/11).

The Independent (2012) 'Tony Nicklinson: right-to-die campaigner who took his case to the High Court', 23 August. Available ay: www.independent.co.uk/news/obituaries/tony-nicklinson-righttodie-campaigner-who-took-his-case-to-the-high-court-8073609.html (accessed 18/04/2013)

Lifenews.com (2012) UK House of Commons Essentially Decriminalizes Euthanasia, 28 March. Available at: www.lifenews.com/2012/03/28/uk-house-of-commons-essentially-decriminalizes-euthanasia/ (accessed 10/04/12).

Lifesitenews (2005) Anglican Church Leader Rowan Williams Says Euthanasia and Assisted Suicide Unacceptable. Available at: www.lifesitenews.com/news/archive/ldn/2005/jan/05012008 (accessed 02/07/11).

Nicklinson v MoJ [Ministry of Justice] (2012) Case No: HQ11X04443 in The High Court of Justice, Queen's Bench Division [UK], 12 March. Available at: www.judiciary.gov.uk/Resources/JCO/ Documents/Judgments/nicklinson-v-moj.pdf (accessed 09/04/12).

Not Dead Yet UK (NDYUK) (2010) Untitled discussion paper. Available at: www.notdeadyetuk.org/notdeadyet-about.html (accessed 21/06/11).

Pratchett, T. (2010) 'When the time comes I'll sit on my lawn, brandy in hand and Thomas Tallis on my iPod. And then I'll shake hands with Death', *Mail Online*, 3 February. Available at: www.dailymail.co.uk/debate/article-1247856/Terry-Pratchett-assisted-suicide-Ill-shake-hands-Death.html (accessed 05/07/11).

Reichel, W. (2009) Naive Choices. Letter to *The Times*, 16 June. Available at: www.timesonline.co.uk/tol/comment/letters/article6513758.ece (accessed 03/07/11).

The Christian Institute (2010) Disability Group to Protest against Assisted Suicide Bill. Available at: www.christian.org.uk/news/disability-group-to-protest-against-assisted-suicide-bill/ (accessed 10/04/12).

The Life Resources Charitable Trust (New Zealand) (undated) Infant Euthanasia. Available at: www.life.org.nz/euthanasia/euthanasiamedicalkeyissues/infant-euthanasia/ (accessed 25/06/11).

The Roman Catholic Church (undated) Catechism of the Catholic Church: Part Three – Life In Christ. Section Two, The Ten Commandments, Chapter Two: 'Ou Shall Love Your Neighbor As Yourself', Article 5, The Fifth Commandment. Available at: www.vatican.va/archive/ccc_css/archive/catechism/ p3s2c2a5.htm (accessed 02/07/11).

UPIAS (1976) *Fundamental Principles of Disability*. London: UPIAS and The Disability Alliance.

Verkaik, R. (2002) 'Diane Pretty loses case, while Miss B "dies with dignity"', *The Independent*, 30 April.

40

Hate Crime and the Criminal Justice System

Pam Thomas

Introduction

The term 'hate crime' is used as a way of describing hostile actions against individuals with certain characteristics. These acts include street crime hostility and violent attacks, such as physical and sexual assault, rape, theft, murder, captivity and damage to people's homes and property (Oliver et al., 2012; Thomas, 2011, 2012). The perpetrators may live in the same neighbourhood, but do not usually have a relationship with their victims, and it is generally considered that they are motivated by hatred of a perceived group.

There are similarities between these types of targeted attacks against disabled people and people in other identity groups, such as Black and Minority Ethnic (BME) communities, lesbians, gay men and transgender people (Macdonald, 2008). Iganski's (2008) study highlighted the opportunistic nature of most racist 'hate crime' – everyday conflicts aggravated by racist hostility, often committed by 'ordinary' people going about their ordinary business. Knowledge developed from racist 'hate crime' forms a useful basis from which to increase an understanding of other forms of 'hate crime', but using a 'race model' as the template for disablist hate crime policy is likely to be misplaced (Roulstone et al., 2011).

There is a growing body of evidence, and growing media interest, which raises the profile of disablist hostility (Sin et al., 2009). These are acts of hostility against disabled people on the street or in neighbourhoods, harassment, which may be verbal, or missile throwing at individuals or their homes. These are similar to incidents which are recognised as 'hate crime' against other groups. These acts of hostility against a disabled person may not amount to crime, but nevertheless hurt psychologically and emotionally. A person who has been attacked because of one or more of their characteristics knows that they are more likely than a person without that characteristic to be targeted again (Macdonald, 2008).

Courts have the power through Section 146 of the CJS Act 2003 to pass enhanced sentences when there is proof that a crime was motivated by hostility immediately prior to, during or following an offence. In 2007, the Crown Prosecution Service (CPS) developed its disability hate crime policy and performance framework (CPS, 2007).

Disablist 'mate crime'

A particular form of hostility which seems to be specific to disabled people is that termed 'mate crime'. This term (like 'hate crime' itself) is not ideal, but this chapter will concentrate on concepts not terms. 'Mate crime' refers to hostile incidents carried out by one or more people the disabled person considers to be their friends – or they may be relatives. Because of the way society disables and segregates people with impairments, disabled people can become isolated from those friends and family members who do care about them. Like anyone else, disabled people desire relationships, friendships, company and belonging to a group. They may therefore fall prey to people who feign friendship. These issues differentiate hostility toward disabled people from the types of hostility directed toward people in other groups known to be subjected to 'hate crime'. The CPS does not use the term 'mate crime', leading Perry (2012) to comment: 'It is likely to be regarded with bewilderment by the criminal justice system, which has already been slow to get to grips with the hate crime concept and disability hate crime in particular' (2012: 48).

Certainly, there is often confusion between 'hate crime' and 'mate crime', but 'mate crime' is not a separate issue – it is a particular type of 'hate crime'. There are identifiable characteristics of 'mate crime' (Thomas, 2011, 2012). It is important to recognise these characteristics, and not to assume that because someone has family or friends who seem to be supporting them, they are safe.

Attacks and theft where the perpetrator and victim share domesticity are features of 'mate crime'. Such instances have been included in cases described as 'hate crime' – in the same way that street attacks by strangers can be conflated with domestic violence. Ridicule, contempt, bullying and harassment are features in both hate and mate crime, yet there are also distinguishing features:

- 'Hate crime' – violent attacks which are perpetrated by 'outsiders', not a part of the disabled person's household. Such outsiders may enter the home purely to carry out the attack. In such cases, there is little or no relationship between the perpetrator and the disabled person; they may both live in the area, but there is no reciprocal arrangement or inter-dependency. The disabled person does not welcome any part of any relationship there may be. These may be opportunistic attacks, or may be long-term repeated, sustained attacks. Examples include Francecca Hardwick, Brent Martin, Colin Greenwood, Christine Lakinski (Scope et al., 2008) and David Askew (Jenkins and Naughton, 2010: unpaginated).
- 'Mate crime' – the hostile acts of perpetrators who are 'insiders', sharing domesticity to some degree; there is a mutual relationship. The disabled person may

cling to the relationship, wanting the hostility to stop but welcoming the company and feeling part of a family or group. These situations are not opportunistic; they are calculated. Disabled people in these situations are less likely to complain to the police or other authorities because they consider the perpetrators to be their friends. They may even justify the violence. Examples include Kevin Davies, Steven Hoskin, Raymond Atherton (House of Lords, 2008: 14) and Michael Gilbert (Sugden, 2010). (Thomas, 2011: 108)

'Hate crime' and 'mate crime' happen in the context of a culture that excludes individuals with impairments, a culture that also allows and maintains structures and practices that disable people with impairments. Young (1990) identified five forms of oppression: exploitation, marginalisation, powerlessness, cultural imperialism and violence. Some authors argue that this hostility is motivated by hatred of disabled people (Sherry, 2010), and the perpetrators may perceive vulnerability – making it easier for them to carry out their acts of hostility (Waxman, 1991). A culture that fosters a society which excludes people with impairments from all areas of life can also persuade individuals that disabled people are worthy of contempt and hostility. This is illustrated by a comment from one of the murderers of Brent Martin: 'I am not going down for a muppet' (BBC, 2008).

Disablist jokes are still considered good material for high-profile comedy while racist and homophobic jokes are no longer tolerated. In response, disabled people have developed their own form of satire which finds the humour in all things disablist whilst maintaining a serious note where required, an example being Laurence Clark's website (www.laurenceclark.co.uk/index.php). Ridiculing a culture, society and individuals that make life difficult for disabled people is challenging, and is experienced as uncomfortable by many non-disabled people.

That disabled people are expected to be vulnerable, dependent and above all grateful, is also a crucial part of our culture which supports systems and practices based on care rather than empowerment. Current practice in welfare and social care conveys an assumption that adults must be vulnerable and dependent to be eligible for social care. So disabled people may find they need to appear vulnerable, dependent and grateful in order to get the support they need – even if they are made to feel excluded and patronised. If disabled people appear independent and assertive, they can lose support services, and even be considered fraudsters.

Combining their widespread exclusion from mainstream life with the expectation that disabled people must be vulnerable and dependent creates a situation where hostility and exploitation are not extraordinary. Some carers have devoted their lives to looking after someone, and it is likely that most are very good carers – and care 'about' as well as 'for' people. However, there are circumstances where carers maintain a dependent relationship for financial reasons; that is, they may be reliant on their family member or friend remaining dependent. As I have discussed elsewhere (Thomas, 2011, 2012), all of this provides a situation that allows carers and pseudo-friends – if they are so minded – to take control of a disabled person's everyday life, to control that person's behaviour through punishment or to take advantage of a situation for personal gain.

These are all ways for one individual to have power over another, and such situations are not out of the ordinary (Barnes, 2006; BBC, 2011; Hague et al., 2008; Hansard, 2008). Such power can be exercised by ordinary people, in ordinary homes. These actions may not be considered unreasonable behaviour by those carrying them out, by the disabled person themselves or by others – and many would probably not consider these activities to be crimes. Such actions can easily be carried out without recourse to violence or even argument – if the disabled person remains passive, uncomplaining and grateful. If the disabled person resists by using agency and objects, claiming independence and control, then the carer might concede willingly. Disabled people do turn things around through gaining control, especially if they secure their own accommodation and an individual budget. However, in the face of arguments, verbal abuse or physical violence, the disabled person might back down for fear of losing the support of their carer or home, especially if they have no other means of support, and have nowhere else to go. Disabled people may resign themselves to a reality that others will have control over their lives (Hague et al., 2008). The use of personal agency is not enough in some situations. There are some carers or pseudo-friends who may enact some or all of the abuses outlined above, and combine these with violence, regardless of the passive or active response of the disabled person. A great deal of this is hidden in the privacy of ordinary home situations, making the whole matter much closer to domestic violence than to street or neighbourhood crimes in the 'hate crime' category.

Research and information

Whilst there is little accurate information about what is happening, or about the extent of hostility toward disabled people across all impairment groups, there is a growing body of evidence showing the increased likelihood of disabled people being the targets of violent crime (Balderston and Morgan, 2009; Roulstone et al., 2011; Roulstone and Thomas, 2009; Scope et al., 2008; Sin et al., 2009; Thomas, 2011). Sin et al. (2009) provide a useful analysis showing eight types of incident against people with learning difficulties and people experiencing mental distress. Hotspots were identified, particularly in relation to housing and transport, and also incidents perpetrated by agency staff. In addition, *Disability Now* has published a dossier of disability 'hate crime', giving brief descriptions of 51 incidents of hostility and violence against disabled people (one of which involved two disabled people). This dossier has many omissions, and is presented as a list of incidents under the impairment headings of learning difficulties, physical impairments, sensory impairment, autism and unnamed disabilities; further analysis of this information is not provided. There are indications that the type of incident may vary according to the type of impairment an individual has. It seems that people with learning difficulties were most likely to die and be held captive, whilst wheelchairs users are likely to be tipped out of their wheelchairs and robbed. Only two of the incidents were treated as 'hate crime' by the police, and in ten cases people were described as vulnerable.

There is also a lack of recognition of disabled people as a group in the British Crime Survey – the closest category in use in major national surveys is 'long-term sick'. A major source of confusion in the information available is that definitions do not differentiate between long-term health conditions and impairments on the one hand, and disability which is the result of discrimination on the other (Roulstone et al., 2011).

Disabled people may be reluctant to report 'hate crime' for fear of not being believed. Furthermore, asking 'disabled people to define themselves individually as objects of hatred in the eyes of the law demands a great deal in a culture which is often unthinkingly disabling' (Piggott, 2011: 32).

The police and CPS acknowledge major under-reporting of anti-social behaviour, which in turn will lead to under-recording. But there is also reporting which is under-recorded, as shown in the case of Fiona Pilkington, where years of reporting of anti-social behaviour (ASB) were not recognised or appropriately recorded (IPCC, 2011).

Her Majesty's Inspectorate of Constabulary (HMIC) undertook a review to determine how well police forces understand and respond to reports of ASB. They interviewed members of the public who had recently reported ASB and found that:

> There are still indications that a significant amount of ASB is targeted at individuals or their families, with 39% of the victims surveyed feeling that their incident was the result of them being personally targeted (rather than a random act). Twelve percent felt the motivation for the incident was due to factors such as race, religion, sexual orientation or disability. It is important to emphasise here that such motivation constitutes 'hate', and therefore these incidents must be considered as hate crimes. (HMIC, 2012: 13)

HMIC also listened to 4400 calls made by victims of ASB to the police and found that disabled people 'are far more susceptible to being harmed by ASB' (2012: 22), yet 'discussions with police officers and police staff during the inspection suggested there might be some reluctance to question callers to find out if they have a disability or long term illness' (2012: 22).

Conclusion

The dominant culture currently allows and supports policies, structures and practices which foster a milieu where 'hate crime' and 'mate crime' are ordinary everyday occurrences. To tackle this, the media needs to take disablism as seriously as racism and homophobia. Current images of disabled people as scroungers and benefit fraudsters are stirring up hatred of disabled people.

Disablism or the experience of disability needs to be the butt of jokes, not impairment. Putting disability comedy into the control of disabled people who ridicule disablism would go a long way to achieving cultural change.

There needs to be change within the legal and community safety system so that hostility toward disabled people, which is triggered by a perception of vulnerability, is recognised as a complication of hatred – but is just as serious as uncomplicated hatred.

Some current social policy is intended to bring about the changes in practice that are needed. Personalisation and the emphasis on independent living, which put power and control on the side of disabled people, will go a long way to shift the dominant expectation of dependence. However, this also needs a change in culture and practice in social care agencies because many are still struggling with handing over control to disabled people or engaging in 'co-production'.

Disabled people's organisations which are controlled by disabled people are well placed to support disabled people to live independently and to resist being drawn into abusive relationships. A key part in this is peer support and capacity building amongst disabled people; this can cascade down to those not involved in organisations, and send out a clear message more broadly: that disabled people are not vulnerable and dependent in the right circumstances (Evans, 2006). The development of disabled people's organisations can also go a long way to shifting the culture away from disabled people not being in control.

References

Balderston, S. and Morgan, T. (2009) Mapping and Tackling Hate Crime in the North East of England. Newcastle: Equality and Human Rights Commission and Vision Sense. Unpublished report.

Barnes, C. (2006) Independent Futures: Policies, Practices and the Illusion of Inclusion. Background notes on a verbal presentation to the European Network for Independent Living, 3 November.

BBC (2008) Disabled Man 'Killed for Sport'. Available at: http://news.bbc.co.uk/1/hi/england/wear/7177716.stm [accessed 11/03/10].

BBC (2011) New Blue Badge Disabled Parking Crackdown in England. Available at: www.bbc.co.uk/news/uk-12435529 [accessed 13/06/11].

Crown Prosecution Service (CPS) (2007) Guidance on Prosecuting Cases of Disability Hate Crime. London: CPS. Available at: www.cps.gov.uk/news/fact_sheets/hate_crime/ [accessed 30/06/12].

Evans, J. (2006) The Importance of CILs in Our Movement. Paper presented to the European Network of Independent Living, 2 November.

Hague, G., Thiara, R.K., Magowan, P. and Mullender, A. (2008) Making the Links: Disabled Women and Domestic Violence. Bristol: Women's Aid Federation of England.

Hansard (2008) Motability: Fraud, 6 October – Column 67W [224091]. Available at: www.publications.parliament.uk/pa/cm200708/cmhansrd/cm081006/text/81006w0015.htm

Her Majesty's Inspectorate of Constabulary (HMIC) (2012) A Step in the Right Direction: The Policing of Anti-social Behaviour. London: HMIC.

House of Lords, House of Commons Joint Committee on Human Rights (2008) A Life Like Any Other? Human Rights of Adults with Learning Disabilities, Seventh Report of Session 2007–08. London: The Stationery Office.

Iganski, B. (2008) Hate Crime and the City. Bristol: Policy Press.

Independent Police Complaints Commission (IPCC) (2011) IPCC Report into the Contact between Fiona Pilkington and Leicestershire Constabulary 2004–2007: Independent Investigation. Final Report IPCC ref: 2009/016872. Available at: www.ipcc.gov.uk/cy/pages/investigation_reports.aspx

Jenkins, R. and Naughton, P. (2010) Footage Shows Plight of 'Tormented to Death' David Askew. Available at: www.timesonline.co.uk/tol/news/uk/crime/article7059812.ece

Macdonald, K. (2008) Prosecuting Disability Hate Crime. Sir Ken Macdonald, QC, DPP speech, October.

Oliver, M., Sapey, B. and Thomas, P. (2012) *Social Work with Disabled People* (2nd edn). Basingstoke: Palgrave.

Perry, J. (2012) 'The wrong war? Critically examining the "fight against disability hate crime"', in R. Roulstone and H. Mason-Bish (eds), *Disability, Hate Crime and Violence*. London: Routledge. pp. 40–51.

Piggott, L. (2011) 'Prosecuting disability hate crime: a disabling solution?', *People, Place and Policy Online*, 5 (1): 25–34. Available at: http://extra.shu.ac.uk/ppp-online/issue_1_130411/issue_downloads/disability_hate_crime_solution.pdf [accessed 13 June 2011].

Roulstone, A. and Thomas, P. (2009) *Hate Crime and Disabled People*. Manchester: Equality and Human Rights Commission and Breakthrough UK.

Roulstone, A., Thomas, P. and Balderston, S. (2011) 'Between hate and vulnerability: unpacking the British criminal justice system's construction of disablist hate crime', *Disability & Society*, 26 (3): 351–64.

Scope, UKCDP and Disability Now (2008) *Getting Away with Murder*. London.

Sherry, M. (2010) *Disability Hate Crimes: Does Anyone Really Hate Disabled People?* Aldershot: Ashgate.

Sin, C.H., Hedges, H., Cook, C., Mguni, N. and Comber, N. (2009) *Disabled People's Experiences of Targeted Violence and Hostility*. Manchester: EHRC.

Sugden, J. (2010) Family who Tortured and Decapitated Michael Gilbert Sent to Jail. Available at: www.timesonline.co.uk/tol/news/uk/crime/article7108473.ece

Thomas, P. (2011) '"Mate crime": ridicule, hostility and targeted attacks against disabled people', *Disability & Society*, 26 (1): 107–11.

Thomas, P. (2012) 'Hate crime or mate crime? Disablist hostility, contempt and ridicule', in R. Roulstone and H. Mason-Bish (eds), *Disability, Hate Crime and Violence*. London: Routledge. pp. 135–46.

Waxman, B. (1991) '"Hatred": the unacknowledged dimension in violence against disabled people', *Sexuality and Disability*, 9 (3): 185–99.

Young, I.M. (1990) *Justice and the Politics of Difference*. Princeton, NJ: Princeton University Press.

41

Human Rights in Context: Making Rights Count

Marcia Rioux and Bonita Heath

Although the 1947 United Nations (UN) Declaration of Human Rights[1] clearly covers all human beings, a human rights approach is a relatively recent phenomenon in disability. Disability is also a relatively recent phenomenon in the field of human rights. For people long viewed as somehow 'deficient', a human rights approach to disability has gained wide acceptance with scholars and activists alike, because it is underpinned by values of human dignity (Basser, 2011) and 'universal inherence, inalienability, inherent self-worth of each individual, autonomy and self-determination, [and] equality and freedom of the individual through social support' (Rioux, 2007: 86). Further, a human rights approach to disability promotes legal and policy reforms as a matter of universal right rather than charity (Oliver, 1990; Quinn and Degener, 2002; Rioux, 2003). This chapter provides a brief description of the relatively short 35-year history of international human rights and disability, culminating with the UN 2006 Convention on the Rights of Persons with Disabilities (CRPD). Some consider the CRPD the beginning of a new era in disability human rights (Harpur, 2012; Rioux et al., 2011), and understanding why illuminates some of the accomplishments and limitations of a human rights approach to disability.

The first recognition of disability as a human right did not occur until the 1970s with the UN Declaration on the Rights of Mentally Retarded [*sic*] Persons (1971) and the 1975 Declaration on the Rights of Disabled Persons. These were not, however, unequivocal statements of rights equivalent to those in the Universal Declaration. They contained many qualifications (Hansen and Malhotra, 2011) that effectively limited entitlements according to both disabled people's capacity to exercise their rights and governments' capacity to fund the implementation of those rights.

The 1980s brought the UN Declaration of the International Year of Disabled Persons (1981), and the establishment of a number of disabled people's international organisations, including Disabled Persons International, powering the shift towards disability rights as an underpinning of action on disability. Those events were followed in 1982 by the World Programme of Action concerning Disabled People, which emphasised equal opportunity, as well as equal access to improved social and economic conditions. The UN declared 1983–1992 as the Decade of Disabled Persons to provide a time frame for governments to implement the World Programme of Action adopted in December 1982 (United Nations General Assembly, Resolution 37/51, 1982).

In 1984, the UN Subcommittee on the Prevention of Discrimination and Protection of Minorities appointed Argentina's Leonardo Despouy as Special Rapporteur for the UN Commission for Social Development. Despouy's mandate was to study the causal connection between violations of disability human rights and people's ability to exercise fundamental freedoms. His 1992 comprehensive report documented widespread human rights abuses of disabled people and called for greater engagement of UN treaty monitoring bodies in addressing abuses.

As early as 1987, an experts' meeting in Sweden recognised the importance of disability rights and recommended a Disability Convention. That led in 1993 to the UN Standard Rules on the Equalization of Opportunities for Persons with Disabilities (UN GA, Res. 48/96, 1993). In 1994, Sweden's Bengt Lindqvist was appointed the second Special Rapporteur on Disability (1994–2002) with a mandate to monitor the Rules.

Still, there were few human rights treaties that specifically mentioned disability until the International Committee on Economic, Social and Cultural Rights in 1994. Finally, in 1998 a UN Commission on Human Rights Resolution (UNCHR, Res. 31, 1998) recognised the UN's general responsibility for disability within its mandate, stating that inequality and discrimination related to disability are violations of human rights. Three UN consultative meetings on International Norms and Standards were held in the following years (Berkeley, California, 1998[2]; Hong Kong, 1999[3]; Almåsa, Sweden, 2000[4]). In 2002, Lindqvist gave his final report, aptly called 'Let the World Know', to the UN Social Development Committee, recommending a two-pronged approach – monitor disability rights under the current international Conventions and work towards a specific UN Convention on disability. Between 2002 and 2006, an Ad Hoc Committee, strongly influenced by disability movements worldwide, drafted the CRPD as the first Convention to explicitly protect the human rights of disabled persons.[5]

A view of disability as deviance, deficiency and disease lingers, but the critique of this perspective within academia (Barnes and Mercer, 2010; Oliver, 1990) and from the disability movement has successfully promoted a view of disability as society's failure to be inclusive, rather than individuals' failure to achieve 'normalcy' (Quinn and Degener, 2002; Rioux and Valentine, 2006). The CRDP is not the first document to adopt this understanding of disability, but it explicitly recognises the characteristics associated with disability as inherent to the human condition, calling for 'respect for difference and acceptance of persons with disabilities as part of human diversity and humanity' (UN, CRPD, Article 3(d)). This perspective

entails moving away from viewing people with disabilities as problems toward viewing them as rights holders. Importantly, it means locating any problems outside the person and *especially in the manner by which various economic and social processes accommodate the difference of disability* ... . The debate about disability rights is therefore connected to a larger debate about the place of difference in society. (Quinn and Degener, 2002: 1, emphasis added)

By emphasising the 'various economic and social processes' in disability, these authors touch on the long-standing tension in the politics of disability and human rights, sometimes characterised as one of 'recognition versus redistribution' (Barnes and Mercer, 2003: 128; Fraser and Gordon, 1994). Historically, civil and political rights have been understood to impose 'negative' duties in that they are to ensure recognition of difference and freedom *from* something (e.g. discrimination). Social and cultural rights, however, impose 'positive' rights and duties, such as entitlement programs that redistribute wealth. Positive rights are vulnerable to the question of 'affordability' (Rioux and Valentine, 2006; Rummery, 2002). This has led to a situation in which 'existing legal protections are either not applied or are applied with much less rigour in the case of persons with disabilities' due to the cost of these interventions (Quinn and Degener, 2002: 23).

The CRPD, however, explicitly adopts a rights-outcome approach, which constructs an analysis of how society creates barriers and how society should address this marginalisation. Thus, the CRPD avoids the dichotomisation of 'civil and political' versus 'social, economic and cultural' rights, recognising the interdependence of all categories of rights as essential in addressing the inequality experienced by disabled persons (Pinto, 2011). 'Understood in this way, rights are entitlements that ground claims against the State and found obligations on the part of the State' (Rioux et al., 2011: 20–1).

Thus, the CRPD's approach to rights addresses the structural violence that disabled people face. Drawing on Galtung's work, Farmer (2005) describes structural violence as a 'host of offensives against human dignity: extreme and relative poverty, social inequalities ranging from racism to gender inequality and the more spectacular forms of violence that are uncontestably human rights abuses' (p. 8). Sen (1999) calls these violations 'unfreedoms'. He advocates social and economic development as a response:

Development requires the removal of major sources of unfreedom: poverty as well as tyranny, poor economic conditions as well as systemic social deprivation, neglect of public facilities as well as intolerance or over-activity of the repressive state. Despite unprecedented increases in overall opulence, the contemporary world denies elementary freedoms to vast numbers – perhaps even the majority – of people. (1999: 3–4)

Moreover, the disability movement's commitment to human rights increasingly extends to other international issues emerging 'as an important discourse of resistance movements all over the world' (Goodale and Merry, 2007: 176). For example, the recent Rio+20 Conference on Sustainable Development Outcome document, 'The Future We Want' (United Nations, 2012), reflects the developing solidarity between the disability rights movement and other movements struggling against 'unfreedoms'. This landmark document specifically refers to disability in five traditional pillars of disadvantage: states' responsibility to respect, protect and promote human rights and fundamental freedom for all (para. 9); the need for participation and access to information and judicial and administrative proceedings for promotion of sustainable development (para. 43); the need for green economic policies for sustainable development and poverty eradication (para. 58(k)); the need for integrated planning and building for sustainable cities; the need for inclusive policies for housing and social services and a safe and healthy living environment for all, particularly disabled persons (para. 135); and the need for ensuring equal access to education for all (para. 229).

UN treaties are only one of a number of international human rights instruments (e.g. the International Labour Organization also promotes human rights through Conventions and Recommendations). These instruments are effective only if they are domesticated and monitored, that is, practised at the local level. Specifically, UN member countries must formally adopt the principles of these Conventions and agree to implement them. Harpur (2012) argues that a unique and promising characteristic of the CRPD is that, for the first time, it reduces the 'scope for interpretation' (p. 5) with 'detail on what states need to do to ensure … rights are realized' (p. 1). Other important innovations are the CRPD's built-in monitoring mechanism which includes the participation of disabled people in follow-up work[6] and its requirements for states to provide 'periodic comprehensive reports' on implementation (Harpur, 2012: 8).

Praise and anticipation for these innovations reflect a concern about the enforceability of human rights. Other legal expressions of human rights such as domestic anti-discrimination legislation like the Americans with Disabilities Act 1990 (ADA) and the British Disability Discrimination Act 1995 are also potentially enforceable. A small number of countries, such as Canada and South Africa, have actually entrenched disability rights into their national Constitutions, which states a strong commitment to equality for disabled people because successful court cases under constitutional laws bind all levels of government and can potentially influence law and policy-making more broadly.

Some argue that 'human rights that cannot be enforced by a sovereign authority are simply abstractions' (Turner, 2009: 71). However, an increasingly competitive, deregulated and globalised labour market threatens to erode 'sovereign authority' in favour of the demands of transnational corporations (Portero, 2012; Rioux, 2011; Teeple, 2005). Although human rights instruments cannot address the imbalance in power between disabled people and entities such as states and transnational corporations, the defence of human rights may be an increasingly important means of protection in this globalised context (Teeple, 2005).

Furthermore, Sen (2004) points to the aspirational nature of human rights, arguing that their legal expression is secondary because they are 'quintessentially ethical articulations … sustainable only by open public reasoning' (p. 321). Thus, '[t]hey may or may not be reflected in a legal framework … but there are also other ways of implementing human rights (including public recognition, agitation and monitoring)' (pp. 355–6).

For disabled people to exercise their human rights, there needs to be an ongoing dialogue and agreement by the public, by governments and by the private sector of disability rights as shared rights – rights that reflect the solidarity between those whose rights are respected and those who have been distinguished and left out. There must be a commitment to implement the spirit and moral intent found in the CRPD, as well as a commitment to disabled people worldwide who fought for this articulation of their rights. This dialogue has to acknowledge the way conventional notions of disability focused on individuals and their impairments and the extent to which this has fundamentally disadvantaged them. It must incorporate ideas of structural violence and solidarity with those who have been marginalised – those caught in the web of precarious social participation (Rioux, 2011) in the post-globalisation era of deregulated labour markets, waning welfare states and social protections, and deleterious changes in development aid. The privatisation of disadvantage of disabled people must be addressed as a public issue. The diminishing accommodation of difference in the current economic conditions pushes towards the need to recognise participation and rights as political issues. The implementation and practice of human rights mandates the recognition that political, economic, social and cultural rights are indivisible; that the inclusion of disability and disadvantage is fundamental to all programmes and policies; that enforceable anti-discrimination legislation must be in place; that segregating policy and affirmative action must be replaced with universal design; and that social action and solidarity are necessary to address the systemic sources of inequality. Governments must now be held accountable to recognise that it is not business as usual. It is time to put in place systems that accommodate difference, and to hold those accountable who do not honour the equality and rights of disabled people.

Notes

1 This and all other UN documents referred to can be found at www.un.org/disabilities/
2 The Berkeley meeting produced the Report of the United Nations Consultative Expert Groups in 1998. Available at: www.un.org/esa/socdev/enable/disberk0.htm
3 The Hong Kong meeting produced the report, Interregional Seminars and Symposium, in 1999. Available at: www.un.org/esa/socdev/enable/comp304.htm
4 The Swedish meeting produced the report, Let the World Know, in 2000. Available at: www.un.org/esa/socdev/enable/stockholmnov2000.htm
5 This was followed by an ongoing project, Disability Rights Promotion International (DRPI), funded by the Swedish International Development Agency (SIDA) and the Social Sciences and Humanities Council of Canada (SSHRC). DRPI continues to monitor rights worldwide funded by the SIDA, Canadian International Development Agency (CIDA) and other agencies of the Canadian government, the Swedish Association of the Visually Impaired (SRF) and York University. See http://drpi.research.yorku.ca/
6 A number of organisations and projects have developed and implemented human rights monitoring mechanisms, including Disability Rights Promotion International (DRPI) at http://drpi.research.yorku.ca/; International Disability Alliance (IDA) at www.internationaldisabilityalliance.org/en; and Mental Disability Rights International (MDRi) at www.disabilityrightsintl.org/

References

Barnes, C. and Mercer, G. (2003) *Disability*. Cambridge, UK and Malden, MA: Polity and Blackwell.

Barnes, C. and Mercer, G. (2010) *Exploring Disability: A Sociological Introduction* (2nd edn). Cambridge: Polity.

Basser, L.A. (2011) 'Human dignity', in M.H. Rioux, L.A. Basser and M. Jones (eds), *Critical Perspectives on Human Rights and Disability Law*. Leiden, Boston, MA: Martinus Nijhoff Publishers. pp. 17–36.

Farmer, P. (2005) *Pathologies of Power: Health, Human Rights and the New War on the Poor*. Los Angeles: University of California Press.

Fraser, N. and Gordon, L. (1994) '"Dependency" demystified: inscriptions of power in a keyword of the welfare state', *Social Politics*, 1 (1): 4–31.

Goodale, M. and Merry, S.E. (2007) *The Practice of Human Rights: Tracking Law between the Global and the Local*. Cambridge: Cambridge University Press.

Hansen, R. and Malhotra, R. (2011) 'The United Nations Convention on the Rights of Persons with Disabilities and its implications for the equality rights of Canadians with disabilities: the case of education', *Windsor Yearbook of Access to Justice*, 29 (1): 73–106.

Harpur, P. (2012) 'Embracing the new disability rights paradigm: the importance of the Convention on the Rights of Persons with Disabilities', *Disability & Society*, 27 (1): 1–14.

Oliver, M. (1990) *The Politics of Disablement*. London: Macmillan.

Pinto, P.C. (2011) 'Monitoring human rights: a holistic approach', in M.H. Rioux, L.A. Basser and M. Jones (eds), *Critical Perspectives on Human Rights and Disability Law*. Leiden: Martinus Nijhoff. pp. 451–77.

Portero, I.B. (2012) 'Are there rights in a time of crisis?', *Disability & Society*, 2 (4): 581–5.

Quinn, G. and Degener, T. (2002) Human Rights and Disability: The Current Use and Future Potential of United Nations Human Rights Instruments in the Context of Disability. New York and Geneva: United Nations. Available at: www.ohchgr.org/Documents/Publications/HRDisabilityen.pdf

Rioux, M.H. (2003) 'On second thought: constructing knowledge, law, disability and inequality', in S. Herr, L. Gostin and H. Koh (eds), *The Human Rights of Persons with Intellectual Disabilities: Different but Equal*. Oxford: Oxford University Press. pp. 287–317.

Rioux, M.H. (2007) 'Human rights approaches to health', in D. Raphael, T. Bryant and M.H. Rioux (eds), *Staying Alive: Critical Perspectives on Health, Illness, and Health Care*. Toronto: Canadian Scholars' Press and Women's Press. pp. 85–138.

Rioux, M.H. (2011) Precarious Participation. Paper presented at Social Participation: Knowledge, Policy and Practice, Institute for Social Participation and La Trobe University, Melbourne, Australia, 28 November. Available at: www.latrobe.edu.au/isp/ISP%20Conference/Rioux.avi

Rioux, M. and Valentine, F. (2006) 'Does theory matter? Exploring the nexus between disability, human rights and public policy', in R.F. Devlin and D. Pothier (eds), *Critical Disability Theory: Essays in Philosophy, Politics, Policy, and Law*. Vancouver: UBC Press. pp. 47–69.

Rioux, M.H., Basser, L.A. and Jones, M. (eds) (2011) *Critical Perspectives on Human Rights and Disability Law*. Leiden: Martinus Nijhoff.

Rummery, K. (2002) 'Social policy, rights and citizenship', *Disability, Citizenship and Community Care: A Case for Welfare Rights?* Aldershot: Ashgate. pp. 7–25.

Sen, A.K. (1999) *Development as Freedom*. Oxford, New York: Oxford University Press.

Sen, A.K. (2004) 'Elements of a theory of human rights', *Philosophy & Public Affairs*, 32 (4): 315–56.

Teeple, G. (2005) *The Riddle of Human Rights*. Aurora, ON: Merlin Press and Garamond Press.

Turner, B.S. (2009) 'T.H. Marshall, social rights and English national identity', *Citizenship Studies*, 13 (1): 65–73.

United Nations (2006) Convention on the Rights of Persons with Disabilities (CRPD). Available at: www.un.org/disabilities/convention/conventionfull.shtml

United Nations (2012) The Future We Want. Outcome document, Conference on Sustainable Development, Rio de Janeiro, Brazil, 20–22 June. Available at: www.un.org/en/sustainablefuture/

United Nations Commission on Human Rights (UNCHR) (1998) Resolution 31/51. Human Rights of Persons with Disabilities. 51st Meeting, 17 April. Available at: www.unhchr.ch/Huridocda/Huridoca.nsf/TestFrame/98beedb1e09478478025667002f9596?Opendocument

United Nations General Assembly (1982) Resolution 37/51. World Programme of Action Concerning Disabled Persons. 37th Session, 3 December. Available at: www.un.org/disabilities/default.asp?id=23#1

United Nations General Assembly (1993) Resolution 48/96. Standard Rules on the Equalization of Opportunities for Persons with Disabilities (A/RES/48/96). 48th Session, 20 December. Available at: www.un.org/esa/socdev/enable/dissre00.htm

42

The Future of Disability Studies

Alison Sheldon

As the chapters in this collection indicate, disability studies is an exciting, vibrant and diverse field. The first edition of *Disabling Barriers – Enabling Environments*, published in 1993, was an important and very welcome addition to a relatively small disability studies section on the shelves of a few university libraries. This – the third edition – will be jostling for space amongst an ever-expanding catalogue of disability studies literature in a growing number of libraries around the globe. If measured by the numbers of new books, academic journals, international conferences, professorial appointments and successfully defended PhDs, it would appear that disability studies has a bright future. For many disabled people though, the future seems less bright. Driven deeper into poverty by government spending cuts, characterised as skivers and scroungers by the media and increasingly subjected to abuse and violence, '(all) of the advances that disabled people have made over the period since 1945 are being reversed' (Edwards, 2012: 4).

Despite this 'climate of fear', there has seen a heartening swing back to direct action as a means of putting people's concerns – including those of disabled people – onto the political agenda. Before the latest recession kicked in, many were grieving the demise of the disabled people's movement (Oliver and Barnes, 2006; Sheldon, 2006). Now, however, the disabled people's movement is coming out of abeyance and finding innovative new ways to oppose austerity. In the UK, disability studies as an academic field was built on foundations laid by disabled activists and has subsequently prided itself on its strong links with the grassroots movement. This is in many respects an uneasy relationship, especially as the aims of the academy and the aims of the movement are often rather different. With the movement in abeyance, these links were severed and disability studies arguably suffered as a consequence. Disability studies now stands accused of losing its soul (Peace, 2010: 343), with the emancipatory struggle taking a back seat to academic career-building. Furthermore, in an increasingly fragmented field of study, concerns have been voiced about a 'possible division of disability studies into two overtly hostile camps' (Oliver and Barnes,

2012: 182). The time is ripe then to take stock of current tensions within disability studies, to re-energise the field's relationship with the disabled people's movement and to think seriously about how we might best face future challenges.

As a contribution to this process, this chapter will consider the emerging tensions within disability studies before proposing possible ways forward. First though, a brief account will be provided of the meteoric rise of disability studies as an academic field (see Chapter 1).

Disability studies: The story so far

The emergence and ascendancy of disability studies is an often told story, which – for the purposes of this chapter – will be recapped only briefly. Before the advent of disability studies, the academic study of disability was confined to fields such as medicine, psychology and medical sociology, with disability conceptualised as a functional deficiency experienced by unfortunate, 'deviant' individuals. Disabled people in the UK and elsewhere, largely excluded from academic debates, began to challenge such thinking along with their disadvantaged position in society. From the 1970s, this dissent accelerated with the formation of radical organisations run and controlled by disabled people such as the Union of the Physically Impaired against Segregation (UPIAS) in the UK. This resulted in the reconceptualisation of disability as a form of social oppression – what is now often referred to as the social interpretation of disability or the social model. Here, disability is something 'imposed on top of our impairments by the way we are unnecessarily isolated and excluded from full participation in society' (UPIAS, 1976: 3). Inspired by this new perspective, different ways of studying disability began to emerge and the seeds of what we now know as 'disability studies' were planted. Disability studies, then, was built on foundations laid by activist 'organic' intellectuals. Its originators were concerned with:

> the study of the various forces, economic, political, and cultural, that support and sustain 'disability', as defined by the disabled people's movement, in order to generate meaningful and practical knowledge with which to further its eradication. (Barnes, 2003: 9)

This early commitment to disabled people's self-emancipation is still in evidence through a continuing emphasis on non-oppressive research methodologies, user-involvement, accountability to the grassroots community and concrete policy outcomes. Through its close ties with the disabled people's movement, disability studies is said to have 'transformed the intellectual scene' and is credited with all manner of successes:

> Disability studies has produced not just an intellectual challenge to the way that disability is understood and theorized but has resulted in the establishment of a new paradigm around disability. Large-scale international organizations such as

the United Nations and the World Health Organization (WHO), national governments and voluntary and third sector organizations everywhere have engaged with – and been influenced by – the ideas that have emerged as a direct result of the way that disability studies scholars and activists have engaged with disability. (Roulstone et al., 2012: 4)

Unfortunately though, the much-vaunted initial links with the disabled people's movement have proved difficult to maintain. There is increasing pressure on academics to produce particular kinds of research outputs and rather than forming genuine partnerships with disabled people, disability studies scholars stand accused of using the 'subject and the experience of disabled people for their own ends and to build their own careers' (Oliver and Barnes, 2010: 551).

Furthermore, as with other similar fields of study, disability studies has developed in a number of new directions. There are possibly as many versions of disability studies as there are academics working in the field and not all seem to have the same priorities, especially when it comes to 'reconciling theoretical advance with emancipatory social change' (Blume and Hiddinga, 2010: 234) . For some, disability studies has become 'an interdisciplinary subject that is at much at home with theory as with pragmatic solutions' (Shildrick, 2012: 30). For others, it is failing to balance theory and political action and thus runs the risk of becoming increasingly irrelevant to the people it once purported to support (Peace, 2010). As will be discussed below, these differences are creating tensions in the academy and are not assisting disabled people and their organisations in their struggles for change.

Where are we now? Disability studies at the crossroads

The approach described above, where disability studies is seen as 'tightly connected to the political activism of disabled people', is considered by Mårten Söder (2009: 67) to constitute a 'narrow definition' of the field. A wider definition of disability studies is also identified. In this version, there is little mention of any relation to grassroots activism, theories and perspectives from other fields are imported 'rather uncritically' (Söder, 2009: 68) and disability studies thus becomes 'a matrix of theories, pedagogies and practices' (Garland-Thomson, 2002, cited in Goodley, 2011: 10). Such developments are not universally welcomed. As one commentator suggests, for example:

we have had too many books ... where academics take it in turn to discuss one highly obscure cultural phenomenon after another, jumbling together dozens of different theoretical or cultural references, in a confusing collage of ideas and concepts and readings, which seems unlikely to have even an indirect impact on the lived experience of disabled people. (Shakespeare, 2012: 894)

Nonetheless, some proponents of this 'wide definition' are now setting themselves apart from 'traditional' disability studies by naming what they do '*critical* disability studies' or simply 'CDS' (Goodley et al., 2012; Shildrick, 2012). It seems then that the boxing gloves are out. In the red corner, we have old-style disability studies; in the blue corner, critical disability studies – drawing on a hotchpotch of social theorists, arguing for the validity of non-disabled people's accounts (Shildrick, 2012) and putting impairment centre-stage in their analyses:

> Critical disability studies takes up the challenge of impaired bodies to highlight the limits of the straight body, calling into question 'the 'givenness' of the 'natural body' ... conceptualised as ... bodies of interconnection and production ... Disabled bodies expand and develop in exciting ways ... offering us critical languages for denaturalising impairment (Goodley, 2001: 159). (Goodley et al., 2012: 321)

Whilst this might sound fresh and interesting, and the need for a 'social theory of impairment' has long been acknowledged (Abberley, 1987), disabled people and their bodies have for too long 'been subjected to the gaze of the interested' (Bailey, 2004). Perhaps I am not alone in feeling a little uncomfortable that my 'expanding and developing', 'disabled' body might be the subject of such scrutiny and fascination.

That said, it may well be the case that such postmodernist accounts have usefully 'reaffirmed the importance of cultural responses to disability' (Oliver and Barnes, 2012: 181). There are concerns though that insight is not provided into 'how the problem of disablism might be resolved in terms of politics, policy or practice' (Oliver and Barnes, 2012: 181) and that an 'overreliance on metaphor at the expense of materiality' might limit the effectiveness of the disability studies enterprise (Erevelles, 2012: 119). Activists in the disabled people's movement have raised similar concerns. According to Robert Williams-Findlay (co-founder of Disabled People Against Cuts), there has been a 'watering down' of the early ideas of disability studies such that disablism:

> is simply reduced to the experience of discriminatory attitudes and practices within society; lost has been our ability to question the actual fabric of society itself and the implications this has for disabled people. I would argue this de-politicisation has weakened our ability to address the current attacks upon disabled people. (Williams-Findlay, 2011: 775)

To remain relevant to the grassroots movement then, rather than 'de-materialising' the problem, disability studies needs to 'hang onto more economically informed interpretations of disabled people's oppression in order to effectively draw links between disability and the capitalist mode of production' (Sheldon, 2009: 669–70). We desperately need theory in order to make such connections and we need to attend to this task urgently, since it has arguably:

never been more important for the link between the global economy and the oppression and grinding poverty of millions of disabled (and indeed non-disabled) people to be acknowledged, recognised and taken seriously at a political and an intellectual level. (Sheldon, 2009: 667–8)

As well as examining the political economy, the disabled people's movement has also recognised the need for research that reveals the full extent of the effects of austerity on disabled people's day-to-day lives, and has begun to generate data in order to support its campaigning (see Briant et al., 2011; Campbell et al., 2012; Edwards, 2012). The grassroots movement then seems to be leading the way in producing research reports that highlight the destructive implications of current austerity measures. The universities are lagging behind in this respect and, in addition, have still not managed to produce 'an adequate social theory of disability' that makes a 'full analysis of the organisation of society' and thus 'leads to the very essence of disability' (UPIAS, 1976: 14, 20).

It is worth noting that many of the key activists in the UK have an academic background in disability studies. Perhaps then, education could be one of the most important functions of disability studies in universities. Vic Finkelstein, whilst acknowledging the danger of a parasitic relationship developing between academics and oppressed people (2001: 16), highlighted that university academics can have a positive influence by 'feed(ing) the hunger for knowledge that accompanies struggles against oppression'. Here too though, disability studies has been found lacking. Concerns have been raised about the 'exclusive nature of disability studies scholarship', since 'those who could benefit the most from disability studies … are unable to read the work intended to empower them' (Peace, 2010: 343). It costs money to access academic books and research papers and whilst online resources like the Disability Archive UK are invaluable for those with Internet access, this is not a luxury that all disabled people can enjoy (see Chapters 23 and 36). The proposed introduction of open access publishing might make academic research more accessible to those outside universities. This development is not universally welcomed however and it remains to be seen what its implications might be in terms of academic freedom (Boffey, 2013). Even when literature *can* be accessed, it is suggested that 'academic jargon' can make information difficult to digest – even for seasoned professors (Swain, 2011). Perhaps then we should curb our tendencies to 'use a lot of awfully long words to say very little that is actually new' (Shakespeare, 2012: 894).

If – as has been suggested – disability studies is at a crossroads (Roulstone et al., 2012), its future will depend on which path or paths we choose to take. Having briefly outlined some key issues, by way of conclusion, the final section will present my thoughts on fruitful ways forward.

Conclusion: The long road to freedom?

Disability studies undoubtedly has a bright future as a field of study in university social science and humanities faculties. Tensions between so-called 'narrow' and 'wide' definitions of the field will doubtless result in ongoing academic debate and a plethora of books, journal articles and conference papers. According to pessimistic predictions though, unless our academic differences are reconciled disability studies will 'become exclusively a matter of academic in-fighting and career advancement' (Oliver and Barnes, 2012: 182–3). It will thus cease to engage meaningfully with the concerns of disabled people – the supposed beneficiaries of our endeavours. Whether or not we are able to bridge the ideological divide that is emerging in the field of disability studies, it is imperative that we begin to address the mismatch between the ascendancy of disability studies in universities and the worsening conditions in which many disabled people are forced to live. We need a self-critical disability studies that is fit for the 'age of austerity' and takes us closer to the original emancipatory goals of the field.

As a starting point, I would argue that those working in disability studies must transform their thinking and actions and reforge their links with the disabled people's movement (Sheldon, 2012). Maintaining relevance to disabled people's immediate and long-term concerns is vital, especially now that we once again have an angry, well-informed and thriving grassroots movement. In order to assist the struggle, academics could work harder at the difficult task of producing an adequate social theory of disability – a theory that does *not* examine aspects of disablement in isolation, seeks causes not symptoms, and aims to think not only of the here and now but also look to the future. Whilst theory for its own sake may be interesting, interesting is not sufficient for the task in hand. In view of the ongoing global recession and the austerity measures being implemented by governments of numerous nation-states, we might be best advised to prioritise economically-informed interpretations of disabled people's oppression. Finally, as disability studies academics, we need to more actively share our skills, knowledge and resources with the people we purport to be representing; and try to provide the political education that might serve to raise levels of social awareness and increase the urge to collectively self-organise and demand change.

If disability studies is to remain true to the ideals of its activist founders, the path ahead will lead to the eventual eradication of disability as a form of social oppression. Without disability, there will be no need for disability studies. Current trends, however, suggest that disability studies will be around for the foreseeable future, since for disabled people – along with other oppressed social groupings – it is predicted that 'the worst is yet to come' (Wood, 2012). Faced with this stark reality, I firmly believe that 'Disability Studies has a continuing duty to seek out new ways in which to assist the struggle towards a better society for all' (Sheldon, 2006: 9).

This may seem an onerous responsibility, but we will shirk it at our peril.

References

Abberley, P. (1987) 'The concept of oppression and the development of a social theory of disability', *Disability & Society*, 2 (1): 5–19.
Bailey, K. (2004) 'Learning more from the social model: linking experience, participation and knowledge production', in C. Barnes and G. Mercer (eds), *Implementing the Social Model of Disability: Theory and Research*. Leeds: The Disability Press. p. 140.

Barnes, C. (2003) Disability Studies: What's the Point? Presentation at the Disability Studies: Theory, Policy and Practice conference, University of Lancaster, 4 September. Available at: www.leeds.ac.uk/disability-studies/archiveuk/ [accessed 02/09/06].

Blume, S. and Hiddinga, A. (2010) 'Disability studies as an academic field: reflections on its development', *Medische Antropologie*, 22 (2): 225–36.

Boffey, D. (2013) 'Historians warn minister: hands off our academic freedoms', *The Guardian*, 26 January. Available at: www.guardian.co.uk/education/2013/jan/26/historians-warn-minister-over-academic-freedom [accessed 28/01/13].

Briant, E., Watson, N. and Philo, G. (2011) Bad News for Disabled People: How the Newspapers are Reporting Disability. Strathclyde Centre for Disability Research and Glasgow Media Group, in association with Inclusion London. Available at: www.inclusionlondon.co.uk/domains/inclusionlondon.co.uk/local/media/downloads/bad_news_for_disabled_people_pdf.pdf [accessed 19/09/12].

Campbell, S.J., Marsh, S., Franklin, K., Gaffney, D., Dixon, M., James, L., et al. (2012) Responsible Reform: A Report on the Proposed Changes to Disability Living Allowance (Diary of a Benefit Scrounger). London: Spartacus. Available at: http://wearespartacus.org.uk/spartacus-report/ [accessed 19/09/12].

Edwards, C. (2012) The Austerity War and the Impoverishment of Disabled People. Norwich: NCODP. Available at: http://documents.ncodp.org.uk/news/3%20September%202012%20The%20Austerity%20War%20and%20the%20impoverishment%20of%20disabled%20people.pdf [accessed 19/09/12].

Erevelles, N. (2012) 'The color of violence: reflecting on gender, race and disability in wartime', in K.Q. Hall (ed.), *Feminist Disability Studies*. Bloomington: Indiana University Press. pp. 117–35.

Finkelstein, V. (2001) A Personal Journey into Disability Politics. Presentation at Leeds University Centre for Disability Studies, Leeds, 7 February. Available at: www.leeds.ac.uk/disability-studies/archiveuk/ [accessed 02/10/12].

Goodley, D. (2011) *Disability Studies: An Interdisciplinary Introduction*. London: SAGE.

Goodley, D., Hughes, B. and Davis, L. (2012) 'Glossary', in D. Goodley, B. Hughes and L. Davis (eds), *Disability and Social Theory: New Developments and Directions*. Basingstoke: Palgrave Macmillan. pp. 318–35.

Oliver, M. and Barnes, C. (2006) 'Disability politics and the disability movement in Britain: Where did it all go wrong?', *Coalition*, August, pp. 8–13.

Oliver, M. and Barnes, C. (2010) 'Disability studies, disabled people and the struggle for inclusion', *British Journal of Sociology of Education*, 31 (5): 547–60.

Oliver, M. and Barnes, C. (2012) *The New Politics of Disablement*. Basingstoke: Palgrave Macmillan.

Peace, W.J. (2010) 'Slippery slopes: media, disability and adaptive sports', in L.J. Moore and M. Kosut (eds), *The Body Reader: Essential Social and Cultural Readings*. New York: New York University Press. pp. 332–48.

Roulstone, A., Thomas, C. and Watson, N. (2012) 'The changing terrain of disability studies', in N. Watson, A. Roulstone and C. Thomas (eds), *Routledge Handbook of Disability Studies*. London: Routledge. pp. 3–11.

Shakespeare, T. (2012) 'Review of Sex and Disability, edited by Robert McRuer and Anna Mollow', *Disability & Society*, 27 (6): 894–5.

Sheldon, A. (2006) Disabling the Disabled People's Movement: The Influence of Disability Studies on the Struggle for Liberation. Keynote address at the Third Disability Studies Association conference, Lancaster, 18–20 September.

Sheldon, A. (2009) 'Recession, radicalism and the road to recovery?', *Disability & Society*, 24 (5): 667–71.

Sheldon, A. (2012) A Disability Studies for the 'Age of Austerity'. Paper presented at Deficiência e emancipação social: para uma crise da normalidade colloquium, Lisbon, Portugal, 13 November.

Shildrick, M. (2012) 'Critical disability studies: rethinking the conventions for the age of postmodernity', in N. Watson, A. Roulstone and C. Thomas (eds), *Routledge Handbook of Disability Studies*. London: Routledge. pp. 30–41.

Söder, M. (2009) 'Tensions, perspectives and themes in disability studies', *Scandinavian Journal of Disability Research*, 11 (2): 67–81.

Swain, J. (2011) 'Review of Disability Studies: An Interdisciplinary Introduction, by Dan Goodley', *Disability & Society*, 26 (4): 503–5.

UPIAS (1976) *Fundamental Principles of Disability*. London: UPIAS.

Williams-Findlay, R. (2011) 'Lifting the lid on Disabled People Against Cuts', *Disability & Society*, 26 (6): 773–8.

Wood, C. (2012) *'For Disabled People the Worst is Yet to Come …'. Destination Unknown: Summer 2012*. London: Demos. Available at: www.demos.co.uk/files/Destination_ Unknown_ Summer_2012_-_web.pdf?1340294386 [accessed 02/10/12].

Index

information gathering 263
information provision
    counselling for disabled people 259, 260
    disability rights 287
    disability studies research findings 330, 331
    Disabled People's User-Led Organisations
        (DPULOs) 209, 210
    for older people 231, 234, 235
    sports and physical activities for disabled
        people 223
    technological change and disability 176
    user involvement in services 199, 201
information society/technology and disability
        173–8, 183, 184, 186–7, 279–85
informational barriers
    counselling for disabled people 258
    housing for disabled people 168
    information technology and disabled
        people 284
    people with aphasia 184
    sexual expression of disabled people
        141–2, 144
    social and leisure activities for visually
        impaired people 215, 218–19
    sports and physical activities for disabled
        people 224
    user involvement in services 201
'inside out' approach to disability studies 21, 22
insiders, and 'mate crime' 313–14
Institute for Human Centered Design 287, 289
institutional barriers 11, 92
institutional power 109
insurance sector 299
intellectual impairment see learning difficulties
inter-dependencies 32, 36, 313
interactionist perspective 19, 21
internalised oppression 64, 95–6, 97, 258, 300
internalised racism 95
International Classification of Functioning,
    Disability and Health (ICF) 40–1, 43
International Guild of Disabled Artists and
    Performers (IGODAP) 118
International Labour Organization 322
international legislation on disability equality
    and rights 50, 272, 273, 287–8, 306, 319,
    320–1, 322, 323
International Monetary Fund (IMF)
    271, 274, 275
international organisations 327–8
    See also individual organisations
International Paralympic Committee 222
international perspectives on disability 45–51,
    143, 240–1, 284, 287, 306, 319–23
    See also global economy of 'care'; international
        legislation on disability equality and
        rights; internationalisation of disability
        arts; Paralympic Games

International Professional Surrogates Association
    (IPSA) 143
international trade agreements 271
internationalisation of disability arts 117, 118
Internet 118, 119, 141–2, 175, 176–7, 178, 183,
    184, 186–7, 281, 282, 283–4
intimate relationships 63, 64, 65, 141, 144
    See also sexuality and disability
iPads 186, 279, 281
iPhones 279, 281
Ireland, C. 181, 185
Islam 125–6, 127, 309
Islam, Z. 122, 124, 125
Islamophobia 125–6

Jaeger, P.T. 284
Jerome, J. 252
Johnson, C. 259
Johnston, D.W. 126
Jolly, D. 40, 43, 252
Jordan 195
Jordan, A. 108, 111
Joseph Rowntree Foundation 38, 232
journals 142, 206, 210–11, 315
Judaism 309

Kafer, A. 142
Kagan, A. 187
Kassah, A.K. 47–8
Keidan, L. 119
Keith, L. 94
Kershaw, Joyce 134
Keyes, S. 150
Khosa, J. 182
knowledge 12, 20, 115, 119–20
Konkkola, Kalle 49–50
Kriegel, L. 79
Kuhse, H. 35
Kuusisto, S. 176, 177
Kvam, M.H. 46

labelling
    disability and impairment 39, 41, 102,
        134, 256
    disability culture 117
    housing for disabled people 166
    parents of disabled children 152
    people with ADHD 65–6
    people with learning difficulties 62–3, 133–4,
        169, 170
    welfare benefit 'scroungers' 96, 265, 301,
        316, 326
labour markets 10, 11, 56, 101, 103–4
    See also employment; unemployment
Labour Party's Public Administration Select
    Committee (UK) 198
Lamp, S. 72